Immunochemistry 2

The Practical Approach Series

SERIES EDITOR

B. D. HAMES
Department of Biochemistry and Molecular Biology
University of Leeds, Leeds LS2 9JT, UK

★ indicates new and forthcoming titles

Affinity Chromatography
★ Affinity Separations
Anaerobic Microbiology
Animal Cell Culture (2nd edition)
Animal Virus Pathogenesis
Antibodies I and II
★ Antibody Engineering
Basic Cell Culture
Behavioural Neuroscience
Biochemical Toxicology
Bioenergetics
Biological Data Analysis
Biological Membranes
Biomechanics—Materials
Biomechanics—Structures and Systems
Biosensors
★ Calcium-PI signalling
Carbohydrate Analysis (2nd edition)
Cell–Cell Interactions
The Cell Cycle
Cell Growth and Apoptosis
Cellular Calcium
Cellular Interactions in Development
Cellular Neurobiology
Clinical Immunology
★ Complement
Crystallization of Nucleic Acids and Proteins
Cytokines (2nd edition)
The Cytoskeleton
Diagnostic Molecular Pathology I and II
Directed Mutagenesis
★ DNA and Protein Sequence Analysis
DNA Cloning 1: Core Techniques (2nd edition)
DNA Cloning 2: Expression Systems (2nd edition)
★ DNA Cloning 3: Complex Genomes (2nd edition)
★ DNA Cloning 4: Mammalian Systems (2nd edition)
Electron Microscopy in Biology

Electron Microscopy in Molecular Biology
Electrophysiology
Enzyme Assays
★ Epithelial Cell Culture
Essential Developmental Biology
Essential Molecular Biology I and II
Experimental Neuroanatomy
★ Extracellular Matrix
Flow Cytometry (2nd edition)
★ Free Radicals
Gas Chromatography
Gel Electrophoresis of Nucleic Acids (2nd edition)
Gel Electrophoresis of Proteins (2nd edition)
Gene Probes 1 and 2
Gene Targeting
Gene Transcription
Glycobiology
Growth Factors
Haemopoiesis
Histocompatibility Testing
HIV Volumes 1 and 2
Human Cytogenetics I and II (2nd edition)
Human Genetic Disease Analysis
★ Immunochemistry 1
★ Immunochemistry 2
Immunocytochemistry
In Situ Hybridization
Iodinated Density Gradient Media
★ Ion Channels
Lipid Analysis
Lipid Modification of Proteins
Lipoprotein Analysis
Liposomes
Mammalian Cell Biotechnology
Medical Bacteriology
Medical Mycology
Medical Parasitology
Medical Virology
★ MHC Volume 1
★ MHC Volume 2
Microcomputers in Biology
Molecular Genetic Analysis of Populations
Molecular Genetics of Yeast
Molecular Imaging in Neuroscience
Molecular Neurobiology
Molecular Plant Pathology I and II
Molecular Virology
Monitoring Neuronal Activity
Mutagenicity Testing
★ Neural Cell Culture
Neural Transplantation
★ Neurochemistry (2nd edition)
Neuronal Cell Lines
NMR of Biological Macromolecules
Non-isotopic Methods in Molecular Biology
Nucleic Acid Hybridization
Nucleic Acid and Protein Sequence Analysis
Oligonucleotides and Analogues
Oligonucleotide Synthesis

PCR 1
PCR 2
Peptide Antigens
Photosynthesis: Energy Transduction
Plant Cell Biology
Plant Cell Culture (2nd edition)
Plant Molecular Biology
Plasmids (2nd edition)
★ Platelets
Pollination Ecology
Postimplantation Mammalian Embryos
Preparative Centrifugation
Prostaglandins and Related Substances
Protein Blotting
Protein Engineering
★ Protein Function (2nd edition)
Protein Phosphorylation
Protein Purification Applications
Protein Purification Methods
Protein Sequencing
★ Protein Structure (2nd edition)
★ Protein Structure Prediction
Protein Targeting
Proteolytic Enzymes
Pulsed Field Gel Electrophoresis
Radioisotopes in Biology
Receptor Biochemistry
Receptor–Ligand Interactions
RNA Processing I and II
★ Subcellular Fractionation
Signal Transduction
Solid Phase Peptide Synthesis
Transcription Factors
Transcription and Translation
Tumour Immunobiology
Virology
Yeast

Immunochemistry 2

A Practical Approach

Edited by

ALAN P. JOHNSTONE
Division of Immunology, St George's Hospital Medical School
London

and

MALCOLM W. TURNER
Immunobiology Unit, Institute of Child Health
London

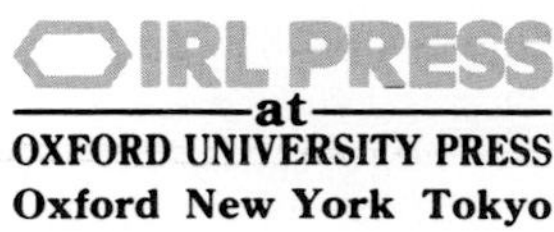

OXFORD UNIVERSITY PRESS
Oxford New York Tokyo

Oxford University Press, Great Clarendon Street, Oxford OX2 6DP

Oxford New York
Athens Auckland Bangkok Bogota Bombay Buenos Aires
Calcutta Cape Town Dar es Salaam Delhi Florence Hong Kong
Istanbul Karachi Kuala Lumpur Madras Madrid Melbourne
Mexico City Nairobi Paris Singapore Taipei Tokyo Toronto

and associated companies in
Berlin Ibadan

Oxford is a trade mark of Oxford University Press

Published in the United States
by Oxford University Press Inc., New York

A catalogue record for this book is available from the British Library

Library of Congress Cataloging in Publication Data
(Data available)

ISBN 0 19 963610 9 (Hbk)
ISBN 0 19 963609 5 (Pbk)

Also available as a two volume set
ISBN 0 19 963608 7 (Hbk)
ISBN 0 19 963607 9 (Pbk)

Typeset by Footnote Graphics, Warminster, Wilts
Printed in Great Britain by Information Press, Ltd, Eynsham, Oxon.

Preface

Immunochemistry is of immense importance to virtually all areas of modern biology and medicine. In its broadest sense, the term has come to mean the structure and function of all molecules of immunological importance. The wide scope of the subject caused our provisional contents list to quickly outgrow the standard Practical Approach size and we were delighted that Oxford University Press agreed to publish the work as two volumes. This space has allowed coverage of a wide range of topics, commensurate with the importance of immunochemistry. However, we realize that many aspects remain uncovered, some of which are covered by other volumes in the Practical Approach series.

The availability of high quality antibodies has been an essential prerequisite for progress in most areas of immunochemistry and various strategies currently used in their production are covered in the first five chapters of *Immunochemistry 1*: G. T. Stevenson and K. S. Kan describe how antibodies may be chemically engineered and R. J. Owens discusses the use of genetic engineering in this field, whilst M. D. Melamed, J. Sutherland, M. D. Thomas, and J. Newton address the continuing difficulties associated with the preparation of human monoclonal antibodies. In contast, J. Chr. Jensenius and C. Koch illustrate the simplicity of production and utility of applications of chicken antibodies. *Immunochemistry 1* also covers some of the uses of antibodies in immunoassays: R. Thorpe, M. Wadhwa, and T. Mire-Sluis give advice on the standardization of antibodies and antigens, whereas D. M. Kemeny and C. H. Self, D. L. Bates, and D. B. Cook cover the latest ELISA techniques in two further chapters. The application of enzyme immunoassays to cells (the cell–ELISA and ELISPOT procedures) are detailed by N. W. Pearce and J. D. Sedgwick, and I. A. Hemmilä presents the latest refinements of photoluminescence immunoassays. *Immunochemistry 1* also describes the incorporation of antibodies and their fragments into immunotoxins (E. J. Derbyshire, C. Gottstein, and P. E. Thorpe) and the use of synthetic peptides in mapping the epitopes of both antibodies and T cells (S. J. Rodda, G. Tribbick, and N. J. Maeji).

Immunochemistry 2 begins with two chapters on affinity and avidity measurements (by H. Saunal, R. Karlsson, and M. H. V. van Regenmortel and by D. Goldblatt). Next, E. Claassen and F. van Iwaarden describe the use of liposomes to modulate immune responses. The use of antibodies in histo- and cytochemistry is presented in three chapters: P. Brandtzaeg, T. S. Halstensen, H. S. Huitfeldt, and K. N. Valnes discuss comprehensively immunofluorescence and immunoenzyme histochemistry; G. D. Johnson explores immunological applications of confocal microscopy; and G. Damgaard, C. H. Nielsen, and R. G. Q. Leslie review various aspects of flow cytometry. *Immunochem-*

istry 2 ends with three chapters focusing on immunochemical aspects of some immunologically important molecules, namely: soluble adhesion molecules (by M. G. Bouma, M. P. Laan, M. A. Dentener, and W. A. Buurman), complement components (by R. Würzner, T. E. Mollnes, and B. P. Morgan); complement receptors (by I. Bartók and M. J. Walport).

We would like to thank all of the authors for their hard work in producing such high quality contributions when they all have so many other competing responsibilities. We are sure that their efforts will contribute significantly to the increasing use of immunochemistry in so many diverse biological fields.

London
Jan 1997

A. P. J.
M. W. T.

Contents

Immunochemistry 1

Immunochemistry 2

5. Confocal laser scanning microscopy 131

G. D. Johnson

6. Flow cytofluorimetry 149

G. Damgaard, C. H. Nielsen, and R. G. Q. Leslie

Contributors

ISTVÁN BARTÓK
Department of Medicine, Royal Postgraduate Medical School, DuCane Road, London W12 0HS, UK.

DAVID L. BATES
Dako Diagnostics Ltd., Denmark House, Angel Grove, Ely, Cambridgeshire CB7 4ET, UK.

M. G. BOUMA
Department of General Surgery, Maastricht University, PO Box 616, Maastricht, The Netherlands.

P. BRANDTZAEG
LIIPAT, Institute of Pathology, Rikshospitalet, N-0027 Oslo, Norway.

W. A. BUURMAN
Department of General Surgery, Maastricht University, PO Box 616, Maastricht, The Netherlands.

ERIC CLAASSEN
Institute for Animal Science and Health, ID-DLO, POB 65 8200 AB Lelystad, The Netherlands.

DAVID B. COOK
Deparment of Clinical Biochemistry, The Medical School, Framlington Place, University of Newcastle, Newcastle upon Tyne NE2 4HH, UK.

G. DAMGAARD
Department of Medical Microbiology, Institute of Medical Biology, University of Odense, J. B. Winslowsvej 19, 5000 Odense C, Denmark.

M. A. DENTENER
Department of General Surgery, Maastricht University, PO Box 616, Maastricht, The Netherlands.

ELAINE J. DERBYSHIRE
Department of Pharmacology, University of Texas South Western Medical Center, Dallas 75235, USA.

DAVID GOLDBLATT
Immunobiology Unit, Institute of Child Health, 30 Guilford Street, London WC1N 1EH, UK.

CLAUDIA GOTTSTEIN
Department of Pharmacology, University of Texas South Western Medical Center, Dallas 75235, USA.

T. S. HALSTENSEN
Department of Environmental Medicine, The National Institute of Public Health, University of Oslo, Oslo, Norway.

I. A. HEMMILÄ
Wallac Oy, PO Box 10, SF-20101 Turku 10, Finland.

H. S. HUITFELDT
Institute of Pathology, Rikshospitalet, N-0027 Oslo, Norway.

JENS CHRISTIAN JENSENIUS
Department of Immunology, Institute of Medical Microbiology, The Bartholin Building, DK-8000 Aarhus C, Denmark.

G. D. JOHNSON
Department of Immunology, University of Birmingham Medical School, Vincent Drive, Birmingham B15 2TJ, UK.

K. S. KAN
Department of Biological Sciences, King Alfred's College, Winchester SO22 4NR, UK.

ROBERT KARLSSON
BIA core AB Pty Ltd, Uppsala, Sweden.

D. M. KEMENY
Department of Immunology, King's College Hospital School of Medicine, London SE5 9PJ, UK.

CLAUS KOCH
Statens Serum Institut, Artillerivej 5, 2300 Copenhagen S, Denmark.

M. P. LAAN
Department of General Surgery, Maastricht University, PO Box 616, Maastricht, The Netherlands.

R. G. Q. LESLIE
Department of Medical Microbiology, Institute of Medical Biology, University of Odense, J. B. Winslowsvej 19, 5000 Odense C, Denmark.

N. JOE MAEJI
Chiron Technologies Pty Ltd., 11 Duerdin Street, Clayton, Victoria 3169, Australia.

M. D. MELAMED
Antibody and Cell Culture Research Unit, Faculty of Science, University of East London, London E15 4LZ, UK.

TONY MIRE-SLUIS
Immunobiology Division, National Institute for Biological Standards and Control, Blanche Lane, Potters Bar EN6 3QG, UK.

T. E. MOLLNES
Department of Immunology and Transfusion Medicine, University of Tromsø, Nordland Centre Hospital, N 8017 BODØ, Norway.

B. P. MORGAN
Department of Medical Biochemistry, University of Wales College of Medicine, Health Park, Cardiff CF4 4XN, UK.

J. NEWTON
Antibody and Cell Culture Research Unit, Faculty of Science, University of East London, London E15 4LZ, UK.

C. H. NIELSEN
Department of Medical Microbiology, Institute of Medical Biology, University of Odense, J. B. Winslowsvej 19, 5000 Odense C, Denmark.

RAYMOND J. OWENS
Celltech Ltd., 216 Bath Road, Slough SL1 4EN, UK.

N. W. PEARCE
Centenary Institute of Cancer Medicine and Cell Biology, Building 93, Royal Prince Alfred Hospital, Missenden Road, Camperdown, Sydney, NSW, Australia.

STUART J. RODDA
Chiron Technologies Pty Ltd., 11 Duerdin Street, Clayton, Victoria 3169, Australia.

HÉLÈNE SAUNAL
UPR 9021, CNRS, IBMC, 15 rue Descartes, Strasbourg, France.

J. D. SEDGWICK
Centenary Institute of Cancer Medicine and Cell Biology, Building 93, Royal Prince Alfred Hospital, Missenden Road, Camperdown, Sydney, NSW, Australia.

COLIN H. SELF
Deparment of Clinical Biochemistry, The Medical School, Framlington Place, University of Newcastle, Newcastle upon Tyne NE2 4HH, UK.

G. T. STEVENSON
Tenovus Research Laboratory, Southampton University Hospitals, Southampton SO16 6YD, UK.

J. SUTHERLAND
Antibody and Cell Culture Research Unit, Faculty of Science, University of East London, London E15 4LZ, UK.

M. D. THOMAS
Antibody and Cell Culture Research Unit, Faculty of Science, University of East London, London E15 4LZ, UK.

PHILIP E. THORPE
Department of Pharmacology, University of Texas South Western Medical Center, Dallas 75235, USA.

ROBIN THORPE
Immunobiology Division, National Institute for Biological Standards and Control, Blanche Lane, Potters Bar EN6 3QG, UK.

GORDON TRIBBICK
Chiron Technologies Pty Ltd., 11 Duerdin Street, Clayton, Victoria 3169, Australia.

K. N. VALNES
Institute of Pathology, Rikshospitalet, N-0027 Oslo, Norway.

FREEK VAN IWAARDEN
Department of Cellbiology, Medical Faculty, Vrije Universiteit, Amsterdam, The Netherlands.

MARC H. V. VAN REGENMORTEL
UPR 9021, CNRS, IBMC, 15 rue Descartes, Strasbourg, France.

MEENU WADHWA
Immunobiology Division, National Institute for Biological Standards and Control, Blanche Lane, Potters Bar EN6 3QG, UK.

MARK J. WALPORT
Department of Medicine, Royal Postgraduate Medical School, DuCane Road, London W12 0HS, UK.

R. WÜRZNER
Institut für Hygiene, University of Innsbruck, Fritz Pregl Strasse 3, A-6020 Innsbruck, Austria.

Abbreviations

2-IT	2-iminothiolane hydrochloride
A/C	alternating current
AAF	2-actylaminofluorene
ABC	avidin–biotin complex
ABTS	2,2′-azino-di[3-ethylbenzthiazoline sulfonate]
ADCC	antibody-dependent cell-mediated cytotoxicity
AEC	3-amino-3-ethylcarbazole
AET	amino ethyl thiouronium bromide
AF	aminofluorene
AMCA	aminomethylcoumarin acetic acid
AP	alkaline phosphatase
APAAP	alkaline phosphatase anti-alkaline phosphatase
APC	antigen-presenting cell
ARDS	acute respiratory distress syndrome
ART-tips	aerosol resistant tips
Az	sodium azide
BALF	broncho-alveolar lavage fluid
BCIP	bromochloroindolyl phosphate
BDHC	benzidine dihydrochloride
BNHS	*N*-hydroxysuccinimidobiotin
BrdU	bromodeoxyuridine
BrdUrd	5-bromodeoxyuridine
BSA	bovine serum albumin
CCD	charge coupled device
CDR	complementarity determining region
CFSE	5-(and-6)-carboxy-2′,7′ dichlorofluorescein diacetate succinimidylester
CHO	Chinese hamster ovary cell
cm	chloramphenicol resistance gene
CN	4-chloro-1-naphthol
CPD	citrate, phosphate, dextrose
CR	complement receptor
CSA	cyclosporin A
CTL	cytotoxic T lymphocyte
Cy	indocarbocyanine/ide
D/C	direct current
DAB	diaminobenzidine
DABCO	1,4-diazobicyclo(2,2,2)-octane
DAF	decay accelerator factor
DAPI	4′6-diamidino-2-phenylindole

DCFH-DA	dichlorofluorescein-diacetate
DEPC	diethyl pyrocarbonate
DHFR	dihydrofolate reductase
DHR	dihydrorhodamine
DIC	diisopropylcarbodiimide
DKP	diketopiperazine
DMEM	Dulbecco's modified Eagles medium
DMF	dimethylformamide
DMSO	dimethyl sulfoxide
dsFv	disulfide linked Fv
DT	diphtheria toxin
DTPA	diethylenetriaminepenta acetic anhydride
DTT	dithiothreitol
DTTA	diethylenetriaminetetra acetic anhydride
EBV	Epstein–Barr virus
ECLIA	enzyme-linked chemiluminescence immunoassay
EDT	ethanedithiol
EDTA	ethylenediaminetetraacetic acid
EF2	elongation factor-2
EIA	enzyme immunoassay
ELFIA	enzyme-linked fluoroimmunoassay
ELISA	enzyme-linked immunosorbent assay
ELISPOT	enzyme-linked immunospot
EPOS	enhanced polymer one-step staining
F:P:	fluorochrome:protein
FC	flow cytofluorimetry
FCS	fetal calf serum
FDNB	fluorodinitrobenzene
FI	fluorescence intensity
FIA	fluoroimmunoassay
FISH	fluorescent *in situ* hybridization
FITC	fluorescein isothiocyanate
FMLP	f-met-leu-phe
FOAM	fluorescent overlay antigen mapping
F:P	fluorochrome-to-protein ratio
FR	framework region
FSC	forward light scatter
Fv	variable domain fragment
GAP	glycine acid peptide
gpt	guanosine phosphoribosyl transferase gene
GS	glutamine synthetase
GTC	guanidinium thiocyanate
H/B	HBSS with 0.01% bovine serum albumin
HAT	hypoxanthine aminopterin thymidine

HBSS	Hanks balanced salt solution
hCMV	human cytamegalovirus major immediate-early gene
HGPRT	hypoxanthine guanine phosphoribosyl transferase
HIFCS	heat inactivated FCS
HOBt	1-hydroxybenzotriazole
HRP	horse-radish peroxidase
HT	hypoxanthine thymidine
IC	immune complex
ICAM-1	intercellular adhesion molecule-1
IFN-γ	interferon-γ
Ig	immunoglobulin
IL-1β	interleukin-1β
IOD	integrated optical density
IPTG	isopropyl-β-D-thiogalactopyranoside
IRMA	immunoradiometric assay
ISC	immunoglobulin-secreting cell
IT	immunotoxin
KLH	keyhole limpet haemocyanin
LAK	lymphokine-activated killer cell
LCL	lymphoblastoid cell line
Leu-leuO-Me	leucyl-leucine-methyl ester
LIA	luminoimmunoassay
LISS	low ionic strength saline
LPS	lipopolysaccharide
LSAB	labelled streptavidin–biotin
mAb	monoclonal antibody
MNC	mononuclear cell
MPS	multiple peptide synthesis
MRI	magnetic resonance imaging
MSX	methionine sulfoximine
MTX	methotrexate
NBT	nitroblue tetrazolium
neo	neomycin resistance gene
NPG	*n*-propyl gallate
NPP	*p*-nitrophenyl phosphate
OD	optical density
ONPG	ortho nitrophenyl-β-D-galactopyranoside
PAP	peroxidase anti-peroxidase
PBMC	peripheral blood mononuclear cell
PBS/BSA	PBS containing 0.5% (w/v) bovine serum albumin
PBS	phosphate-buffered saline
PBSe	PBS containing 1 mM EDTA
PBST	PBS with 0.1% (w/v) added Tween 20
PBSTA	PBST with 0.1% (w/v) added sodium azide

PCNA	proliferating cellular nuclear antigen
PCR	polymerase chain reaction
PE	pseudomonas exotoxin
PEG	polyethylene glycol
PFC	plaque-forming cell
PHA	phytohaemagglutinin
PI	propidium iodide
PLP	periodate–lysine–paraformaldehyde
PMSF	phenylmethylsulfonyl fluoride
PMT	photomultiplier tube
PPD	paraphenylenediamine
PRINS	primed *in situ* labelling
PVA	polyvinyl alcohol
PWM	pokeweed mitogen
Px	peroxidase
rDNA	recombinant DNA
rbs	ribosome binding site
RB200SC	lissamine rhodamine B sulfonyl chloride
RGB	red, green, and blue
RIP	ribosome-inactivating protein
R-PE	R-phycoerythrin
RPMI	Roswell Park Memorial Institute
sE-selectin	soluble E-selectin
SFE	specific fluorescence equivalent
sFv	single chain Fv
sICAM-1	soluble intercellular adhesion molecule-1
SIF	specificity interval factor
SIT	silicone-intensified tube
SMCC	*N*-succinimidyl-4-(*N*-maleimidomethylcyclohexane)-1-carboxylate
SMPT	succinimidyloxycarbonyl-α-methyl-α-(2-pyridyldithio)-toluene
SNARF	carboxy-seminaphthorhodafluor
SPDP	*N*-succinimidyl-3(2-pyridyldithio) propionate
SRBC	sheep red blood cell
SSC	side light scatter
sVCAM-1	soluble vascular cell adhesion molecule-1
TBS	tris-buffered saline
Tc	cytotoxic T cell
TCA	trichloroacetic acid
TCM	tissue culture media
TCR	T cell receptor
Th	helper T cell
TNF-α	tumour necrosis factor-α

TOPO	tri-*n*-octylphosphineoxide
TRITC	tetramethylrhodamine isothiocyanate
U	relative units
VCAM-1	vascular cell adhesion molecule-1
V_H	heavy chain variable domain
V_L	light chain variable domain

1

Antibody affinity measurements

HÉLÈNE SAUNAL, ROBERT KARLSSON, and
MARC H. V. VAN REGENMORTEL

1. Introduction

In order to assess the biological activity of antibody (Ab) molecules, it is necessary to measure the strength of their interaction with the antigen (Ag) in terms of the equilibrium constant K_A (1). This constant corresponds to the inverse of the Ab concentration which is needed to obtain 50% of complexed species. Since formation and dissociation of complexes continuously occur the equilibrium state is dynamic. The rates of association and dissociation are of considerable interest since they give information on the way the equilibrium is reached. Changes in reaction rate and affinity can be used to probe structure–activity correlations in one of the reactants (2–4) and to select appropriate reagents for the immunodetection of biological substances.

Several techniques are available to measure the equilibrium constant K_A of Ag–Ab interactions but there are only very few methods for kinetic analysis. At present the easiest and most reliable way to measure binding kinetics is by means of a biosensor instrument based on surface plasmon resonance (5).

Three widely used methods for measuring affinity constants will be described. All three methods are based on the separation of bound and free reactants and the molecular weight of the Ag determines which method is most appropriate. The technique of equilibrium dialysis is suitable for measuring the affinity of Abs to haptens whereas precipitation with ammonium sulfate can be used with small haptens as well as with protein Ags. For large Ags such as viruses, ultracentrifugation can be used for separating free from bound Ab. A fourth method used for measuring affinity constants but which does not require the separation of free from bound Abs will be described.

The recently developed biosensor technique for measuring binding kinetics will be described in detail since it offers many advantages over other methods.

2. General theory

When two interacting molecular species A and B are mixed in solution, the formation of complexes will proceed until an equilibrium is reached. At equilibrium, the Ab–Ag interaction may be expressed as follows:

$$A + B \underset{k_d}{\overset{k_a}{\Leftrightarrow}} AB$$

where A represents free Ag; B free Ab; AB the Ag–Ab complex; k_a (M^{-1} sec^{-1}) and k_d (sec^{-1}) the association and dissociation rate constants respectively.

According to the law of mass action, the equilibrium constant can be expressed in terms of the concentrations of A, B, and AB either as an association equilibrium constant K_A (unit M^{-1}) or a dissociation equilibrium constant K_D (unit M). At equilibrium:

$$k_a[A][B] = k_d[AB]$$
$$k_a/k_d = K_A = [AB]/[A][B]$$
$$\text{and } k_d/k_a = K_D = [A][B]/[AB].$$

It should be noted that these formulae for the affinity constant are correct only when interactions between Ab and Ag combining sites are independent of each other. When both reactants are binding in a multivalent manner, the binding events will be linked and no longer independent of each other.

The increase in concentration of AB complexes over time can be written as:

$$d[AB]/dt = k_a[A][B].$$

The decrease in concentration of AB complexes over time can be written as:

$$d[AB]/dt = -k_d[AB].$$

The observed net rate of formation or dissociation of AB complexes when approaching equilibrium is the sum of the two rate expressions:

$$d[AB]/dt = k_a[A][B] - k_d[AB].$$

At equilibrium, the association rate will offset the dissociation rate and the net rate of complex formation will be zero:

$$d[AB]/dt = 0 \quad \text{and} \quad k_a[A][B] = k_d[AB].$$

3. Equilibrium constant *K* measurement

A variety of symbols have been employed to express the different parameters used in affinity calculations. When the symbols used by Hardie and Van

Regenmortel (6) are employed, the association equilibrium constant K of an Ab may be expressed in terms of the mass action law as follows:

$$K_A = \frac{sx}{(As - sx)(Bn - sx)} = \frac{ny}{(As - ny)(Bn - ny)} \qquad [1]$$

where: A = total antigen concentration (mol/litre); B = total antibody concentration (mol/litre); s = antigen valence; n = antibody valence; y = bound antibody concentration (mol/litre); Bn = total antibody sites (mol/litre); and $ny = sx$ = total bound sites. *Equation 1* can be rearranged into forms suitable for Scatchard representation of binding data, e.g.

$$f/d = K_A\,(s - nf) \qquad [2]$$

where $f = y/A$ and $d = B - y$.

The Scatchard plot of f/d versus nf gives the value of K_A as the slope and the value of the antigen valence s by extrapolation of the abscissa at the origin (7–9).

3.1 Equilibrium dialysis

For determining the affinity constant of an Ab directed to a monovalent hapten, the usual procedure consists of measuring the free Ag concentration after having separated the small hapten molecules from the larger Ag–Ab complex by equilibrium dialysis (10–12). The principle of the technique is indicated in *Figure 1*.

The reaction vessel is divided into two compartments A and B of equal size (usually about 1 ml volume) separated by a cellophane membrane that allows only the hapten molecules to pass through in either direction. Radioactively

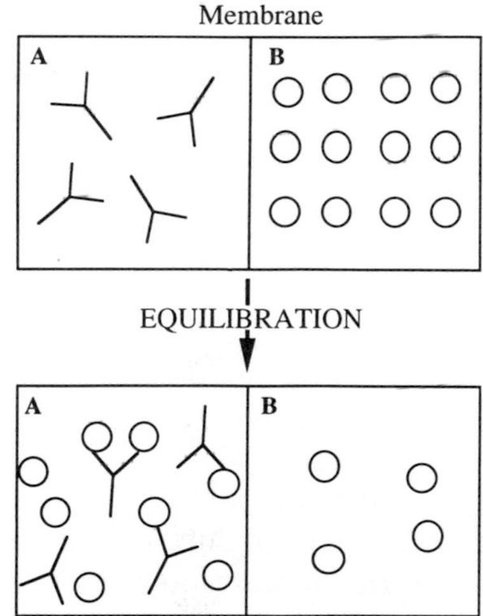

Figure 1. The principle of the method of equilibrium dialysis.

labelled haptens are commonly used. The Ab and the hapten are introduced into compartments A and B respectively. The Ab molecules, because of their large size, remain in compartment A. When equilibrium has been established, usually after 24–48 hours, the concentration of free hapten on both sides of the cellophane membrane is the same. However, there is a larger number of hapten molecules in compartment A since this compartment also contains hapten molecules bound to the Ab. From a knowledge of the initial hapten concentration in compartment B and after measuring the remaining free hapten concentration after equilibrium has been reached, it is possible to calculate the concentration of bound hapten. A series of experiments at different Ag and Ab concentrations are carried out and the equilibrium constant is derived from Scatchard plots. It is necessary to check for the possible adsorption of Ag or Ab to the membrane. The method is applicable to Ag with $M_r < 3000$ Da (12).

3.2 Ammonium sulfate precipitation

The ammonium sulfate precipitation method also known as the Farr method (13) involves precipitating Ag–Ab complexes with 50% saturated ammonium sulfate and measuring the amount of free Ag in the supernatant after centrifugation. Usually the Ag is labelled with a radioactive or fluorescent probe. This makes it possible to quantify the amount of free Ag in the supernatant or the amount of bound Ag in the pellet. The method requires that the Ag be soluble in 50% saturated ammonium sulfate and that all free and bound Ab molecules be precipitated. This method is no longer widely used because of several disadvantages. The equilibrium may be disturbed by the addition of salts (14), Ag molecules may be precipitated together with the complexes (15), and not all classes of Ab molecules may be equally precipitable (16).

3.3 Measurement of free Ab at equilibrium by ELISA titration

In order to calculate the binding affinity of Ab raised against large multivalent Ags such as viruses, it is necessary to measure the amount of free Ab present in an Ag–Ab mixture under equilibrium conditions.

Free Ab can be separated from Ag–Ab complexes by various procedures such as ultracentrifugation (6,17,18), equilibrium filtration (19,20), or simple washing when the multivalent Ag is immobilized on plastic in a solid phase assay (see Chapter 2). Ultracentrifugation can be used if there is a significant difference between the sedimentation coefficient of the Ag and the Ab. The amount of free Ab present in the supernatant after centrifugation of Ag–Ab complexes can be determined by absorbance readings at 280 nm (6,17,21) but this necessitates the use of high concentrations of Ag and Ab which are prohibitive for many applications. Azimzadeh and Van Regenmortel (22) described the use of a simple ELISA titration method for quantifying the amount of the free monoclonal Ab present in the supernatant after ultracentrifugation of tobacco mosaic virus (TMV)–Ab complexes. The absorbance measured by ELISA at various dilutions of supernatants is expressed as free Ab using a calibration curve established with known Ab concentrations. This allows the affinity constant (or avidity) of anti-viral Abs to be measured at low concentrations under conditions where the Ab binds in either a monovalent or a bivalent fashion. This method is described below using data from Azimzadeh and Van Regenmortel (22).

Optimal ultracentrifugation conditions for separating the Ag from free Ab has to be determined in preliminary experiments. Under the conditions used the supernatant should be free of residual Ag and the pellet should contain no significant free Ab. It is also necessary to determine the range of concentrations that must be used in order to obtain linear plots of absorbance versus standard Ab concentration. Monoclonal antibodies (Mabs) contained in supernatants (see *Protocol 1*) must be diluted in order to fall within this predetermined linear range of the plot. Mabs of known concentration for establishing the calibration curve and Mabs from supernatants are incubated on the same plate (see *Protocol 2*).

Protocol 1. Binding tests

Equipment and reagents

- 200 μl centrifuge tubes (Beckman No. 343775)
- Beckman TL-100 ultracentrifuge
- TLA-100 Beckman rotor
- PE buffer: 10 mM sodium phosphate pH 7.2, 1 mM EDTA

Method

1. Mix into 200 μl centrifuge tubes 75 μl of different dilutions of virus (20–100 μg/ml TMV) in PE buffer and 75 μl of a constant concentration of Mab 253P in PE buffer containing 0.05% Tween 20 and 1% BSA (bovine serum albumin).
2. Incubate the tubes for 1 h at 25 °C. Centrifuge for 10 min at 109 000 *g*.
3. Remove 70 μl of supernatant from each tube. Store in silicone treated tubes at 4 °C.

The calibration curve is drawn by plotting log [Ab concentration] versus absorbance. The amount of free Ab remaining in the supernatant is measured by ELISA (see *Protocol 2*) and is used to calculate $y = B - d$ and $f = y/A$ (see *Table 1*). The exact concentration of active antibody (B) introduced in a binding assay is usually unknown and the need to correct for the presence of inactive antibody, especially in the case of bivalent Ab binding, is discussed below.

Protocol 2. Measurement of free Ab concentration by ELISA

Equipment and reagents

- Polyvinyl microtitre plates (Falcon, 3912)
- Rabbit anti-mouse Ab (RAM/Ig/7S, Nordic)
- Horse-radish peroxidase (HRP)-conjugated rabbit anti-mouse Ab (RAM/IgG(H + L)/PO) (Nordic)
- PBS-T buffer: PBS buffer, 0.05% Tween 20
- PBS buffer: 150 mM NaCl, 10 mM KH_2PO_4, 10 mM Na_2HPO_4, 2.7 mM KCl, 3 mM NaN_3 pH 7.4
- ABTS substrate: 2,2′-azino-bis(3-ethylbenzthiazoline-6)sulfonic acid (Bœrhinger 102946)

Method

1. Coat the wells by overnight incubation at 37 °C with 150 μl of RAM/Ig/7S diluted 1/2000 in 0.05 M carbonate buffer pH 9.6.
2. Wash the plate thoroughly with PBS-T.
3. Shake the plate dry, saturate the wells by adding 200 μl of PBS-T containing 0.1% BSA (PBS-T-BSA). Incubate for 1 h at 37 °C.
4. Wash the plate, shake it dry, add 100 μl of different dilutions of the monoclonal Ab in PBS-T-BSA to the plate in duplicate. Incubate for 2 h at 37 °C.
5. Wash the plate, shake it dry, add 150 μl of RAM/IgG(H + L)/PO diluted 1/2000 in PBS-T. Incubate for 2 h at 37 °C.
6. Add to each well of the washed plates 100 μl of ABTS substrate. After 70–80 min incubation at 37 °C, stop the reaction by adding to each well 50 μl of 0.1 M citric acid containing 1.5 mM sodium azide.
7. Read the absorbance at 405 nm.

Binding data are represented according to *Equation 2* without any knowledge of Ag and Ab valence (*Figure 2*). In this plot of f/d versus f, two populations of points represented by open and black symbols were observed corresponding to high and low values of f respectively. The points situated in the zone $400 < f < 800$ correspond to Ab molecules binding in a monovalent manner whereas points in the region where $f < 400$ correspond to Ab molecules binding increasingly in a bivalent manner (9). For these last points, a positive slope was obtained from which a meaningful value of K_A could not be calculated. This positive slope is due to the presence of a certain proportion of inactive molecules in the Ab preparation.

A very similar method for measuring the Ab affinity to cell surface Ags has been described by Bator and Reading (23). In this study, however, the authors limited their analysis to the region where bivalent binding predominated.

Table 1. Example of experimental data of a binding test between TMV and Mab 253[a]

A^b (10^{-9} M)	$OD_{405\ nm}$[c]	Supernatant dilution	d^d (μg/ml)	d (10^{-9} M)	$y = sx^e$ ($n = 1$)	$f = y/A$	f/d	As^f	$2y = sx$ ($n = 2$)	$sc = As - y^g$ ($n = 1$)	$sc = As - 2y$ ($n = 2$)
0.5	0.765	1000	29.90	199.333	400.667	801.334	4.021	338	801.334	<0	<0
0.625	0.878	500	20.50	136.667	463.333	741.333	5.424	485	926.666	21.667	<0
0.75	0.881	250	10.30	68.667	531.333	708.444	10.317	582	1062.666	50.667	<0
0.875	0.839	125	4.60	30.667	569.333	650.666	21.217	679	1138.666	109.667	<0
1	0.411	125	1.40	9.333	590.667	590.667	63.238	776	1181.334	185.333	<0
1.125	0.785	31.25	0.98	6.533	593.467	527.526	80.748	873	1186.934	279.533	<0
1.25	0.712	31.25	0.81	5.333	594.667	475.734	89.206	970	1189.334	375.333	<0
1.375	0.653	31.25	0.68	4.533	595.467	433.067	95.537	1.067	1190.934	471.533	<0
1.5	0.595	31.25	0.58	3.867	596.133	397.422	102.773	1.164	1192.266	567.867	<0
1.625	0.573	31.25	0.62	4.133	595.867	366.687	88.722	1.261	1191.734	665.133	69.266
1.75	0.554	31.25	0.59	3.933	596.067	340.611	86.603	1.358	1192.134	761.933	165.866
1.875	0.558	31.25	0.59	3.933	596.067	317.902	80.829	1.455	1192.134	858.933	262.866
2	0.526	31.25	0.54	3.601	596.401	298.201	82.833	1.552	1192.801	955.601	359.201
2.125	0.521	31.25	0.53	3.533	596.467	280.691	79.448	1.649	1192.934	1052.533	456.066
2.25	0.542	31.25	0.57	3.801	596.201	264.978	69.731	1.746	1192.401	1149.801	553.601
2.375	0.484	31.25	0.48	3.201	596.801	251.284	78.526	1843	1193.601	1246.201	649.401
2.5	0.496	31.25	0.49	3.267	596.733	238.693	73.062	1940	1193.466	1343.267	746.534

[a] Data from ref. 22.
[b] A = TMV concentration.
[c] $OD_{405\ nm}$ = average of duplicate values obtained from ELISA.
[d] d = free igG concentration.
[e] y = bound IgG concentration, y is obtained from the relation $y = B - d$.
[f] As = total antigen sites concentration ($s = 789$).
[g] sc = free antigen sites concentration.

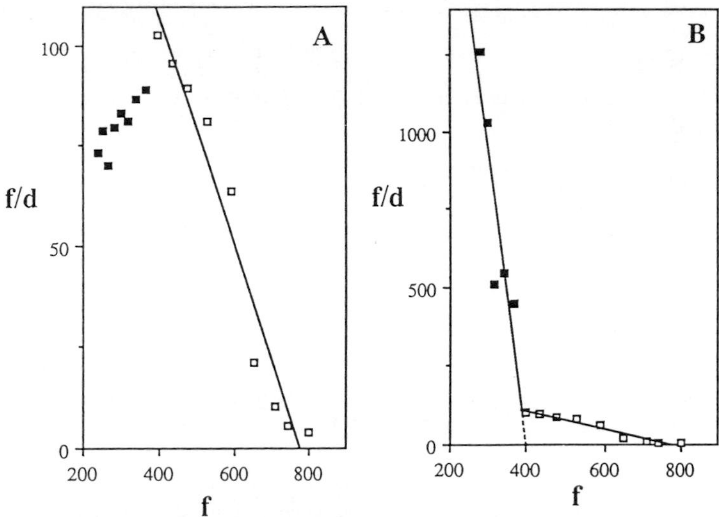

Figure 2. TMV–Mab binding data plotted according to *Equation 2* before (A) and after (B) correcting for the presence of 0.55% inactive antibody molecules. Open and black symbols correspond, respectively, to monovalent and bivalent binding of IgG molecules (from ref. 22).

3.3.1 Correction for the presence of inactive molecules in the Ab preparation

Two transformations of the mass action law are useful for assessing the extent to which the real value of *Bn* differs from the amount of Ab supposedly introduced in the test. These are:

$$sc = Bn\left(\frac{sc}{sx}\right) - \frac{1}{K_A} \qquad [3]$$

$$\frac{sc}{sx} = \frac{1}{Bn}(sc) + \frac{1}{K_A.Bn} \qquad [4]$$

Both representations make it possible to derive the *Bn* value from the slope and to calculate the proportion of inactive Ab molecules present in the test.

The parameter*s*, *x*, *r*, and *c* used in these equations can be calculated as follows. The amount of bound Ab (y) is calculated from the binding data (*Table 1*) and the bound Ab sites are expressed as Ag sites using the relation $ny = sx$. However, this requires that an hypothesis be made regarding the values of s and n. In the example shown in *Table 1* and *Figure 2* the value of $s = 789$ obtained by extrapolation in *Figure 2A* was used. As far as the Ab is concerned, the value of n could be one or two depending of whether IgG is bound in a monovalent or divalent manner. In order to assess which of these two situations is likely to be the case, calculations are carried out with both

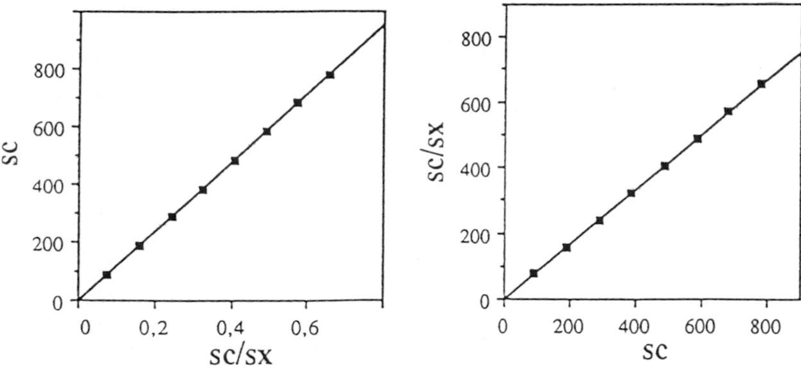

Figure 3. TMV–Mab 253P binding data corresponding to monovalent antibody binding plotted according to *Equations 3* and *4* (from ref. 22).

values of n. For some of the points it was found that negative values of sc were obtained when the value $n = 2$ (*Table 1*) was used. In this case it was assumed that the Ab was binding in a monovalent manner. All others points were assumed to correspond to bivalent binding. Bn values obtained from plots according to *Equations 3* and *4* corresponding to bivalent binding (*Figure 3*) were significantly lower than the theoretical Bn value. The percentage of inactive Ab (0.55%) obtained from *Equation 3* was found to correspond to 3.31×10^{-9} M inactive Ab sites. When this amount was subtracted from d, the plot f/d versus f shown in *Figure 2B* was obtained and the points produced a line with a normal negative slope. The extrapolation of the abscissa at the origin corresponded to a value of $s/2$ while the slope was twice the value of K_A (4.7×10^9 M^{-1}). Modelling studies (*Figure 4*) have demonstrated that in the case of Abs of increasing affinity, it becomes increasingly important to correct for the presence of inactive Ab in the binding assay. The avidity of the Mab when binding in a bivalent manner was about 15 times higher (4.6×10^9 M^{-1}) than the affinity corresponding to monovalent binding (3.2×10^8 M^{-1}). In the case of monovalent binding, it was not necessary to correct the Bn value.

3.4 Measurement of free Ab at equilibrium using BIAcore

This method described by Zeder-Lutz *et al.* (24) is based on the same principle as the method described above. The amount of free Ab is determined by means of the biosensor technique described in Section 4.1. The Ag is immobilized on the sensor surface and the Ab is introduced in a flow passing over the surface. The binding of Ab is visualized in real time and is expressed in RU (resonance units). The data are presented in the form of a sensorgram visualized on a computer screen which plots RU versus time. A calibration curve of response level in RU versus Ab concentration is established using a

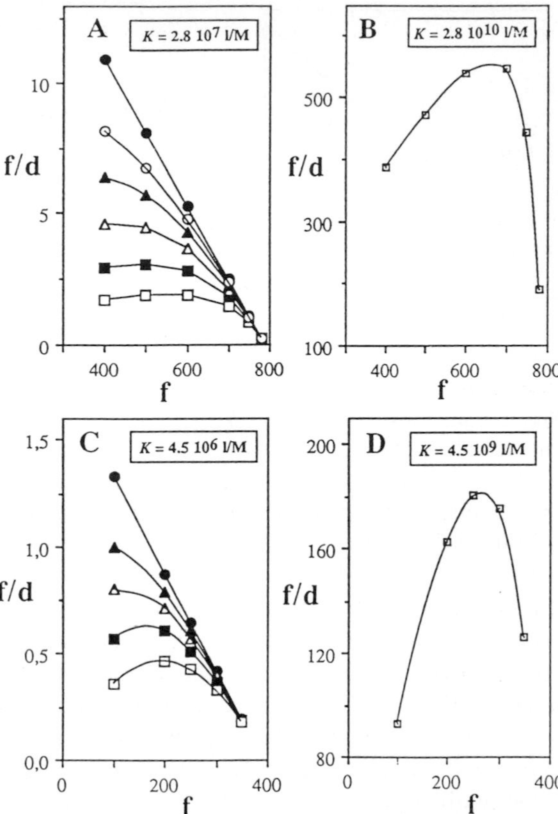

Figure 4. Modelling studies showing the influence of various percentages of inactive antibody molecules on the *f/d* versus *f* plot in the case of antibodies of different K_A. Theoretical plots for monovalent binding of TMV antibody of $K_A = 2.8 \times 10^7$ M^{-1} (A) and $K_A = 2.8 \times 10^{10}$ M^{-1} (B). Theoretical plots for bivalent binding of TMV antibody of $K_A = 4.5 \times 10^6$ M^{-1} (C) and $K_A = 4.5 \times 10^9$ M^{-1} (D). The following percentages of inactive antibody were introduced: 0.17% (□) for B and D, and 0% (●); 2% (○); 4% (▲); 8% (△); 17% (■); 33% (□) for A and C (from ref. 22).

series of dilutions of an Ab of known concentration. A constant amount of Ag is mixed with increasing amounts of Ab and incubated for one hour. The mixture is injected on the surface containing immobilized Ag and free Ab will bind to this surface. The method does not require the preliminary separation of free from bound Ab and it can therefore be used with Ags of any size. It should be stressed that the sensitivity of the BIAcore makes it possible to determine free Ab concentrations down to at least 0.1 nM. A large range of affinities (from 10^4 to at least 10^9 M^{-1}) can then be measured, provided that the assay gives RU values that fall within the predetermined calibration curve.

4. Measurement of the kinetic rate constants k_a and k_d

4.1 Principles and technology of real time biosensor measurements

The BIAcore™ (Pharmacia, Uppsala), a biosensor system based on surface plasmon resonance (SPR) detection permits the quantitative analysis of biospecific interactions in real time. SPR is a quantum phenomenon which detects changes in optical properties at the surface of a thin gold film on a glass support (sensor surface). The instrument contains the SPR detector and a microfluidic cartridge that together with an autosampler, controls the delivery of sample plugs into a transport buffer that continuously passes over the sensor surface.

The sensor surface carries a dextran matrix to which one of the two reactants is covalently attached. The other is introduced in a flow passing over the surface. SPR detects changes in refractive index and this allows the concentration of the reactants to be measured. The dextran matrix extends out from the sensor surface and this permits proteins to be immobilized, for instance through amine groups. The interacting components do not need to be labelled. The reaction between immobilized ligand and injected analyte takes place in the hydrophilic environment defined by the dextran matrix. The reaction is monitored continuously in real time and the binding curve presented in a sensorgram is directly visualized on a computer screen. The y axis of the sensorgram corresponds to the resonance signal and is measured in resonance units (RU). The running buffer defines the baseline and all responses are expressed relative to this level.

At a given time the relative response R can be expressed as:

$$R = R_R + R_A + R_L$$

where R_R is the refractive index component for the buffer or sample, R_L corresponds to amount of immobilized ligand, and R_A corresponds to amount of analyte bound to immobilized ligand.

The change in signal level with respect to time is:

$$dR/dt = dR_R/dt + dR_A/dt + dR_L/dt.$$

Except for the 10–20 sec in the beginning and at the end of an injection, where running buffer is exchanged for samples and vice versa, $dR_R/dt = 0$. For covalently or biospecifically immobilized ligands, dR_L/dt is in most cases zero or close to zero and is always measurable. The change in response level reflects the binding of analyte to the immobilized ligand:

$$dR/dt = dR_A/dt.$$

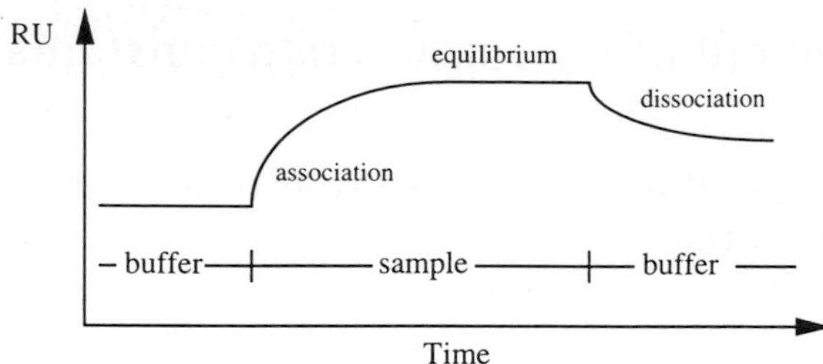

Figure 5. Schematic sensorgram showing association, equilibrium, and dissociation phase.

4.2 Principle of the method

When analyte is injected across a ligand surface, the resulting sensorgram (*Figure 5*) can be divided into three essential phases:

(a) Injection of analyte.
(b) Equilibrium or steady state during sample injection, where the rate of analyte binding is balanced by dissociation from the complex.
(c) A post-injection phase where buffer flows over the surface and where the concentration of analyte is zero.

Response values and binding curves are presented on a computer screen. Recorded data can later be processed, transformed, and analysed using BIAevaluation software.

4.2.1 Theoretical equations describing the interactions in BIAcore

When analyte A reacts with ligand B to form the complex AB, the net rate of complex formation depends on the free concentration of the A and B components and on the stability of the formed complex:

$$d[AB]/dt = k_a[A][B] - k_d[AB].$$

One can substitute [B] for $[B]_0 - [AB]$, where $[B]_0$ is the total concentration of reactant B:

$$d[AB]/dt = k_a[A]([B]_0 - [AB]) - k_d[AB].$$

In the biosensor, one of the reactants is immobilized on the sensor surface and the other is continuously replenished from a solution flowing over the sensor surface. The response R will correspond to the amount of AB complexes formed and the maximum response R_{max} will correspond to the surface concentration of the immobilized ligand $[B]_0$ which can be expressed in terms of the maximum analyte binding capacity of the surface. All concentration terms can then be expressed as an SPR response in RU, eliminating the need to convert from mass to molar concentration. The rate equation can thus be rewritten as:

$$dR/dt = k_aC(R_{max} - R) - k_dR$$

where dR/dt is the rate of formation of surface complexes (i.e. the rate of change of the SPR signal); C, which is kept constant is the concentration of analyte in free solution; R_{max} is the maximum analyte binding capacity in RU; R is the SPR signal in RU at time t.

During the post-injection phase $C = 0$, and

$$dR/dt = -k_d R.$$

During the injection phase, interaction kinetics measured in the BIAcore depend on both association and dissociation rate constants (k_a and k_d) whereas during the post-injection phase, only the dissociation rate constant (k_d) operates.

In the first reports describing BIAcore experiments, the interaction was analysed by means of a linear transformation of the interaction kinetics equation (5,25). Subsequently new software was introduced which analyses data by a non-linear regression method. This software calculates the dissociation rate constant (k_d) from the post-injection phase after the sample has been replaced by buffer and does not make use of the injection phase (26,27).

4.2.2 Processing of the post-injection phase data

The post-injection phase data are analysed first since the value of k_d is required in order to analyse the injection phase and calculate k_a.

After the pulse of analyte has passed over the sensor chip surface, the surface-bound complex dissociates according to a zero-order reaction. Assuming that reassociation of released analyte is negligible:

$$dR/dt = -k_d R$$

integrating with respect to time gives:

$$\ln R_1/Rt = k_d(t-t_1)$$

where Rt is the response at time t, and R_1 is the response at an arbitrary starting time t_1.

It is therefore informative to plot $\ln(R_1/Rt)$ versus t since this should give a straight line with slope k_d. The value of k_d is calculated using the untransformed signal by fitting experimental data to the fully integrated rate equation:

$$R_t = R_1\, e^{-kd\,(t - t_1)}.$$

In order to assess the reliability of the k_d value it is essential to perform a control experiment by introducing free ligand in the buffer used during the post-injection phase using the available 'kinject' program. The free ligand competes with the immobilized ligand, preventing the rebinding of the released analyte. The way in which the apparent dissociation rate may be affected by mass transfer is discussed in Section 4.3.

4.2.3 Processing of the injection phase data

During the injection phase, the observed rate of complex formation is described by:

$$\mathrm{d}R/\mathrm{d}t = k_a C(R_{max} - R) - k_d R.$$

This equation may be rearranged to give:

$$\mathrm{d}R/\mathrm{d}t = k_a C R_{max} - (k_a c + k_d)R$$
$$\text{or } \ln(\mathrm{d}R/\mathrm{d}t) = \ln(k_a C R_{max}) - (k_a c + k_d)t.$$

Thus plots of $\mathrm{d}R/\mathrm{d}t$ against R or of $\ln(\mathrm{d}R/\mathrm{d}t)$ against t will be a straight line with slope:

$$k_s = -(k_a C + k_d).$$

The rate constants k_s are then determined using non-transformed data and the integrated rate equation:

$$R(t) = R_{eq}(1 - e^{-k_s t}).$$

A first approach to obtain k_a is to measure the association sensorgram at several different analyte concentrations. Then a plot of k_s against C will give a straight line with slope k_a. In theory the dissociation rate constant k_d could be obtained from the intercept on the y axis. However, this intercept cannot be determined accurately, especially when k_d is low. Another approach consists of calculating the k_a value from a single k_s value, using k_d derived from the post-injection phase. In theory, only one analyte concentration could be run to obtain the k_a value. However, it is advisable to perform experiments at several concentrations and to compare k_a values obtained at each concentration.

If R_{max} is known, both k_a and k_d can be determined from a single association sensorgram. In practice R_{max} is sometimes difficult to determine experimentally, since a high analyte concentration may be required to saturate the surface.

4.3 Mass transfer during BIAcore experiments

The above analysis assumes that the observed rate of binding reflects only the interaction kinetics between analyte and ligand and not the transport of analyte to the surface (28). This means that the interaction kinetics should not be limited by the mass transfer of the analyte to the surface.

To take account of this factor, the reaction should be written:

$$A_{bulk} \underset{k_m}{\overset{k_m}{\Leftrightarrow}} A_{surface} + B \underset{k_d}{\overset{k_a}{\Leftrightarrow}} AB$$

where k_m is the rate constant for mass transfer to and from the surface.

$$k_m = 0.98(D/h)^{2/3}\,(f/0.3.b.l)^{1/3}$$

where D is the diffusion coefficient of the analyte, f is the bulk flow rate, and h, b, and l are the flow cell dimensions. In the flow cell the dimensions are fixed and the only variables affecting the mass transfer coefficient k_m are the flow rate and the diffusion coefficient.

The experimental parameters which determine whether the association rate is limited by mass transfer or by the propensity of the analyte to bind to the ligand are the flow rate and the concentration of surface binding sites (B). The flow rate affects the mass transfer constant k_m but has no effect on the interaction kinetics. The effect of the flow rate on the mass transfer is relatively small, since k_m is proportional to the cube root of the flow rate. In contrast, decreasing the surface binding capacity may significantly reduce mass transfer limitations by decreasing the initial interaction rate. With increasing time of interaction the concentration of surface binding sites falls and, in general, the mass transfer affects the binding rate more in the initial phase. Mass transfer-controlled and interaction-controlled kinetics correspond to extreme cases and most systems show an intermediate behaviour over a significant range of experimental conditions.

The mass transfer rate also depends on the diffusion coefficient of the analyte, which in turn depends on the molecular weight. A large analyte with a low diffusion coefficient will be more subject to mass transfer limitations than a small analyte with the same kinetic parameters. However, the detection is mass-sensitive and the range of rate constants that can be resolved becomes larger when the analyte molecular weight increases and this more than compensates for the effect of the low diffusion coefficient.

For a correct interpretation of association data, it is necessary to check whether the reaction rate is limited in a significant manner by mass transfer. The kinetics operating in BIAcore have been numerically described using an iterative computer model (28). From these data, and in order to assign the degree of mass transfer effect on the observed binding rate, a limit coefficient was defined as (29):

$$LC = k_m/k_a[B].$$

Using simulated sensorgrams for association and dissociation with different values of the limit coefficient, it was shown that for values of $LC > 5$ (when the calculated mass transfer rate is at least five times the interaction rate), the observed binding kinetics provide a good approximation to the interaction kinetics (29). When the limit coefficient is < 5 the contribution of mass transfer to the observed kinetics become more significant (see *Figure 6*).

In most interactions, mass transfer affects the binding rate only in the initial phase (see *Figure 7*) and the BIA evaluation software offers the possibility of selecting a suitable portion of the injection phase for evaluating of data.

During the post-injection phase, the mass transfer coefficient is also an important parameter for the observed rate of dissociation (see *Figure 8*). Continuous flow of buffer over the surface maintains zero analyte concentrations

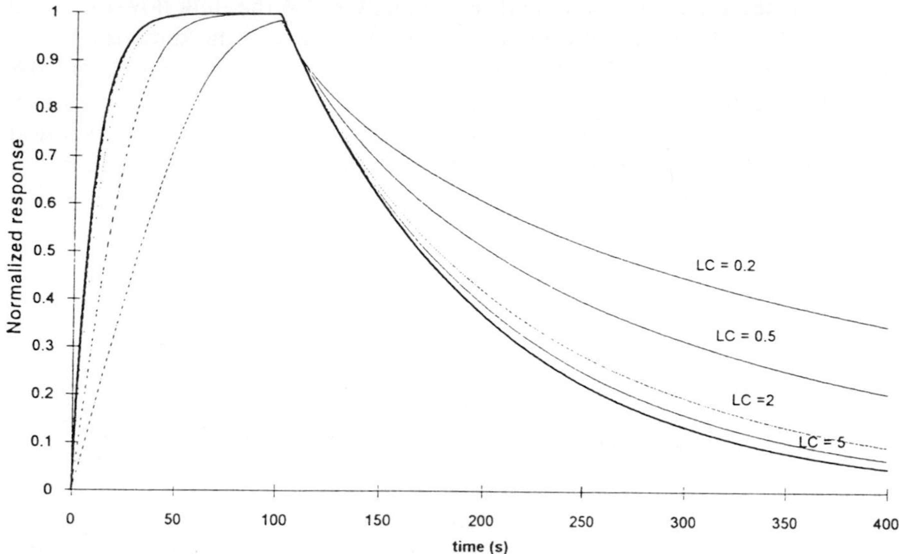

Figure 6. Simulated sensorgrams for association and dissociation with different values of the mass transport limit coefficient (from ref. 29).

in bulk solution during the post-injection phase. Analyte molecules released at the surface by dissociation of the complex can either be removed by mass transfer to the bulk solution or rebind to free ligand sites on the surface. This means that the observed rate of dissociation will reflect the dissociation constant for the interaction only if mass transfer is fast enough to avoid rebinding. The limitation by mass transfer will be most apparent at the end of the dissociation. Consequently, the observed k_d is most reliable at the beginning of the post-injection phase when the surface saturation is high and few ligand molecules are available for rebinding. In most cases, it is advisable to determine association and dissociation rate constants from different experiments, using a very high analyte concentration for k_d measurements. The surface is saturated as much as possible. This minimizes the potential rebinding effects and gives a high signal level thereby decreasing the percentage of error. Mass transfer limitations during dissociation could also be reduced by including free ligand in the buffer used during the post-injection phase (see Section 4.2.2). When mass transfer is an issue, the procedures described so far have been introduced to reduce its influence. Alternatively it is possible to include mass transfer into the calculations (see the rate equations for different interaction models in Section 4.4.5). This would require numerical integration of a set of differential equations. In combination with non-linear analysis of data, such a procedure is calculation intense. Due to the rapid development of computer technology it is now possible to perform these calculations on a PC (30). This should lead to more reliable analysis since all the data can be

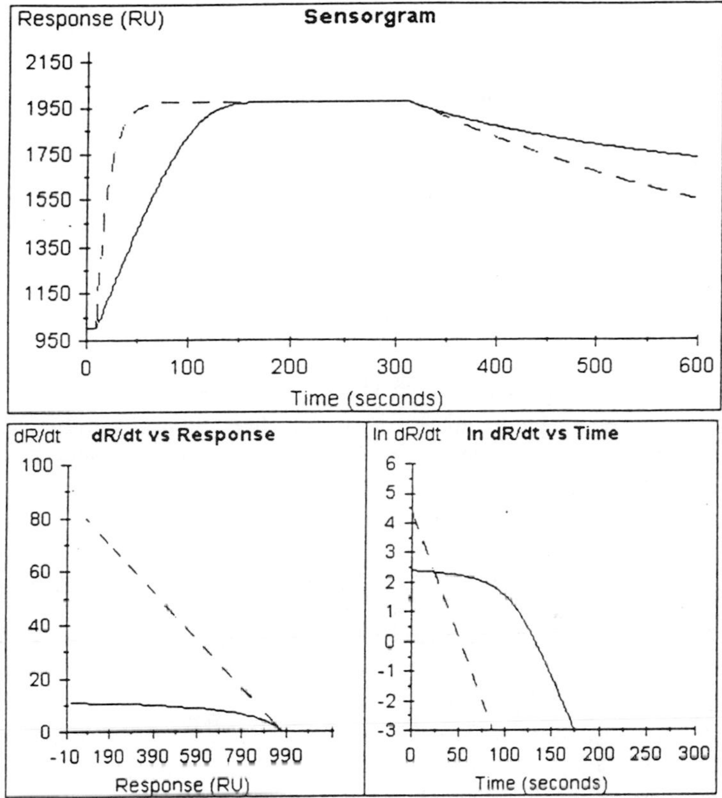

Figure 7. Sensorgram and association plots for binding under strongly mass transport-controlled conditions (from BIA simulation software). The broken lines show the corresponding results for the same interaction without mass transport limitation.

analysed, and it will not be necessary to make subjective selections of sensorgram data. It will still be of interest to minimize the effects of mass transfer when high quality kinetic data are needed and in particular this will be important when the interaction mechanism is complex.

4.4 More complex interactions

In some cases deviations from the pseudo-first order interaction model A + B $\Leftrightarrow$ AB are observed. They can be observed in both injection and post-injection phases but they are most often observed in the post-injection phase (*Figure 9*). Deviations can be due to a number of reasons. Mass transfer has already been mentioned. Non-specific binding, steric hindrance, and release of immobilized or captured ligand may also lead to such deviations. Here control experiments will often be helpful. Another reason for deviation is

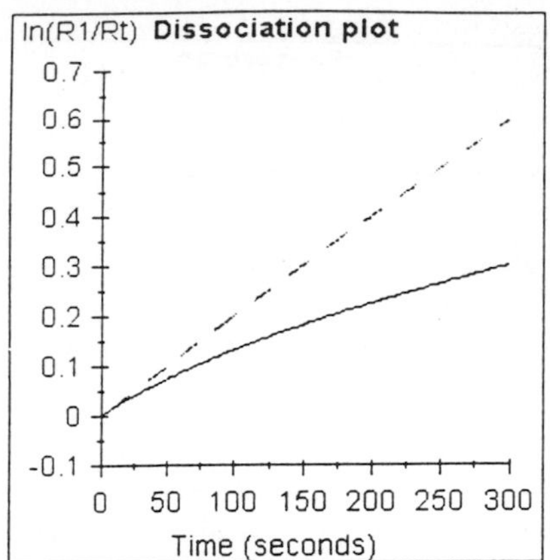

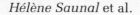

Figure 8. Dissociation plot for mass transport-limited dissociation. The broken line shows the plot for the same interaction without mass transport limitation.

Experimental data

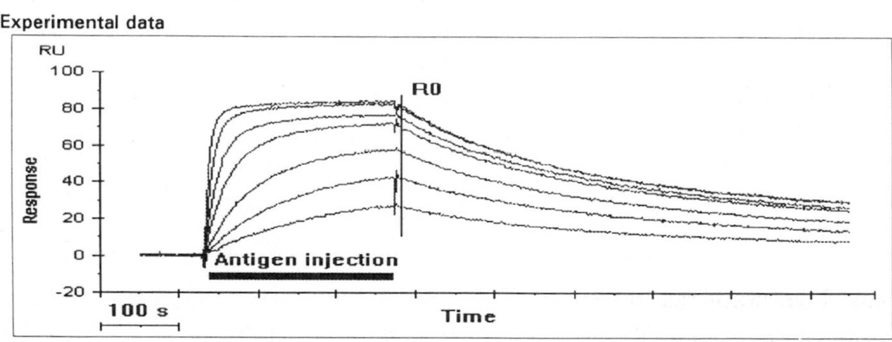

Transformed data

Injection phase data

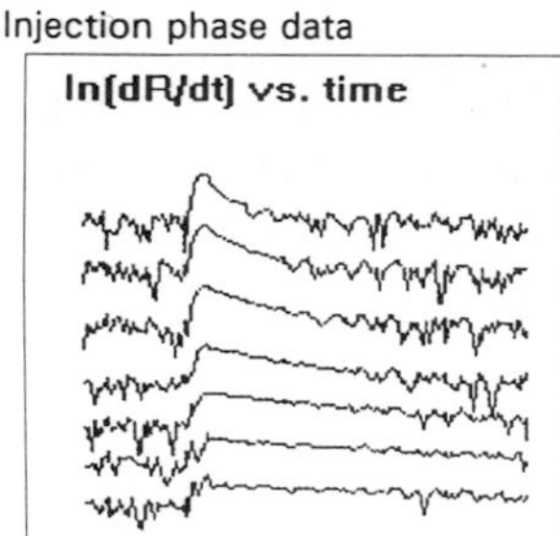

Post injection phase data

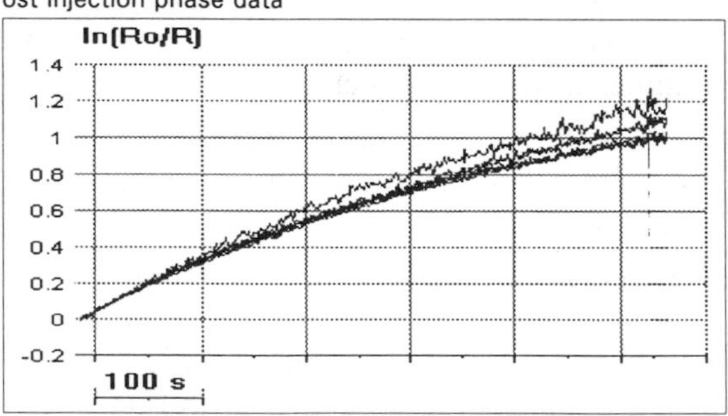

Figure 9. Sensorgrams obtained for interaction between an antibody and an antigen. Transformed data aids the selection of an appropriate interaction model. The deviation from linearity in the post-injection phase data indicates an interaction mechanism that is more complex than described by a one to one reaction.

that the interaction itself is more complex. The underlying assumption for using the pseudo-first order interaction model is that both interaction partners are homogeneous and that only single binding sites are involved.

4.4.1 Parallel reactions

If the immobilized ligand is heterogeneous, or if heterogeneity is introduced during the immobilization procedure, this may give rise to parallel interactions (*Figure 10a*). Each interaction can be viewed as a pseudo-first order interaction.

4.4.2 Competing reactions

If the analyte is heterogeneous two or more forms of the analyte compete for the binding sites of the immobilized ligand (*Figure 10b*). During the injection this means that the binding of one form of the analyte will influence the binding of another form and these interactions are linked to each other. As soon as injection stops, and the analyte concentration drops to zero, the dissociation of the different forms of the analyte from the complexes formed will be independent events.

4.4.3 Reaction with multivalent analyte

If the analyte has more than one binding site it may be appropriate to consider a multivalent interaction (*Figure 10c*). Different complexes are formed on the surface and the reactions are linked to each other during both injection and post-injection phases.

4.4.4 Two-state reaction

In some cases the initially formed AB complex may undergo conformational change leading to a more stable complex. This reaction is described by a two-state model (*Figure 10d*). The conformation change will take place as soon as the first complex has been formed and the shift from one complex to another continues in the post-injection phase.

4.4.5 Discriminating between interaction models

The rate equations for different interaction models are:

(a) One-to-one reaction:

$$\mathrm{A} + \mathrm{B} \Leftrightarrow \mathrm{AB}$$
$$\mathrm{d}R/\mathrm{d}t = k_\mathrm{a} C_\mathrm{A}(R_\mathrm{max} - R) - k_\mathrm{d} R$$

B is immobilized and R_{max} corresponds to the concentration of B. C_A is the concentration of A. R corresponds to the concentration of AB complex. Parallel reactions are treated as the sum of several one to one reactions.

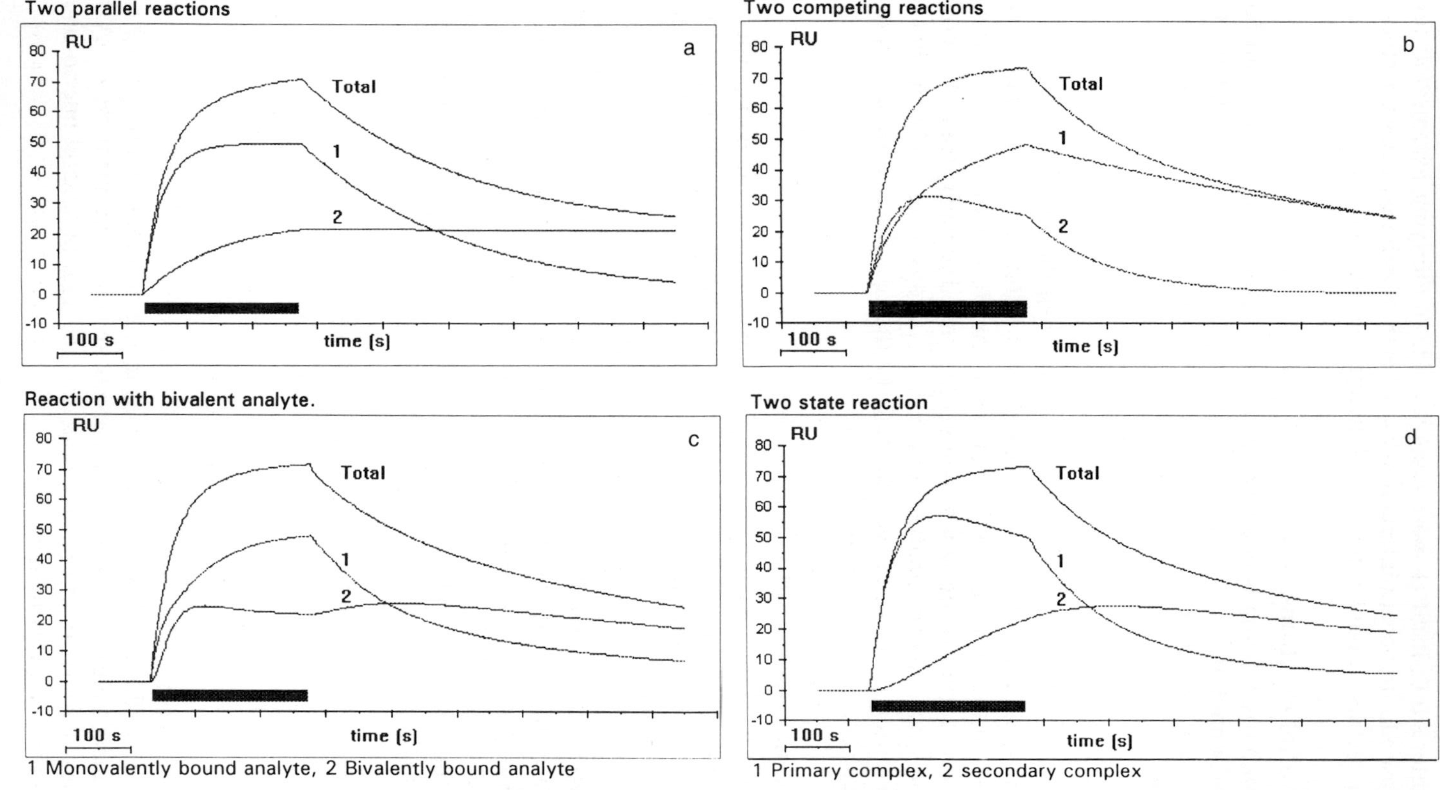

Figure 10. Analysis of one sensorgram in which the total response curve is presented in terms of interaction models describing (a) parallel reactions, (b) competing reactions, (c) reaction with bivalent analyte, and (d) a two-state reaction (see text).

(b) One-to-one reaction including mass transfer. To correct for sample depletion the actual concentration of analyte close to the surface, C_S, can be calculated and linked to the rate equation by introducing the transfer coefficient k_T.

$$dC_S/dt = k_T(C_A - C_S) - k_aC_S(R_{max} - R) + k_dR$$
$$dR/dt = k_aC_S(R_{max} - R) - k_dR$$

(c) Competing reactions:

$$A + B \Leftrightarrow AB$$
$$C + B \Leftrightarrow CB$$
$$dR_1/dt = k_{a1}C_A(R_{max} - R_1 - R_2p) - k_{d1}R_1$$
$$dR_2/dt = k_{a2}C_C.(R_{max}(1/p - R_1)(1/p - R_2)) - k_{d2}R_2$$

B is immobilized and R_{max} corresponds to the concentration of B. C_A is the concentration of A and C_C is the concentration of C. R_1 corresponds to the concentration of AB complex and R_2 to the concentration of CB complex. p is introduced in order to compare response values for analytes of different molecular weight since such analytes give rise to different responses.

(d) Reaction with bivalent analyte:

$$A + B \Leftrightarrow AB$$
$$AB + B \Leftrightarrow AB_2$$
$$dR_1/dt = k_{a1}C_A(R_{max} - R_1 - 2R_2) - k_{d1}R_1 - k_{a2}(R_1(R_{max} - R_1 - 2R_2) + k_{d2}R_2)$$
$$dR_2/dt = k_{a2}(R_1(R_{max} - R_1 - 2R_2) - k_{d2}R_2)$$

B is immobilized and R_{max} corresponds to the concentration of B. C_A is the concentration of A. R_1 corresponds to the concentration of AB complex and R_2 to the concentration of AB_2 complex.

(e) Two-state reaction:

$$A + B \Leftrightarrow AB$$
$$AB \Leftrightarrow AB^*$$
$$dR_1/dt = k_{a1}C_A(R_{max} - R_1 - R_2) - k_{d1}R_1 - k_{a2}R_1 + k_{d2}R_2$$
$$dR_2/dt = k_{a2}R_1 - k_{d2}R_2$$

B is immobilized and R_{max} corresponds to the concentration of B. C_A is the concentration of A. R_1 corresponds to the concentration of AB complex and R_2 to the concentration of AB* complex.

The total response curve in *Figure 10* is actually one of the binding curves from *Figure 9* and it demonstrates the binding of myoglobin to captured anti-myoglobin Mab. *Figures 10a–d* were obtained by analysing these data using the parallel, the competitive, the bivalent, and the two-state interaction models, and software combining numerical integration and global analysis.

The results clearly demonstrate that a single interaction curve can be analysed with equal success using several different interaction models. Using a series of analyte concentrations, heterogeneity may often be identified. To discriminate between independent and linked interactions it is also very useful to vary the analyte injection time (*Figure 11*). In such an experiment the concentration of analyte should be high so that antibody binding sites rapidly become saturated. If the reactions are independent the composition of Ab–Ag complexes on the surface will not change during the injection. Consequently the binding curves after the injection should be identical and reflect the dissociation of these complexes. When the interactions are linked, the composition of Ab–Ag complexes will change over time, and the apparent dissociation rate decreases as more stable complexes are formed. Once the existence of linked interactions has been demonstrated it is evident that a model based on parallel and independent binding sites cannot be used to interpret the data. A multivalent interaction will give rise to a different stoichiometry from a monovalent interaction since each analyte can consume several binding sites. The ratio between analyte and ligand response values will thus give a clear indication whether a multivalent interaction is at hand or not. To discriminate between competitive and two-state reactions is more difficult. Evidence obtained from other techniques such as calorimetry or chromatography where conformation change or heterogeneity can be observed could then be used in combination with kinetic data in order to determine the least likely interaction mechanism.

4.4.6 Simulation using different interaction models

Just as interaction data can be directly evaluated it is also possible to simulate interaction curves using different interaction models. If a data set can be evaluated equally well using several models, simulation using parameters obtained in the evaluation procedure may be used to identify experimental

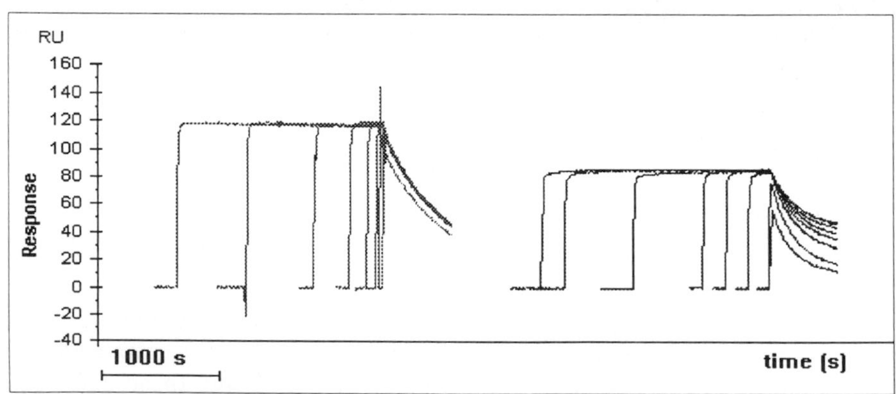

Figure 11. Sensorgrams obtained using variable injection times to demonstrate difference in behaviour for independent and linked interactions.

conditions where it is possible to distinguish between these models. Simulation thus becomes a tool for experimental design.

4.4.7 Reporting rate and affinity constants

The complex nature of Ab–Ag interactions and the increasing awareness that it is sometimes difficult to validate an interaction model, makes it important to interpret and report kinetic rate constants and affinity constants as apparent constants. The interaction model used to obtain the values must be clearly stated. Rate and affinity constants are often used to predict the outcome of an interaction and they also provide a basis for the comparison of different biological systems in terms of the speed, sensitivity, and stability of the interaction. If this is the aim of the investigation, the apparent rate constants calculated using a simple interaction model (although all data are not explained) are often meaningful. When insight into the reaction mechanism is the aim of the investigation more detailed analysis becomes necessary. Thus the purpose of the investigation will determine how detailed the analysis must be. True rate and affinity constants can only be cited when the interaction mechanism is determined and described in an appropriate model.

4.5 Range of kinetic rate constants measurable with the BIAcore system

The range of kinetic constants that can be measured with precision using the BIAcore is 10^2 to 5×10^6 M^{-1} sec^{-1} for k_a and 10^{-5} to 10^{-2} sec^{-1} for k_d. In most biological interactions, values for k_a and k_d typically range from 10^3 to 10^7 M^{-1} sec^{-1} and 10^{-5} to 10^{-2} sec^{-1} respectively. When conditions for determining one or both rate constants are unfavourable, equilibrium measurements can be performed. The limiting factor which determines whether equilibrium determinations can be performed is the injection time required. The maximum time that can be used with the BIAcore is approximatively 40 min at a flow of 1 μl/min, 2 h in the BIAlite system, and about 12 h in the BIAcore 2000. The time to reach equilibrium at a given concentration is only dependent on the k_d value (*Table 2*).

Table 2. Approximate calculated times required to reach 99.9% of the steady state level at analyte concentrations ranging from 0.01 to 100 × K_D[a]

Concentrations	kd			
	10^{-1}	10^{-2}	10^{-3}	10^{-4}
$K_D \cdot 10^{-2}$	68 sec	11.5 min	114 min	–
$K_D \cdot 10^{-1}$	63 sec	10.5 min	105 min	–
K_D	34 sec	6 min	57 min	9.6 h
$K_D \cdot 10^{1}$	–	63 sec	10.5 min	105 min
$K_D \cdot 10^{2}$	–	–	68 sec	11 min

[a]Data from the BIAapplication handbook.

4.6 Experimental aspects of the determination of rate and equilibrium constants

4.6.1 Choice of immobilized ligand and injected analyte

The choice of immobilizing reactant depends on the following parameters.

The injected analyte should be large enough to give RU responses of sufficient magnitude. In practice direct kinetic measurements of analytes of molecular weight smaller than 10000 tend to be difficult with the BIAcore. The increased sensitivity of the BIAcore 2000 instrument makes it possible to perform kinetic measurements of analyte of M_r as low as 1000. The ligand should consist of a homogeneous population of molecules since kinetic data are otherwise difficult to interpret. In addition the immobilized ligand should be easily and reproducibly regenerated since a range of analyte concentrations must be tested for accurate determination of rate constants.

4.6.2 Choice of immobilization method

Ligands can be immobilized via primary amine groups using reactive esters (31). Other immobilization chemistries (coupling by thiol–disulfide exchange, binding biotinylated ligands to immobilized streptavidin, aldehyde coupling to a hydrazine-activated surface) are available (32), and immobilization procedures are described in the BIAapplications handbook. Thiol–disulfide exchange is more specific than the amine coupling chemistry and may provide a more homogeneous ligand. Moreover the thiol coupling is useful for immobilizing peptides or other small ligands when amine groups are lacking or may be required for biological activity.

Indirect immobilization of ligand employing a capture molecule can often be used to advantage for instance to give a uniform orientation of ligand molecules on the surface, to serve as a significant purification step for the ligand, or when any regeneration condition has a deleterious effect on ligand activity. However, the ligand should not dissociate from the capturing agent to any significant extent compared to the dissociation of the analyte.

4.6.3 Amount of immobilized ligand

In order to reduce mass transfer limitations, the amount of immobilized ligand should be kept as low as possible while ensuring that the binding of analyte gives a measurable response (R_{max} 100–1000 RU). A low level of immobilized ligand also minimizes the risk of steric hindrance influencing the reaction rate.

4.6.4 Analyte conditions

Analyte concentration should be high enough to ensure that the reaction is not limited by mass transfer. In general k_a measurements should be made at an analyte concentration well above the equilibrium dissociation constant K_D. This will ensure that the equilibrium level of analyte binding is close to the maximum surface capacity, so that the free ligand concentration approaches very low levels and the binding is not limited by mass transfer. In most cases, analyte concentrations ranging from about 1–100 nM in five to six steps will cover K_D values from about 2×10^{-7} to 2×10^{-10} M. Suitable injection times are from less than a minute to half an hour. The injection of analyte should not lead to a significant bulk refractive index contribution which could introduce errors in the rate determination.

4.7 Example of kinetic measurements in BIAcore analyses and interpretation of experimental data

The measurement of kinetic rate constants between an injected Fab fragment and an immobilized peptide will be described in this section. The Fab fragment was obtained by papain cleavage from Mab 174P, an antibody recognizing tobacco mosaic virus (TMV) protein. The peptide corresponds to residues 134–151 of TMV protein.

4.7.1 Immobilization of peptides on the sensor surface

The peptide was synthesized with an additional N-terminal cysteine in order to immobilize the peptide to the sensor chip via thiol groups (see *Protocol 3*).

Protocol 3. Immobilization of peptides on the sensor surface

Equipment and reagents

- BIAcore system (Pharmacia biosensor, Uppsala, Sweden)
- Amine coupling kit containing *N*-hydroxysuccinimide (NHS), *N*-ethyl-*N'*-(3-diethylaminopropyl), and 1 M ethanolamine hydrochloride (Pharmacia biosensor)
- Sensor chip CM5 (Pharmacia biosensor)
- HBS buffer: 10 mM Hepes pH 7.4, 0.15 M NaCl, 3.4 mM EDTA, 0.05% surfactant P20 (Pharmacia biosensor)

Method[a]

1. Activate the carboxylated dextran matrix by injecting 4 μl of a mixture of EDC 0.2 M and NHS 0.05 M prepared as described in the instructions to Amine coupling kit.
2. Introduce a reactive disulfide group on to carboxyl groups of the dextran layer by injecting 25 μl of PDEA 80 mM in 0.1 M borate buffer pH 8.5.
3. Block remaining reactive ester groups in the matrix by injecting 35 μl of 1 M ethanolamine hydrochloride pH 8.5.
4. Inject 10 μl of peptide at 20 μg/ml[b] in 10 mM acetate buffer pH 4.
5. Saturate the remaining reactive disulfide groups by injecting 20 μl of 1 M NaCl and 50 mM cysteine in 0.1 M formate buffer pH 4.3.
6. Wash the surface by injecting 15 μl of 100 mM HCl.

Protocol 3. *Continued*

7. Check the completeness of the regeneration by injecting repeatedly the same Ab. The amount of captured Ab should be reproducible within a few per cent.[c]

[a]A continuous flow of HBS buffer passing over the sensor surface at 5 μl/min is maintained during the entire experiment.
[b]A concentration of 20 μg/ml was chosen in order to achieve optimal immobilization as described in Section 4.6.3.
[c]This means that the sensor surface can be regenerated and reused without loss of Ab binding capacity.

4.7.2 Kinetic analyses

Analyses were performed at 25 °C, at a flow rate of 5 μl/min taking report points (for R and dR/dt values) every 0.5 sec. *Figure 12* represents overlay sensorgrams of runs performed with Fab concentrations ranging from 40–140 nM. Fab diluted in HBS was injected and became bound to the covalently immobilized peptide (phase A to B, 40 μl injection). After stopping the antigen injection the dissociation of bound Fab in continuous flow was monitored over 200 sec (phase B to C). The surface was then regenerated by an injection of 15 μl 100 mM HCl (phase C to D).

4.7.3 Interpretation of experimental data with the software BIAevaluation 2.0 (non-linear regression method analysis)

The six sensorgrams corresponding to runs performed at different Fab concentrations were transformed for data evaluation. The curves were first displayed in an overlay plot and their baseline adjusted to zero (*Figure 12*).

To assess the association and dissociation data, the most suitable function is $\ln(dR/dt)$ against t. The software allows the plots to be displayed in a split window, with the original data in the top panel (see *Figure 13*).

Data corresponding to the post-injection phase are first processed. According to the discussion above concerning the mass transfer limitations during the post-injection phase, a linear section of 100 sec was selected immediately after the slight fall of RU at the beginning of the post-injection phase on the plot $\ln(dR/dt)$ against t. This part of the curve corresponded to the difference in refractive index between buffer and Fab fragments solution (*Figure 13*). The software calculated the k_d value and its standard error from the selected data and according to the equation $R_t = R_1 e^{-k_d(t - t_1)}$. The average of the k_d values obtained from the six runs is 1.01×10^{-3} sec^{-1} with a standard deviation of 0.3×10^{-3}.

The analysis of the injection phase starts with the selection of the suitable section of each sensorgram individually for analysis. As in the post-injection phase analysis, the plot $\ln(dR/dt)$ against t is very useful for the selection. The selected section has to be chosen in order not to include a part close to the

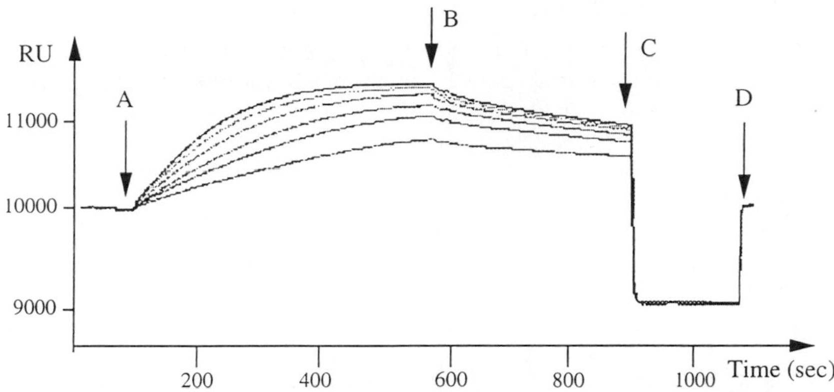

Figure 12. Overlay sensorgrams presenting measurements performed during interaction between the immobilized peptide and Fab fragments at concentrations ranging from 10–140 nM. The Fab fragments diluted in HBS were injected and bound to the covalently immobilized peptide (phase A to B, 40 μl injection). After antigen injection was complete the dissociation of bound Fab fragment in continuous buffer flow was monitored during 200 sec (phase B to C). After the run the surface was regenerated by an injection of 15 μl 100 mM HCl (phase C to D).

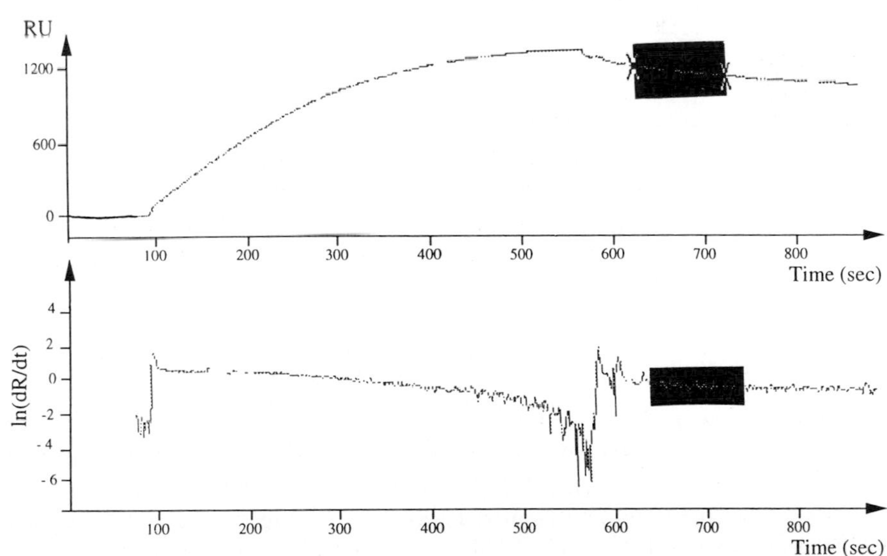

Figure 13. Transformed sensorgram (baseline adjusted to zero) and its plot ln(d*R*/d*t*) against *t*. The dark area corresponds to the section used to calculate the k_d value.

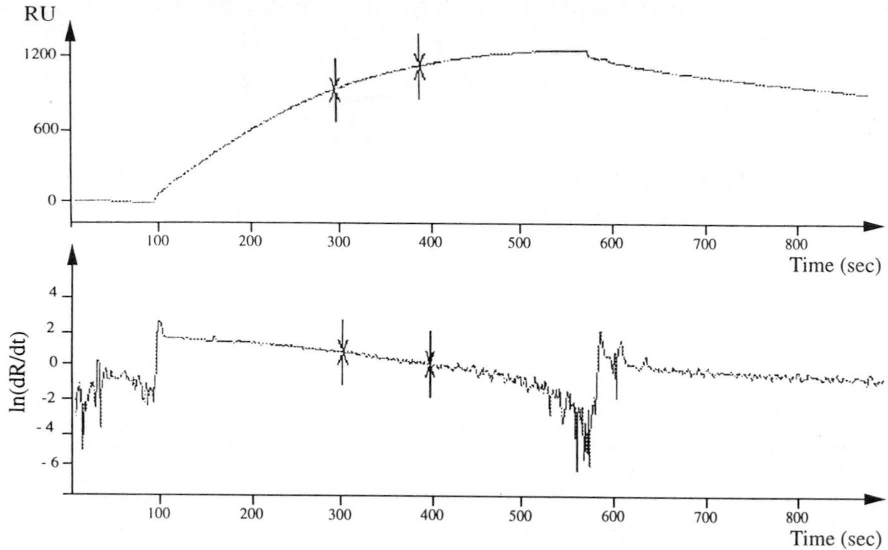

Figure 14. Sensorgram and the plot ln(dR/dt) against t derived from it. The arrows show the section selected for k_a calculations.

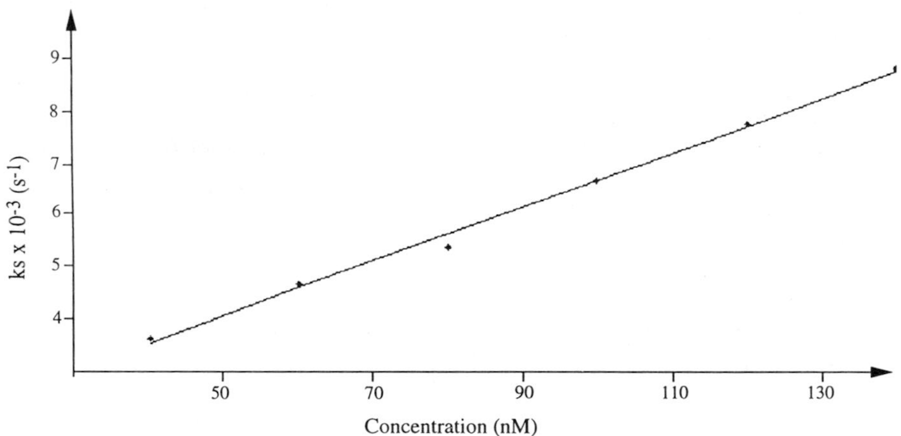

Figure 15. Plot of s against C used to obtain the k_a value as the slope.

horizontal; such a plot indicates that the interaction is mass transfer controlled. Moreover the selected section must not include a region where noise levels are too high (see *Figure 14*). Then the analyte concentration (C) values are entered and the plot of s against C gives a k_a value of 5.12×10^4 M^{-1} sec^{-1} as the slope (*Figure 15*).

Moreover the k_a value for each run could be obtained from s and the calculated k_d value. The average of the k_a values obtained in this way is 6.1×10^4

M^{-1} sec^{-1} with a standard deviation of 0.99×10^4 which is similar to the k_a value obtained above.

References

1. Steward, M. W. and Steensgaard, J. (1983). *Antibody affinity. Thermodynamic aspects and biological significance.* CRC Press, Boca Raton, Florida.
2. Altschuh, D. and Van Regenmortel, M. H. V. (1982). *J. Immunol. Methods*, **50**, 99.
3. Kelley, R. F. and O'Connell, M. P. (1993). *Biochemistry*, **32**, 6828.
4. Rauffer, N., Zeder-Lutz, G., Wenger, R. M., Van Regenmortel, M. H. V., and Altschuh, D. (1994). *Mol. Immunol.*, **31**, 913.
5. Karlsson, R., Michaelsson, A., and Mattsson, L. (1991). *J. Immunol. Methods*, **145**, 229.
6. Hardie, G. and Van Regenmortel, M. H. V. (1975). *Immunochemistry*, **12**, 903.
7. Day, E. D. (1972). *Advanced immunochemistry*. Williams & Wilkins, Baltimore, Maryland.
8. Rappaport, I. (1959). *J. Immunol.*, **82**, 526.
9. Van Regenmortel, M. H. V. and Hardie, G. (1976). *Immunochemistry*, **13**, 503.
10. Eisen, H. N. and Karush, F. (1949). *J. Am. Chem. Soc.*, **71**, 363.
11. Giles, B., Klapper, D. G., and Clem, L. W. (1983). *Mol. Immunol.*, **20**, 737.
12. Pascual, D. and Clem, L. W. (1988). *Mol. Immunol.*, **25**, 87.
13. Minden, P. and Farr, R. S. (1978). In *Handbook of experimental immunology. Immunochemistry*, (ed. D. M. Weir), Vol. 1, p. 13. Blackwell, Oxford.
14. Seppälä, I. J. (1975). *J. Immunol. Methods*, **9**, 135.
15. Berzofsky, J. A. and Berkower, I. J. (1984). In *Fundamental immunology* (ed. W. E. Paul), p. 595. Raven Press, New York.
16. Wagener, C., Clark, B. R., Rickard, K. J., and Shively J. E. (1983). *J. Immunol.*, **130**, 2302.
17. Mamet-Bratley, M. D. (1966). *Immunochemistry*, **3**, 155.
18. Day, E. (1990). *Advanced immunochemistry*. Wiley, New York.
19. Fazekas de St Groth, S. and Webster, R. G. (1961). *Aust. J. Exp. Biol. Med. Sci.*, **39**, 549.
20. Fazekas de St.Groth, S. (1979). In *Immunological methods* (ed. I. Lefkovits and B. Pernis), p. 1. Academic Press, New York.
21. Anderer, F. A., Koch, M. A., and Hirschle, S. D. (1971). *Eur. J. Immunol.*, **1**, 81.
22. Azimzadeh, A. and Van Regenmortel, M. H. V. (1991). *J. Immunol. Methods*, **141**, 199.
23. Bator, J. M. and Reading, C. L. (1989). *J. Immunol. Methods*, **125**, 167.
24. Zeder-Lutz, G., Wenger, R., Van Regenmortel, M. H. V., and Altschuh, D. (1993). *FEBS Lett.*, **326**, 153.
25. Karlsson, R., Altschuh, D., and Van Regenmortel, M. H. V. (1992). In *Structure of antigens* (ed. M. H. V. Van Regenmortel), Vol. 1, p. 127. CRC Press, Boca Raton, Florida.
26. O'Shannessy, D. J., Brigham-Burke, M., Soneson, K. K., Hensley, P., and Brooks, I. (1993). *Anal. Biochem.*, **212**, 457.
27. Malmqvist, M. (1993). *Curr. Opin. Immunol.*, **5**, 282.

28. Glaser, R. W. (1993). *Anal. Biochem.*, **213**, 152.
29. Karlsson, R., Roos, H., Fägerstam, L., and Persson, B. (1994). *Methods: a companion to methods in enzymology*, **6**, 99.
30. Morton, T. A., Myszka, D. G., and Chaiken, I. M. (1995). *Anal. Biochem.*, **227**, 176.
31. Löfas, S. and Johnsson, B. J. (1990). *J. Chem. Soc. Chem. Commun.*, **21**, 1526.
32. Johnsson, B., Löfas, S., Linquist, G., Edström, Å., Müller Hillgren, R.-M., and Hansson, A. (1995). *J. Mol. Recognit.*, **8**, 125.

2

Simple solid phase assays of avidity

DAVID GOLDBLATT

1. Introduction

The affinity of antibody for its antigen refers to the precise physico-chemical interaction between a single antibody combining site and a hapten. Affinity may be expressed as the equilibrium association constant (K) and is defined by the law of mass action which can be calculated from the following equation:

$$K = \frac{K_a}{K_d} = \frac{[AgAb]}{[Ag] \times [Ab]}$$

where Ag represents free antigen, Ab represents free antibody, and AgAb the antigen–antibody complex. Strictly, K can be interpreted accurately only for equilibrium in homogeneous solution and requires purified hapten and relatively pure antibody. The measurement of affinity has been described in detail in Chapter 1.

In contrast to affinity, avidity or functional affinity (1) is defined as the interaction between a complex antigen and bivalent antibody. Bivalent binding increases the avidity of any given interaction because it represents a summation of individual monovalent affinities. A variety of biological functions may be mediated by antibodies on the basis of their functional affinity/avidity (2). When investigating the interaction between large, complex antigens, such as bacteria or whole viruses, and complementary antibody, binding is likely to be complex hence measures of avidity may be relevant. This chapter will focus on techniques that measure the relative avidity of such antibody–antigen interactions.

1.1 The measurement of avidity

The measurement of complex antigen–antibody kinetics using solid phase assays is faced with a number of theoretical problems illustrated in *Figure 1*. In particular these relate to the conformational changes induced in antigen following binding to a solid phase and to the problems of antibody binding to

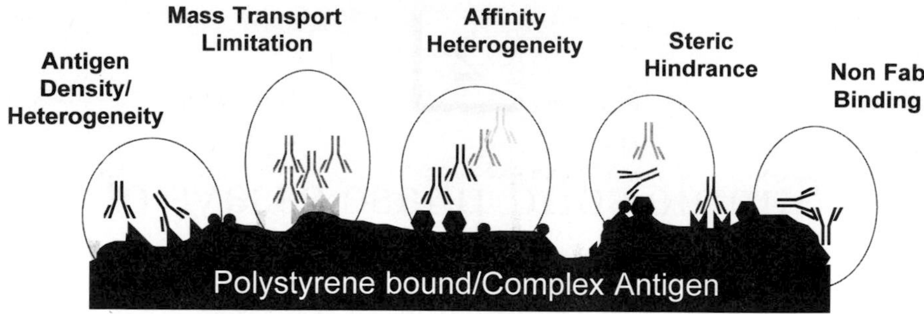

Figure 1. Theoretical interactions between polystyrene-bound or complex antigen and serum-derived antibody which complicate the measurement of equilibrium constants.

bound antigen where binding may be complicated by mass transport limitation, antigen density, or steric hindrance (3,4). In addition, when the solid phase antigen is large, complex, or relatively impure, binding of antibody may be further complicated by antigen heterogeneity and non-Fab binding. When serum-derived antibodies are measured in solid phase assays, the presence of populations of antibodies specific for the same antigen but differing in affinity (affinity heterogeneity) may complicate the interpretation of results and certain populations of antibody, such as small populations of low avidity antibodies, may be masked by higher avidity antibodies (5).

Historically, true affinity measurements have been made under experimental conditions where the antigen and antibody are both in solution thereby avoiding the confounding factors outlined above. Furthermore, pure haptenic antigen is required to ensure monovalent binding and relatively pure preparations of antibody are desirable. Such conditions, in particular the requirement for large amounts of relatively pure antibody preparations, precludes the use of such techniques for the measurement of affinity of small quantities of serum-derived antibody specific for complex antigens such as viral particles, bacterial cell walls, or cell surface antigens. The need to measure affinity/avidity under the latter conditions has led to the development of a variety of ELISA-based techniques.

Despite the theoretical problems outlined above, solid phase assays for the measurement of monoclonal antibody affinity for its hapten appear to correlate well with equilibrium dialysis (6,7) and assays adapted for the measurement of avidity of both monoclonal antibodies and antigen-specific antibodies in serum have been shown to rank antibodies with predetermined affinity values in the correct order (8). Such assays measure bivalent antibody binding to relatively complex antigens in the presence of heterogeneous populations of antibody. While such experimental conditions preclude the measurement of 'true' antibody affinity (9), they may, in fact, approximate the condition of *in vivo* antibody binding to complex antigens more closely than the conditions necessary for the derivation of equilibrium constants.

Table 1. Conditions required for the measurement of antibody affinity/avidity by equilibrium dialysis or modified solid phase assays

Reagent	**Equilibrium dialysis**	**Modified solid phase assays**
Antigen	Purified	Crude
Antibody	Pure monoclonal (preferable)	Monoclonal or polyclonal
Dependent on antibody concentration?	Yes	No
Labelling	Antibody or antigen	Not required
Read out	Absolute affinity constant (*K*)	Relative avidity estimation

While increasing use is being made of simplified assays for the measurement of avidity it is important to recognize the limitations of such assays. Most importantly they do not permit the derivation of an affinity constant (*K*) but permit the ranking of antibodies specific for the same antigen. While this may limit the applicability of such assays, the ability to derive comparative avidity measurements of serum-derived antibody has been shown to be valuable for a variety of antigen–antibody interactions and for a broad range of disciplines including veterinary science, vaccinology, and infectious disease. A comparison of the conditions required for the measurement of affinity by equilibrium dialysis and avidity by solid phase ELISAs is shown in *Table 1*. A major advantage of the modified ELISAs is the fact that they are relatively simple to perform, do not require the purification of the antibody of interest, do not require the labelling of reagents with radioactivity, and thus are within the scope of most laboratories. Furthermore their rapidity permits the evaluation of large numbers of sera.

Assays for the measurement of avidity can be divided into two broad types; those that rely on the principle of competitive inhibition and those that rely on an eluting agent. The former use various concentrations of free antigen in solution to inhibit antibody in solution binding to immobilized antigen. Elution techniques use chaotropic agents to inhibit antibody binding or to disrupt antibody bound to immobilized antigen. Such assays require validation and careful consideration of the effect of chaotrope/denaturant on the integrity of the reagents and this is discussed more fully in Section 2. Both types of assay require careful validation, particularly in choosing an appropriate epitope density for the test antigen (5,10). Furthermore, both types of assay, when analysing serum-derived antibodies, give a measure of the average antibody avidity since serum probably contains a mixture of high and low avidity antibodies (5,8).

2. Competition inhibition assays

Assays designed to derive an affinity constant value (*K*) by means of ELISA have been described by a number of authors (6,7,11). Such assays continue to attract much critical attention and a full discussion of these techniques is beyond the scope of this chapter. The reader is directed to a number of excellent reviews and discussions of the problems in deriving affinity constants from solid phase assays (3,7,9,12,13). ELISAs designed to measure the relative antibody avidity have been developed for a number of antigens and are described fully below.

These assays are modelled on a plaque-forming cell inhibition assay originally described by Anderson, where increasing concentrations of free antigens were used to competitively inhibit the binding of antibodies of decreasing affinity (14). This technique was adapted for the measurement of relative functional affinity (avidity) of serum-derived antibody, a situation where only small amounts of the antigen-specific antibody of interest may be available. The assay was originally validated by the analysis of a panel of dinitrophenol (DNP)-specific monoclonal antibodies of known affinity and was shown to rank these antibodies in the same order as equilibrium dialysis (8). It has subsequently been used to rank the avidity of serum-derived antibody specific for a number of different antigens including tetanus toxoid (15), keyhole limpet haemocyanin (16), streptococcal proteins (17), HIV-derived peptides (18), and type II collagen (19). This technique employs a fixed concentration of antibody and various concentrations of antigen to determine the amount of antigen which will inhibit solid phase binding by 50%. While some of the theoretical objections to solid phase assays and the derivation of affinity constants apply to this methodology, the techniques are used to derive relative avidity constants for a given antibody–antigen system and to rank antibodies according to their avidity rather than to determine the absolute K value. As such they are particularly well suited to studies where a comparison of the avidity of antigen-specific sera derived from different sources is desired.

Protocol 1. Competition inhibition assays

Equipment and reagents

- 96-well flat-bottomed polystyrene microtitre plates
- Phosphate-buffered saline (PBS): 140 mM NaCl (8 g/litre), 2.7 mM KCl (0.2 g/litre), 8.0 mM Na_2HPO_4 (1.15g/litre), 1.5 mM NaH_2PO_4 (0.2 g/litre)
- Phosphate-buffered saline–Tween (PBS-T): PBS with 0.05% (v/v) Tween 20
- 1% bovine serum albumin (Sigma) in PBS-T: PBS-T with 10 g/litre BSA
- Antigen of interest

Method

This method is designed to modify existing antigen-specific ELISAs and, as such, individual coating conditions, blocking procedures, incubation times and temperatures, and substrates used will differ between assays.

1. Coat the microtitre plate with the antigen of interest. The coating conditions will vary for each antigen.

2. Wash the plate with PBS-T.
3. Make doubling dilutions of free antigen in 1% BSA PBS-T and add to two rows on the microtitre plate adding only 1% BSA PBS-T to the final two wells.
4. Dilute the sera in 1% BSA PBS-T to a predetermined concentration which, when diluted 1/2 with antigen in 1% BSA PBS-T will give an A_{280} of approx. 1.0 or, if known, a predetermined gravimetric concentration. Add the serum to the wells containing free antigen or 1% BSA PBS-T and mix. Leave for 2 h at room temperature (time and temperature will differ for different antigens).[a]
5. Wash the plate four times with PBS-T.
6. Add the labelled detector antibody. Leave for 2 h at room temperature (time and temperature will differ for different antigens).
7. Wash the plate four times with PBS-T.
8. Add the substrate.
9. Stop the enzyme reaction by the addition of 2 M H_2SO_4.
10. Read the absorbance at the wavelength appropriate to the substrate used, for example: A_{405} for alkaline phosphate and A_{490} for ortho-phenylene diamine (OPD).

[a] An alternative approach is to mix antibody and antigen prior to adding to the microtitre plate allowing the antigen–antibody to remain in contact for various periods of time.

The relative avidity can be expressed as the amount of antigen required to inhibit binding of antibody by 50%. To express this figure plot the absorbance on the *y* axis versus the free antigen concentration (see *Figure 2*). At the point corresponding to half the absorbance obtained from control wells (no antigen), drop a perpendicular to the *x* axis. This point corresponds to the amount of antigen that will inhibit antibody binding by 50% and is a measure of the average antibody avidity. The figure can be expressed as the log of the free antigen concentration required to produce 50% inhibition, the I_{50}. Antibodies with high avidity will be inhibited by less antigen than low avidity antibodies and consequently will have a lower I_{50}. *Figure 2* illustrates the results obtained from the inhibition of serum-derived IgG1, IgG2, and IgG3 specific for *Moraxella catarrhalis*. IgG3 has the highest avidity and requires the least free antigen to inhibit binding by 50%. In contrast IgG2 is of lowest avidity and cannot be fully inhibited from binding to the solid phase.

3. Elution assays

Elution assays for the derivation of relative antibody avidity have become increasingly popular and have been applied to a wide variety of antigens. A

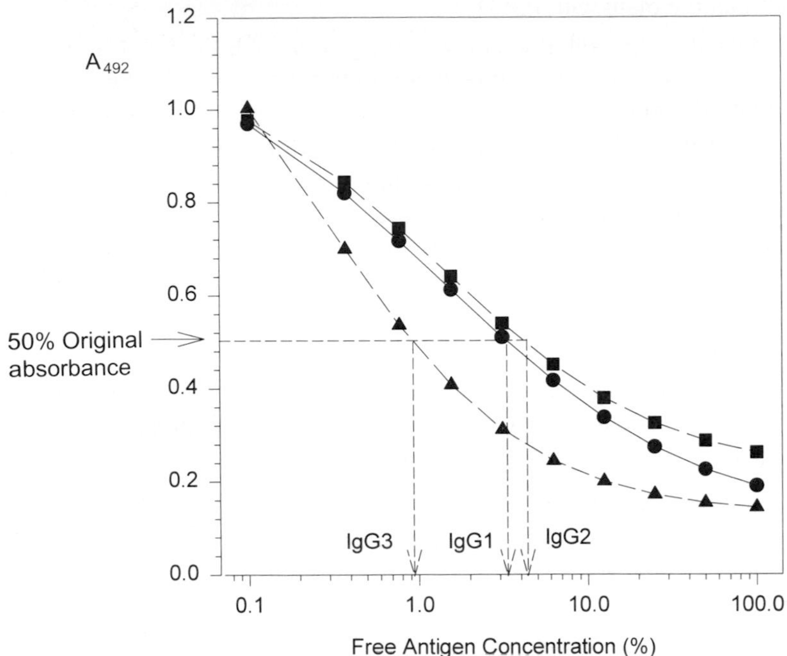

Figure 2. Antigen inhibition assay for the derivation of relative avidity constants for IgG1, IgG2, and IgG3 specific for *M. catarrhalis* (see text for details).

summary of antigen–antibody systems to which such methods have been applied is shown in *Table 2*.

The principle behind elution assays is that the elution of low avidity antibodies from antigen may take place at a lower concentration of chaotrope/denaturant than that of high avidity antigen. It is important to recognize that such assays do not permit the derivation of a *K* value as they do not fulfil the strict criteria required for measuring equilibrium constants. In particular they analyse antibody-bound antigen which in turn has been bound to polystyrene. Such binding may change the conformation of antigen thus altering binding characteristics of the antibody. Elution assays permit the ranking of the avidity of an antibody for a particular antigen but care must be taken in extrapolating between antigen–antibody systems. Three major types of elution assays are described and are shown schematically in *Figure 3*.

In *Figure 3*, method A, antigen is bound to the solid phase and the unknown serum/antibody is then allowed to bind to the antigen. Following this incubation, a chaotrope is added at increasing molarity which strips antibody from antigen. After this step bound antibody is detected by the appropriate detector antibody. In method B the chaotrope or denaturant is incorporated in the sample buffer at different concentrations, preventing antibody binding

Table 2. Published elution assays for the derivation of relative antibody avidity measurements

Antigen	Antibody detected	Elution method
Soybean protein	IgA	Thiocyanate (20)
Myeloperoxidase	IgG	DEA (21)
Moraxella catarrhalis	IgG	DEA/thiocyanate (22)
Alpha 3 chain of type IV collagen	IgG	DEA (23)
Actinobacillus actinomycetemcomitans	IgG	DEA (24)
Rubella	IgG1	DEA/urea (25)
CMV	IgG	Urea (26)
Respiratory syncitial virus	IgG	Urea (27)
Coxiella burnetti	IgG/IgM	Urea (28)
Varicella zoster virus	IgG	Urea (29,30)
Epstein–Barr virus infection	IgG	Urea (31)
Toxoplasma gondii	IgG	Urea (32)
Enterovirus	IgG	Urea (33)
Haemophilus influenzae type b	IgG	Urea (34)
Poliovirus	IgG	Thiocyanate (35)
Anti-mitochondrial antibodies	IgG	Thiocyanate (36)
Group B *Streptococcus* type III	IgG	Thiocyanate (37)
Pophyromonas gingivalis	IgM	Thiocyanate (38)
Retinal S antigen	IgG	Thiocyanate (39)
HIV p17 and p24 protein	IgG	Urea (40)
Tetanus toxoid	IgG1/IgG4	DEA (15)
Casein and β-lactoglobulin	IgA	Thiocyanate (41)

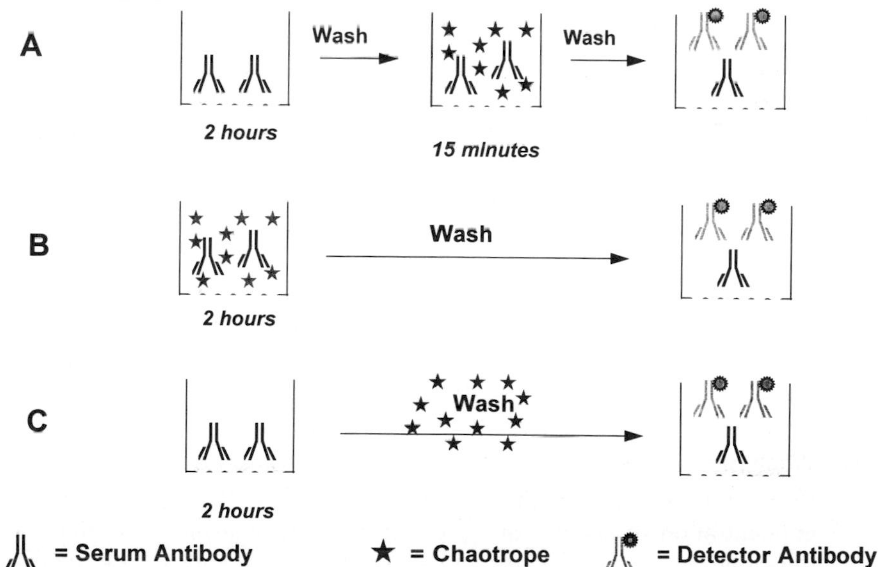

Figure 3. Three schemes for the estimation of relative antibody avidity using elution techniques.

to antigen. In method C a protein denaturant is used in the wash buffer to elute antibody of low avidity. No prolonged contact between the denaturant and the bound antigen is permitted. The protocols in the following sections describe each assay in detail.

3.1 Thiocyanate elution assays

Chaotropic ions are known to exert their effect on antibody–antigen binding by interfering with non-covalent binding. This is achieved primarily through the disruption of hydrophobic bonds and through electrostatic shielding of charged groups which decreases the strength of ionic binding and alters the folding of proteins (42,43). Ultracentrifuge studies have shown that thiocyanate (one of the anionic chaotropic ions) is able to dissociate antigen–antibody complexes without producing irreversible gross structural changes (44). Edgington described the use of thiocyanate to dissociate antibody from the surface of red cells (45) and noted that the membrane antigens were denatured by concentrations of thiocyanate required for the complete removal of antibody but that the there was no denaturation of antibody. Subsequently thiocyanate has been incorporated by a number of researchers into assays designed to measure antibody avidity (see *Table 2*).

Protocol 2. Thiocyanate elution assays

Equipment and reagents

- 96-well flat-bottomed polystyrene microtitre plates (Dynatech)
- Phosphate-buffered saline (PBS) (see *Protocol 1*)
- Phosphate-buffered saline–Tween (PBS-T) (see *Protocol 1*)
- 1% bovine serum albumin (Sigma) in PBS-T (see *Protocol 1*)
- KSCN, NH_4SCN, or NaSCN (Sigma) diluted in PBS to provide a range of molarities (0.5–4 M)

Method

This method is designed to modify existing antigen-specific ELISAs and as such individual coating conditions, blocking procedures, incubation times and temperatures, and substrates used will differ between assays.

1. Coat the microtitre plate with the antigen of interest. The coating conditions will differ for each antigen.
2. Wash the plate with PBS-T.
3. Dilute the sera for avidity testing in 1% BSA PBS-T to a similar concentration (if known) or by predetermined analysis to a dilution designed to give an absorbance of 1.0 at the appropriate wavelength for the substrate used (A_{405} for alkaline phosphate and A_{490} for OPD).

4. Add the sera in duplicate to the wells of the microtitre plate leaving all the outer wells blank. With the outer wells blank the 96-well microtitre plate template illustrated in *Figure 4* would permit the analysis of avidity of five different sera.
5. Following the serum incubation wash the plate with PBS-T and add SCN^- diluted in 1% BSA PBS-T at a range of different molarities which may differ depending on the assay. In the template shown in *Figure 4* add the following concentrations of SCN^-:
   - Row B: 1% BSA PBS-T, no SCN^-
   - Row C : 0.5 M SCN^-
   - Row D: 1.0 M SCN^-
   - Row E: 2.0 M SCN^-
   - Row F: 3.0 M SCN^-
   - Row G: 4.0 M SCN^-
6. After a 15 min SCN^- incubation, wash the plate with PBS-T and add detector antibody in appropriate concentration.
7. Complete the rest of the ELISA as described in *Protocol 1*. Store the absorbance data in an ASCII file if the ELISA plate reader is unable to perform the calculations shown in *Protocol 3*.

A/1	2	3	4	5	6	7	8	9	10	11	12
B	Serum A		Serum B		Serum C		Serum D		Serum E		
C	"		"		"		"		"		
D	"		"		"		"		"		
E	"		"		"		"		"		
F	"		"		"		"		"		
G	"		"		"		"		"		
H											

Figure 4. Template of a 96-well microtitre ELISA plate used for the thiocyanate elution assay (see *Protocol 2*).

Protocol 3. Derivation of an avidity index from data obtained in the thiocyanate elution assay

Equipment

- Computer spreadsheet or calculator

Method

1. To obtain the percentage change in absorbance for each serum at

Protocol 3. *Continued*

different molarities of SCN, perform the following calculation for each of the wells containing SCN^-:

$$\frac{\text{(Mean absorbance of wells containing 1\% BSA PBS-T only)} - \text{(Mean absorbance of wells containing [}SCN^-\text{])}}{\text{Mean absorbance of wells containing 1\% BSA PBS-T only}} \times 100$$

This yields a figure which is equivalent to the percentage of antibody eluted by the SCN^-.

2. Derive the log value of the percentage of antibody eluted.
3. Plot the values for each serum against the molar concentration of SCN^-.
4. Draw a line on the graph at the log of 50 ($y = 1.69$) which is the point equivalent to 50% elution of antibody.
5. At the point where the line of 50% inhibition crosses the curves for individual sera assayed, drop a perpendicular and read off the *x* axis. This figure gives the molarity of thiocyanate required to elute 50% of bound antibody. This figure is the avidity index.

An example of a graph obtained in an experiment described in *Protocol 2* is shown in *Figure 5* and the derivation of the avidity index is displayed.

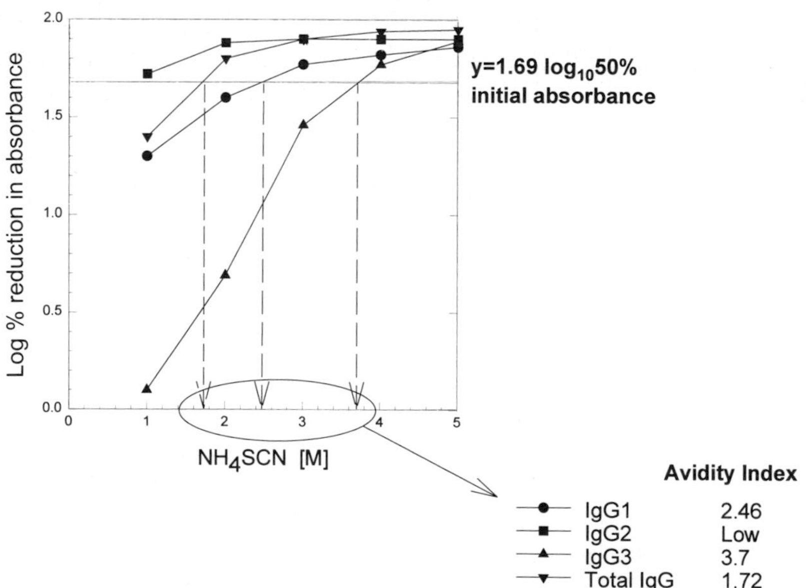

Figure 5. The derivation of the avidity index from data obtained by thiocyanate elution of *M. catarrhalis* specific IgG1, IgG2, and IgG3 (see *Protocol 3* for details).

A number of parameters need to be defined for individual antibody–antigen systems prior to the use of the thiocyanate elution assays. One of the crucial parameters is the stability of the antigen bound to the solid phase during the incubation of the chaotrope. This can be simply tested as illustrated in *Protocol 4*.

Protocol 4. Antigen stability following thiocyanate incubation

Equipment and reagents

- As for *Protocol 2*

Method

1. Coat the microtitre plate with the antigen of interest as for *Protocol 2*.
2. Wash the plate with PBS-T.
3. Incubate half of the plate with SCN^- diluted in sample buffer and half with sample buffer alone for 15 min at room temperature.
4. Wash the plate with PBS-T and perform the standard antigen-specific ELISA with identical standard curves and unknown sera on the two halves of the plate.
5. Compare the standard curves and the derivation of unknown sera from the two halves of the plate.

An example of two standard curves obtained following an experiment similar to that described in *Protocol 4* is shown in *Figure 6*. Pre-incubation with SCN^- in the example shown has no effect on the subsequent binding of antibody to the bound antigen.

Validation of the thiocyanate elution method has been reported by a number of authors and in general, studies using this technique have been able to show the expected increase in avidity of antibody following encounter with an antigen. MacDonald *et al.* (46) compared the affinity ranking of six anti-dinitrophenol monoclonal antibodies by thiocyanate elution to values obtained for the same antibodies by equilibrium dialysis and showed a good correlation between the two assays. Hall and Heckel (47), however, report discrepancies between avidity ranking by thiocyanate elution and affinity estimation by hapten inhibition in their system utilizing monoclonal antibodies specific for phosphocholine. Gray and Shaw (48) describe the apparent increase in binding of one of two human monoclonal antibodies to pneumococcal polysaccharides at low concentrations of thiocyanate. The possible effects of thiocyanate on the bound IgM may account for this phenomenon. It is important that each antigen–antibody system to which the thiocyanate elution methodology is applied should be carefully evaluated.

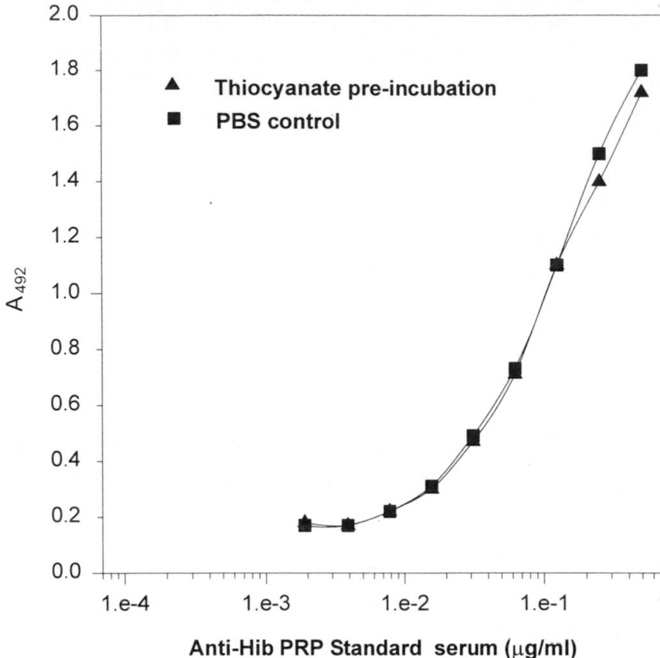

Figure 6. Standard curves obtained for the binding of serum-derived IgG specific for the *Haemophilus influenzae* type b capsular polysaccharide (Hib PRP) following the pre-incubation of antigen coated plates with 5 M NH_4SCN/PBS or PBS alone (see *Protocol 4* for details).

3.2 Urea elution assays

The ability of urea to dissociate antibody–antigen complexes was first described in the late 1950s (49) and is now known to be due to the disruption of hydrophobic rather than hydrogen bonds (50). Bata *et al.* (51) showed that the ability of antibody to bind to antigen could be restored following the removal of urea by dialysis, illustrating the reversible nature of the disruption brought about by urea. Hedman and Seppälä were the first to adapt urea for use in ELISAs and were able to demonstrate differences in the urea elution of rubella-specific antibodies of different avidity (52). The urea elution assay appears to be favoured by clinical laboratories for the estimation of the avidity of clinically relevant antibodies. Because of the rapidity of the assay and the requirement for small amounts of sera, this assay has proven to be particularly applicable to laboratories running routine diagnostic assays for the serological diagnosis of infectious diseases. The importance of distinguishing between primary infection and reactivation on the basis of avidity has made such assays popular in clinical virology (see *Table 2*). Protocols for the use of urea are similar to those for thiocyanate and are summarized in *Protocol 5*.

Protocol 5. Urea elution assays

Equipment and reagents

- As for *Protocol 2*
- PBS-T containing 6 M or 8 M urea[a]

Method

1. Coat the microtitre plate with the antigen of interest. The coating conditions will differ for each antigen.
2. Wash the plate with PBS-T.
3. Add the sera in duplicate at a single dilution to two different rows of the microtitre plate. Include on each plate sera of known high and low avidity.
4. After incubating sera (time and temperature will differ according to the antigen) wash individual rows with PBS-T or PBS-T containing 6 M or 8 M urea. Allow 5 min soaking time for each of three washes.[b]
5. Complete ELISA as described in *Protocol 1*.

[a] Individual assays differ and the molarity of urea producing the most discriminating shift may also differ for each antigen assayed. 6 M or 8 M urea are used most widely when the assay is performed as described here.
[b] Some studies leave 100 μl of 8 M urea/well for 15 min (compare with *Protocol 2*) followed by normal washing of the plate.

The same caveats regarding the stability of polystyrene-bound antigen in the presence of a chaotrope apply to the urea elution assays, and the procedure described in *Protocol 3* to test the stability of bound antigen in the presence of a denaturant/chaotrope should be applied to the urea elution assay.

The avidity index for the urea elution assay may be calculated in two different ways. The following equation derives an avidity index (AI) based on the reduction in absorbance:

$$\frac{\text{Mean absorbance of serum washed with 8 M urea}}{\text{Mean absorbance of serum washed with PBS-T}} \times 100 = \text{AI}$$

Using this equation most authors divide sera into low, moderate, or high avidity according to the reduction in optical density. Thomas *et al.* (53) studied rubella-specific IgG1 using the above equation to derive an avidity index. They reported their results as positive, equivocal, or negative for low avidity IgG1 when the AI was $< 30\%$, between 30% and 50%, or $> 50\%$ respectively. The exact cut-off points, however, differ according to the assay described (29,53–55).

The second method for deriving an avidity index is based on a shift in the end-point titre when incorporating urea in the PBS-T wash buffer and is expressed as an end-point ratio (EPR) (56). The end-point titre is defined as the serum dilution at which the test is negative. Negative results are often defined as those giving an absorbance value below 0.2. The effect of urea is to shift the dilution at which the end-point titre is achieved. This can be expressed as the end-point ratio using the following formula:

$$\mathrm{EPR} = 100 \times \frac{\text{End-point titre with urea/PBS-T wash}}{\text{End-point titre with PBS-T wash}}$$

Validation of the urea elution assays has been accomplished by extrapolation from the analysis of sera derived from individuals with known pre-existing long-standing immunity, and consequently an expectation of high avidity antibody, as compared to serum from non-immune individuals, or those with recent onset of infection in whom the antibody is expected to be low. Such techniques have been used to evaluate assays for the measurement of the avidity of antibody specific for toxoplasmosis (55), varicella zoster (29), cytomegalovirus (54), and rubella (53).

3.3 Diethylamine elution assays

The diethylamine (DEA) elution assay was originally based on an assay described by Inouye and colleagues (57) in which a low concentration (0.5 M–1.0 M) of a protein denaturing agent, guanidine hydrochloride, was included in the serum diluent to prevent the binding of low avidity antibody.

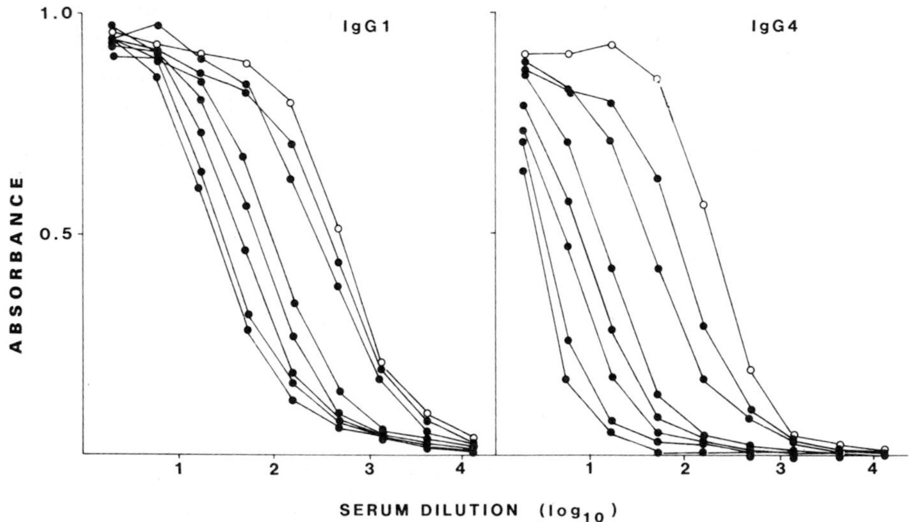

Figure 7. Effect of 0–35 mM DEA on the dose–response curve of IgG1 and IgG4 antibodies to tetanus toxoid in a single serum. Dose–response curve without DEA (open circles) and increasing concentrations of DEA from 5 mM are shown from right to left (from ref. 15 with permission).

Devey *et al.* (15) modified this assay and incorporated DEA as the protein denaturant in their study of antibody avidity to tetanus toxoid. The effect of increasing concentrations of DEA incorporated in the serum diluent results in a shift in the standard curve. *Figure 7* illustrates an example of the antibody binding curves obtained with increasing amounts of DEA incorporated in the serum diluent for serum-derived IgG1 and IgG4 specific for tetanus toxoid.

Protocol 6. DEA shift ELISA

Equipment and reagents

- As for *Protocol 2*

Method

1. Coat the microtitre plate with the antigen of interest. The coating conditions will differ for each antigen.
2. Wash the plate with PBS-T.
3. Make serial dilutions of the sera in 1% BSA PBS-T in the presence and absence of previously determined concentrations of DEA. The usual working range of DEA is between 5–50 mM. The starting dilution of all sera should be adjusted to give an absorbance at the appropriate wavelength for the individual assay of approx. 1.0.
4. Following the incubation of serum (time and temperature will vary according to assay) wash the plates with PBS-T.
5. Complete the ELISA as for *Protocol 1*.
6. To derive the DEA shift index (see *Figure 8*):
   (a) Plot the binding curve for each serum in the presence and absence of DEA.
   (b) Determine the amount of leftward shift in the binding curves at an absorbance 50% that of the starting absorbance.
   (c) Express this leftward shift as a millimolar concentration of DEA. Low avidity antibody will have a greater leftward shift than that of high avidity antibody.
7. The derivation of an avidity index for the DEA assay is similar to that described for urea. The following formula can be used:

$$\text{AI} = 100 \times \frac{\text{Mean absorbance of serum with DEA}}{\text{Mean absorbance of serum without DEA}}$$

The stability of polystyrene-bound antigen in the presence of DEA needs to be determined as described in *Protocol 3*. The validation of the DEA assay

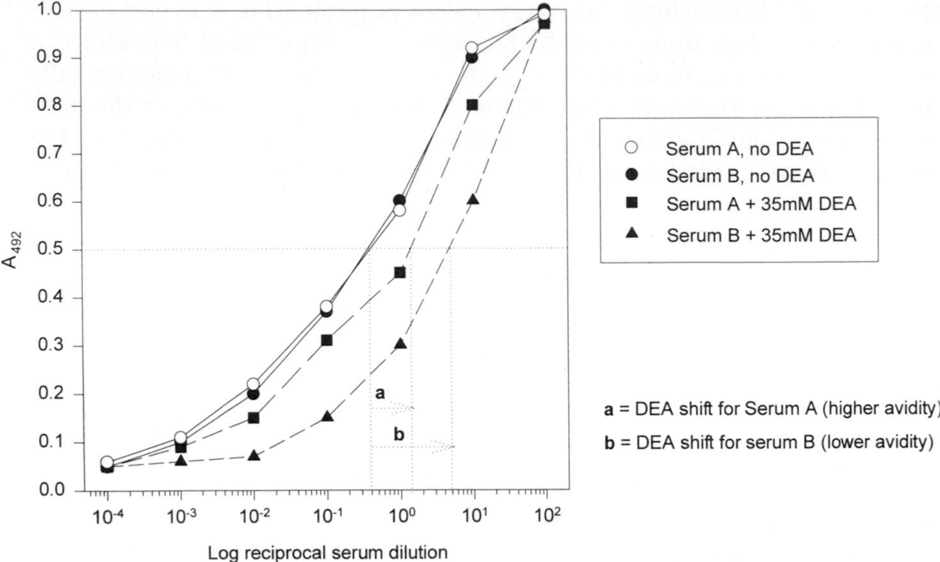

Figure 8. The derivation of the DEA shift index (see *Protocol 6* for details).

has usually been accomplished by the comparison with results obtained from other techniques. Devey *et al.* (15) compared their results with those obtained by competition inhibition and showed good correlation between the two techniques .

4. Comparison of elution techniques

Several studies have compared different elution techniques within their antigen-specific systems. Thomas *et al.* compared urea elution assay with the DEA shift technique for antibodies to rubella (53) and varicella zoster virus (58). In both systems they found the DEA shift technique was more sensitive

Table 3. The pH of 1% BSA PBS-T containing increasing amounts of diethylamine, NH_4SCN, and KSCN

Molarity [mM]	Diethylamine	Molarity [M]	NH_4SCN	KSCN
0	7.2	0	7.3	7.2
5	8.0	0.75	6.32	6.64
10	10.0	1.25	6.24	6.63
20	10.8	2.5	6.04	6.60
30	11.3	5.	5.78	6.69
40	11.44	7.5	5.49	6.82

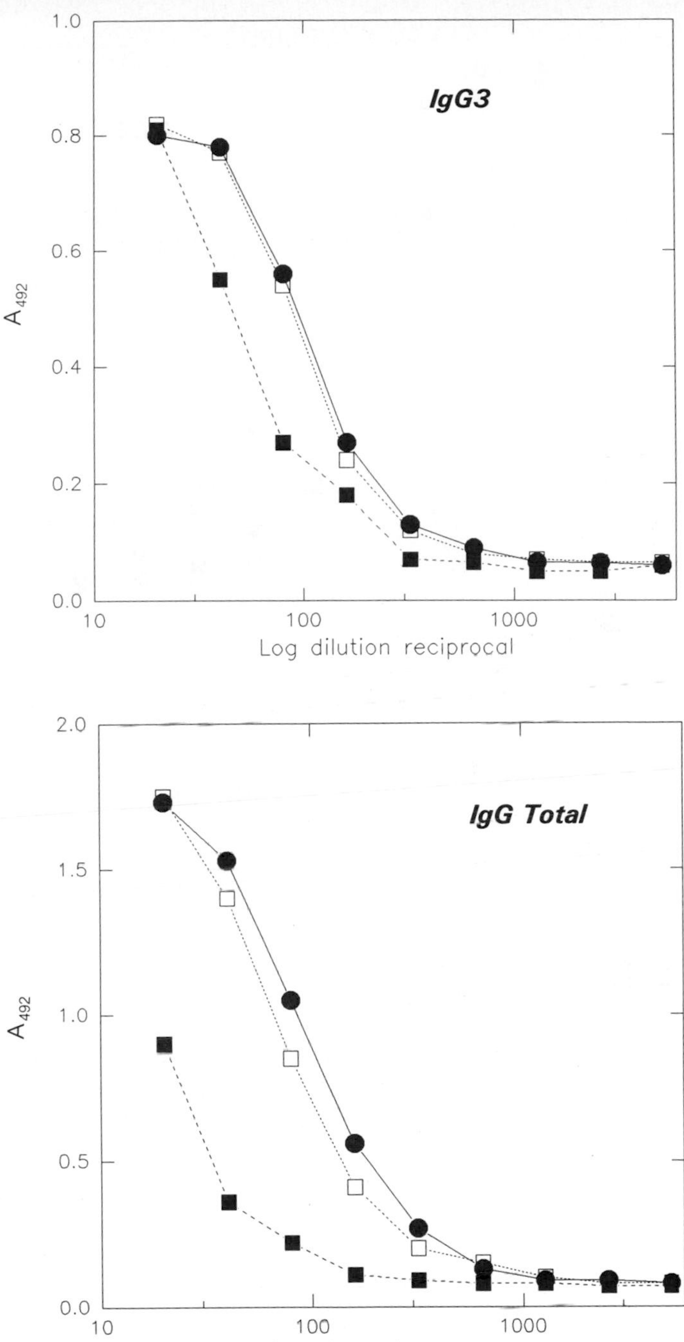

Figure 9. Standard curves obtained for the binding of standard serum IgG3 and total IgG specific for *M. catarrhalis* in BSA PBS-T pH 7.2 (●), 40 mM DEA BSA PBS-T pH 11.44 (■), or neutralized 40 mM DEA BSA PBS-T pH 7.2 (□). Neutralizing 40 mM DEA abolishes the effect of DEA on the binding of antigen (from ref. 22 with permission).

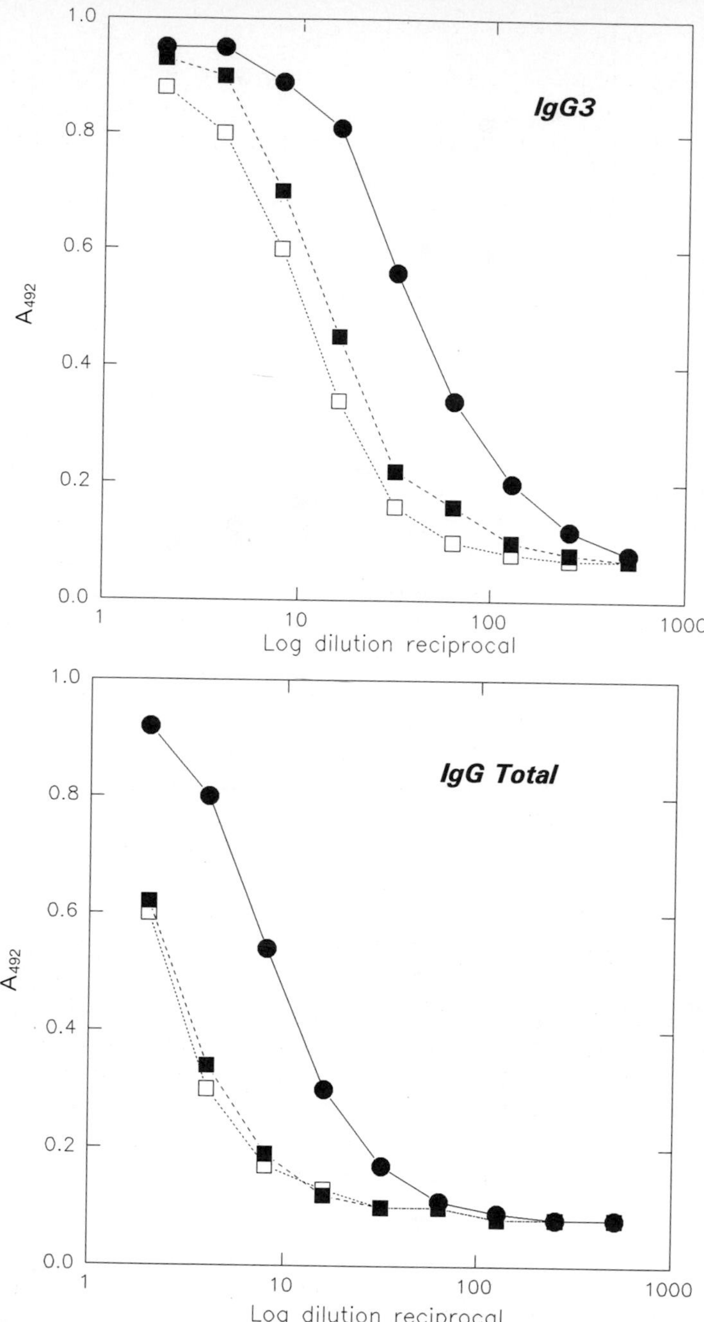

Figure 10. Standard curves obtained for the binding of standard serum IgG3 and total IgG specific for *M. catarrhalis* in BSA PBS-T pH 7.2 (●), BSA PBS-T pH 11.3 (■), and 30 mM DEA BSA PBS-T pH 11.3 (□). The BSA PBS-T pH 11.3 was able to mimic the apparent 'chaotropic' effect of 30 mM DEA and produce a similar leftward shift in the binding curve (from ref. 22 with permission).

in detecting low avidity antibody. They attribute this to the difference in methodology between the two assays, preventing antibody binding by adding denaturant to the serum diluent compared to eluting bound antibody, rather than intrinsic differences between the denaturants used. When DEA was used in an elution assay the elution assay was still less sensitive than the shift technique.

Goldblatt *et al.* studied the role of pH in the DEA and thiocyanate elution assays (22). Increasing concentrations of DEA raised the pH of PBS-T significantly while the addition of increasing amounts of NH_4SCN or KSCN decreased the pH slightly (see *Table 3*). The pH of 8 M urea was 6.8.

The relevance of the increased pH in the DEA avidity assays was demonstrated by comparing the effect of 40 mM DEA and neutral 40 mM DEA on the ability to shift antibody binding curves. *Figure 9* shows how the effect of DEA was abolished by neutralizing DEA with 1 M HCl.

The pH of 1% BSA PBS-T was adjusted to 11.3 by the addition of NaOH and the effects of DEA were reproduced indicating the importance of pH for the shift effect seen with DEA (*Figure 10*). The chaotropic effect of thiocyanate was shown to be independent of pH and hence more reliably used in elution assays. It is possible that the highly basic DEA solution may affect the integrity of the antibody molecule leading to denaturation of the antibody. Despite these theoretical concerns, the DEA assay and the thiocyanate elution assay both gave similar results for the avidity of the IgG subclasses specific for *M. catarrhalis* and both ranked the avidity of the IgG subclasses in the same order as an antigen inhibition assay (*Figure 2*).

Polanec and colleagues (59), using a rubella assay as a model, have compared eluting assays and serum diluent assays as well as evaluating the four chaotropes/denaturants: DEA, guanidine hydrochloride, thiocyanate, and urea. They have evaluated the assays by measuring the avidity of serum pools made from recent seroconverters (low avidity), or individuals with past immunity (higher avidity), as well as sera from well characterized individuals with recent or remote infection. In contrast to the findings of Thomas *et al.* (53), the elution techniques, irrespective of denaturant, proved superior to assays where the denaturant/chaotrope was added to the serum diluent. This study also confirmed that the apparent denaturing/chaotropic effect of DEA was due to the increase pH of PBS-T when DEA was added.

References

1. Karush, F. (1978). In *Comprehensive immunology* (ed. G. W. Litman and R. A. Good), p. 85. Plenum Press, New York.
2. Steward, M. W. (1981). *Immunol. Today*, **2**, 134.
3. Stenberg, M. and Nygren, H. (1988). *J. Immunol. Methods*, **113**, 3.
4. Pesce, A. J. and Michael, J.G. (1992). *J. Immunol. Methods*, **150**, 111.
5. Bruderer, U., Deusinger, M., Schürch, U., and Lang, A. B. (1992). *J. Immunol. Methods*, **151**, 157.

6. Nieto, A., Jansa, G. M., and Moreno, C. (1984). *Mol. Immunol.*, **21**, 537.
7. Friguet, B., Chaffotte, A. F., Djavadi-Ohaniance, L., and Goldberg, M. E. (1985). *J. Immunol. Methods*, **77**, 305.
8. Rath, S., Stanley, C. M., and Steward, M. W. (1988). *J. Immunol. Methods*, **106**, 245.
9. Underwood, P. A. (1993). *J. Immunol. Methods*, **164**, 119.
10. Holland, G. P. and Steward, M. W. (1991). *J. Immunol. Methods*, **138**, 245.
11. Janoff, E. N., Hardy, W. D., Smith, P. D., and Wahl, S. M. (1991). *J. Immunol.*, **147**, 2130.
12. Schwab, C. and Bosshard, R. (1992). *J. Immunol. Methods*, **147**, 125.
13. van Regenmortel, M. H. V. and Azimzadeh, A. (1994). In *Immunochemistry* (ed. C. J. van Oss and M. H. V. van Regenmortel), p. 805. Marcel Dekker, Inc. New York, Basel, Hong Kong.
14. Anderson, B. (1970). *J. Exp. Med.*, **132**, 77.
15. Devey, M. E., Bleasdale, K., Lee, S., and Rath, S. (1988). *J. Immunol. Methods*, **106**, 119.
16. Devey, M. E., Bleasdale Barr, K. M., Bird, P., and Amlot, P. L. (1990). *Immunology*, **70**, 168.
17. Devash, Y., Calvelli, T. A., Wood, D. G., Reagan, K. J., and Rubinstein, A. (1990). *Proc. Natl. Acad. Sci. USA*, **87**, 3445.
18. Falconer, A. E., Carson, R., Johnstone, R., Bird, P., Kehoe, M., and Calvert, J. E. (1993). *Immunology*, **79**, 89.
19. Staines, N. A., Ekong, T. A., Thompson, H. S., Isaacs, A. B., Loryman, B., Major, P. J., *et al.* (1990). *J. Autoimmun.*, **3**, 643.
20. Morikawa, A., Dahlgren, U., Carlsson, B., Narayanan, I., Hahn Zoric, M., Hanson, L. A., *et al.* (1991). *Int. Arch. Allergy Appl. Immunol.*, **95**, 13.
21. Esnault, V. L., Jayne, D. R., Weetman, A. P., and Lockwood, C. M. (1991). *Immunology*, **74**, 714.
22. Goldblatt, D., van Etten, L., van Milligen, F. J., Aalberse, R. C., and Turner, M. W. (1993). *J. Immunol. Methods*, **166**, 281.
23. Marriott, J. B. and Oliveira, D. B. (1994). *Clin. Exp. Immunol.*, **95**, 498.
24. Saito, A., Hosaka, Y., Nakagawa, T., Yamada, S., and Okuda, K. (1993). *Infect. Immunol.*, **61**, 332.
25. Thomas, H. I., Morgan Capner, P., Enders, G., O'Shea, S., Caldicott, D., and Best, J. M. (1992). *J. Virol. Methods*, **39**, 149.
26. Blackburn, N. K., Besselaar, T. G., Schoub, B. D., and O'Connell, K. F. (1991). *J. Med. Virol.*, **33**, 6.
27. Meurman, O., Waris, M., and Hedman, K. (1992). *J. Clin. Microbiol.*, **30**, 1479.
28. Guigno, D., Coupland, B., Smith, E. G., Farrell, I. D., Desselberger, U., and Caul, E. O. (1992). *J. Clin. Microbiol.*, **30**, 1958.
29. Schoub, B. D., Blackburn, N. K., Johnson, S., McAnerney, J. M., and Miller, B. (1992). *J. Med. Virol.*, **37**, 113.
30. Junker, A. K. and Tilley, P. (1994). *J. Med. Virol.*, **43**, 119.
31. de Ory, F., Antonaya, J., Fernandez, M. V., and Echevarria, J. M. (1993). *J. Clin. Microbiol.*, **31**, 1669.
32. Vinhal, F. A., Pena, J. D., Katina, J. H., Brandao, E. O., Silva, D. A., Orefice, F., *et al.* (1994). *Appl. Parasitol.*, **35**, 1.
33. Dahlquist, G. G., Ivarsson, S., Lindberg, B., and Forsgren, M. (1995). *Diabetes*, **44**, 408.

34. Agbarakwe, A. E., Griffiths, H., Begg, N., and Chapel, H. M. (1995). *J. Clin. Pathol.*, **48**, 206.
35. Mellander, L., Bottiger, M., Hanson, L. A., Taranger, J., and Carlsson, B. (1993). *Acta Paediatr.*, **82**, 552.
36. Robertson, C. A., Coppel, R. L., Prindiville, T., Fregeau, D., Kaplan, M., Dickson, E. R., *et al.* (1990). *Hepatology*, **11**, 717.
37. Feldman, R. G., Hamel, M. E., Breukels, M. A., Concepcion, N. F., and Anthony, B. F. (1994). *J. Immunol. Methods*, **170**, 37.
38. Mooney, J. and Kinane, D. F. (1994). *Oral Microbiol. Immunol.*, **9**, 321.
39. Kasp, E., Whiston, R., Dumonde, D., Graham, E., Stanford, M., and Sanders, M. (1992). *Am. J. Ophthalmol.*, **113**, 697.
40. Chargelegue, D., Stanley, C. M., O'Toole, C. M., Colvin, B. T., and Steward, M. W. (1995). *Clin. Exp. Immunol.*, **99**, 175.
41. Jones, C. L., MacDonald, R. A., Hosking, C. S., and Roberton, D. M. (1987). *J. Immunol. Methods*, **105**, 111.
42. Dandliker, W. B., Alonso, R., De Saussure, V. A., Kierszenbaum, F., Levison, S. A., and Schapiro, H. C. (1967). *Biochemistry*, **6**, 1460.
43. Levison, S. A., Kierszenbaum, F., and Dandliker, W. B. (1970). *Biochemistry*, **9**, 322.
44. Saussure, V. A. and Dandliker, W. B. (1969). *Immunochemistry*, **6**, 77.
45. Edgington, T. E. (1971). *J. Immunol.*, **106**, 673.
46. MacDonald, R. A., Hosking, C. S., and Jones, C. L. (1988). *J. Immunol. Methods*, **106**, 191.
47. Hall, T. J. and Heckel, C. (1988). *J. Immunol. Methods*, **115**, 153.
48. Gray, B. M. and Shaw, D. R. (1993). *J. Immunol. Methods*, **157**, 269.
49. Nisonoff, A. and Pressman, D. (1959). *Arch Biochem. Biophys.*, **80**, 464.
50. Kamoun, P. P. (1988). *Trends Biochem. Sci.*, **13**, 424.
51. Bata, J. E., Gyenes, L., and Sehon, A. H. (1964). *Immunochemistry*, **1**, 289.
52. Hedman, K. and Seppälä, I. (1988). *J. Clin. Immunol.*, **8**, 214.
53. Thomas, H. I. and Morgan Capner, P. (1991). *J. Virol. Methods*, **31**, 219.
54. Lutz, E., Ward, K. N., and Gray, J. J. (1994). *J. Med. Virol.*, **44**, 317.
55. Holliman, R. E., Raymond, R., Renton, N., and Johnson, J. D. (1994). *Epidemiol. Infect.*, **112**, 399.
56. Hedman, K., Lappalainen, M., Seppala, I., and Makela, O. (1989). *J. Infect. Dis.*, **159**, 736.
57. Inouye, S., Hasegawa, A., Matsuno, S., and Katow, S. (1984). *J. Clin. Microbiol.*, **20**, 525.
58. Thomas, H. I., Morgan-Capner, P., and Meurisse, E. V. (1990). *Serodiagnosis Immunother. Infect. Dis.*, **4**, 371.
59. Polanec, J., Seppala, I., Rousseau, S., and Hedman, K. (1994). *J. Clin. Lab. Anal.*, **8**, 16.

3

Liposomes

ERIC CLAASSEN and FREEK VAN IWAARDEN

1. Introduction

Liposomes can be used in a number of different ways to influence the homeostasis of a given organism. Typical examples include their use as vaccine, adjuvant, drug delivery system, immunomodulator, imaging agent, or as a cosmetic. Liposomes in their most basic form consist of spontaneously formed phospholipid bilayers enveloping an aqueous phase. When preparing liposomes from naturally occurring (phospho)lipids, in the correct concentrations and without adding foreign substances to the preparation, one can assume that the ensuing vesicles are non-immunogenic (i.e. not a target for antibodies or specific T cells) and biodegradable. However, this type of vesicle can still be a target for immune attack by the innate branch of the immune system embodied in most cases by macrophages which will take up almost any particulate matter not bearing the proper MHC molecules. As reviewed recently (1) the innate immune response which is very swift and efficient in removing non-self does not receive enough attention in the design of liposomes. Consequently, 'natural' liposomes can be used to influence macrophages in several ways. First, by the inclusion of a toxic substance the macrophages can be killed or temporarily suppressed. The latter can also be achieved by overloading the macrophages with large doses of 'empty natural' liposomes. Secondly, by the inclusion of immunomodulators, both in the aqueous or lipid phase, one can stimulate the macrophages. The efficiency of elimination, stimulation, or suppression is critically dependent on factors such as: liposome size, charge, stability, content, and membrane composition. Minor variations in these factors may have major consequences for the eventual outcome.

Obviously, the modulation of macrophage function is only a small aspect of the use of liposomes *in vivo*, but it should never be discounted in any application or experiment. The most visionary, and probably also the most quixotic, application of liposomes is their use as a magic bullet for the targeting of therapeutic substances to defined sites and cells in the body. Basically, for targeting one should design liposomes in such a way that they are not eliminated by the innate or adaptive immune system but remain in the circulation until they have bound to their target. Once bound they can then fuse, depending on the membrane characteristics, and release their toxic or stimulating content in the target cell. Again, the efficacy of such vesicles is critically dependent on factors such as those mentioned above, and the inclusion of receptor/ligand molecules in the liposomal membrane always proves to be an additional complicating factor (mostly by rendering the liposome immunogenic). Furthermore, changes in vesicle characteristics and composition necessary for enhanced targeting can be detrimental to their *in vivo* half-life. However, the same factors that hamper the use of liposomes in drug targeting can be used to advantage when designing liposomes for the induction of humoral or cellular immune responses. Recent developments in liposome technology have led to immunogenic vesicles for tumour and infectious disease vaccines inducing both specific antibodies and cytotoxic T cells under the right circumstances.

In this chapter a choice of methods for the preparation of different types of liposomes are given. Each type has intrinsic advantages and problems, but these may differ depending on the specific application and liposomal constituents. Therefore a standard vesicle composition for a desired application is not always easy to give. Apart from selected methods for liposome preparation a fast and simple method for the fluorescent labelling of liposomes is described in detail. This method can be used to trace liposomes in any *in vivo* animal model by making use of frozen tissue sections and fluorescence microscopy. By studying lipsome targeting and distribution in this way the effects of changes in liposomal composition or characteristics on *in vivo* behaviour can be screened rapidly and liposomes can be optimized accordingly for any desired application. Here we present some selected methods for the preparation of liposomes without the need for expensive or very specialized reagents or equipment. We hope this chapter will serve as a technical stepping stone for those who would like to enter the exciting field of *in vivo* immunomodulation and drug targeting mediated by liposomes. More detailed information about the concepts, usage, and pitfalls of liposome technology can be found elsewhere (reviewed in ref. 1).

2. Lipids

Liposomes prepared with (phospho)lipids, which can also be found in the host, will not readily evoke an adaptive immune response (2). In fact, liposomes prepared with high concentrations of cholesterol have been shown to suppress T cell-mediated responses by exchange of cholesterol between cells and liposomes (3–6). The introduction of synthetic (phospho)lipids or bacterial compounds such as lipid A drastically alters this intrinsic immunosilence and has been used to enhance the intrinsic adjuvant activity of liposomes (7,8). However, concurrent with this increase in non-specific immunostimulating properties an autoimmune response against the 'natural' phospholipids has been observed (7). The importance of this observation is not immediately clear since auto-antibodies directed against phospholipids can also be found in normal serum (9,10), or during particular infections (11), and do not always induce damage (10). Liposomes containing 'stabilizing' lipids such as stearylamine, cardiolipin, phosphatidylglycerol, phosphatidylserine, and/or sphingomyelin have been shown to be toxic under certain conditions and are therefore not ideal for adjuvant liposomes (12,13). In contrast, the incorporation of monosialoganglioside-GM1 eliminated the toxicity of liposomally-associated cholera toxin completely (14) and antigenicity was enhanced (15). Moreover, incorporation of a cationic lipid (lipofectin reagent) has been shown to enhance the induction of T cell-dependent cytotoxicity against *Plasmodium falciparum* epitopes (16).

In view of the fact that lipid composition determines *in vivo* stability (e.g. less cholesterol less stable) and the distibution (net charge, cell fusion behaviour) of liposomes one will have to balance the beneficial and undesirable properties of lipids to be incorporated in the liposomal membrane. This implies that any change in size or composition should lead to re-evaluation and experimental confirmation of the desired biological effect and undesirable properties of the liposomes. This again emphasizes the need for further studies of the innate immune response.

3. Multilamellar vesicles

The type of liposome found after mixing phospholipids with an aqueous phase is dubbed multilamellar because of the numerous concentric phospholipid bilayers found in those vesicles. Hydrophilic compounds can be trapped in the aqueous phase between the bilayers and in the relatively small core. These vesicles are easy to prepare and retain their content relatively well since damage to the outer membrane only results in loss of the outer aqueous compartment (*Figure 1*). Depending on size and lipid composition these vesicles are well suited for targeting to macrophages, either as an immunoadjuvant or as a vehicle for antigen delivery in humoral (antibody) responses (17,18).

We have developed and applied a liposome-suicide technique for the actual elimination of macrophages *in vivo* (19). The method is based on the incorporation of dichloromethylene diphosphonate in large multilamellar reverse-phase evaporation vesicles consisting of cholesterol and phosphatidylcholine (20). This type of liposome is readily taken up by all types of macrophage and even by monocytes. Although it was established that DMDP liposomes also eliminated circulating monocytes this did not apply to bone marrow macrophage precursors (21). After uptake the liposomal bilayer is disrupted, the drug is released, and accumulates in the macrophage which then dies. The route of administration is effectively the only determinant in deciding which macrophage population (or subset) is eliminated (1,22). Intravenous administration of DMDP–liposomes leads to elimination

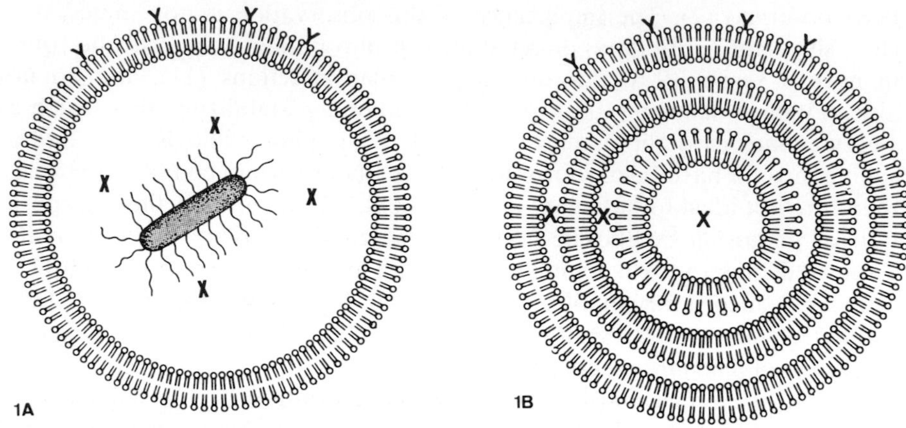

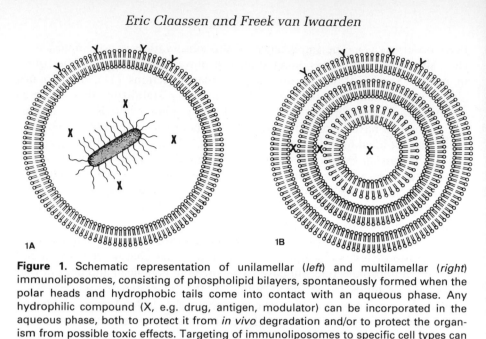

Figure 1. Schematic representation of unilamellar (*left*) and multilamellar (*right*) immunoliposomes, consisting of phospholipid bilayers, spontaneously formed when the polar heads and hydrophobic tails come into contact with an aqueous phase. Any hydrophilic compound (X, e.g. drug, antigen, modulator) can be incorporated in the aqueous phase, both to protect it from *in vivo* degradation and/or to protect the organism from possible toxic effects. Targeting of immunoliposomes to specific cell types can be enhanced by coupling target-specific antibodies, receptors, or ligands (Y) to the surface. Intact pathogens or other substances of large size can be incorporated in the relatively large space of (giant) unilamellar liposomes.

of all splenic (*Figure 2b*) and liver macrophages. Various subsets of macrophages will repopulate at different time intervals enabling subset-specific function studies.

Protocol 1. Reverse-phase liposomes (multilamellar) (22)

Equipment and reagents

- PBS: 10 mM phosphate buffer pH 7.4, 150 mM NaCl
- 100 mg egg phosphatidylcholine/ml chloroform (PC)
- Cholesterol
- 500 ml round-bottom flask
- Water-bath sonicator
- Argon or nitrogen (N_2) gas
- Rotary evaporator

Method

1. Dissolve 8 mg of cholesterol in 10 ml chloroform in a 500 ml round-bottom flask.
2. Add 0.86 ml of egg PC to the cholesterol solution.
3. Transfer the flask to the evaporator. Remove the chloroform by low vacuum (150 mbar) rotation (150 r.p.m.) evaporation. At completion a thin milky white lipid film is formed on the inner wall of the flask.

4. To the coated flask add 10 ml of PBS containing the hydrophilic agent to be entrapped. The lipid film is dispersed by gentle rotation (150–200 r.p.m.) at room temperature for 20 min.
5. Keep the milky white suspension at room temperature for 2 h under nitrogen or argon gas (to prevent denaturation and oxidation of the liposomes).
6. Sonicate the suspension in a water-bath sonicator for 3 min at room temperature. Maintain the liposome suspension at room temperature for 2 h (or overnight at 4°C) under nitrogen or argon gas to facilitate rehydration of the liposomes.
7. Separate the free material from the entrapped material by centrifugation (10 000 *g*, 20 min, room temperature) or size-exclusion chromatography (see *Protocol 3*).

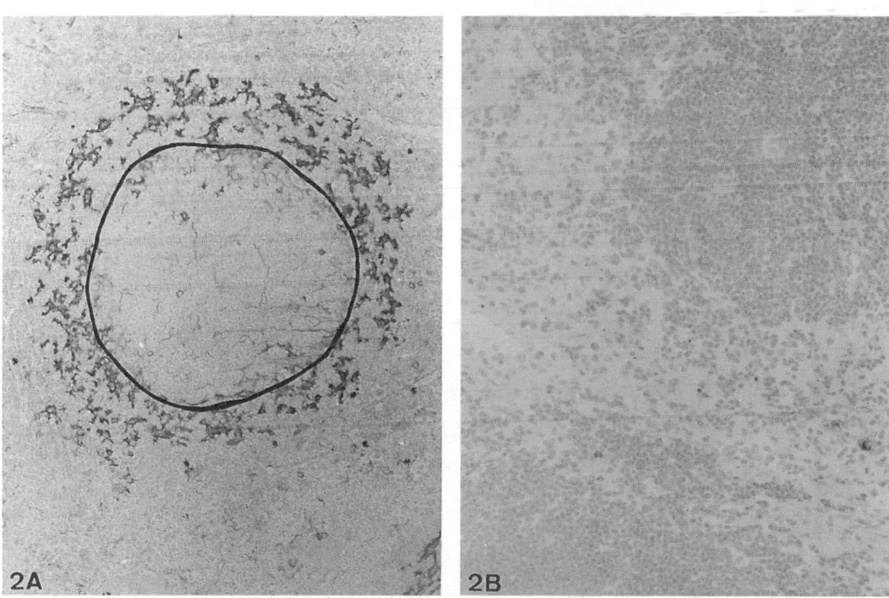

Figure 2. (A) Immunohistochemical staining for splenic marginal zone macrophages (with ERTR-9, compare with ref. 13) outside the black ring, and marginal metallophillic macrophages (with MOMA-1, compare with ref. 46) inside the black ring, on the border of marginal zone and periarteriolar lymphocyte sheath, in a control mouse treated by intravenous administration of empty liposomes. (B) Splenic section stained as in (A), 48 hours after administration of dichloromethylene diphosphonate liposomes. Note all macrophages in marginal zone, PALS, and red pulp have disappeared (empty spaces), and no staining is observed.

4. Unilamellar liposomes

When the content of the liposome is separated from the external milieu by only one bilayer the vesicle is dubbed unilamellar. Obviously these vesicles contain more aqueous phase than their (equal size) multilamellar counterparts (*Figure 1*). Especially in cases where molarity restrictions (i.e. difference inside and outside of liposome) prohibit incorporation of sufficient material, these larger vesicles can be beneficial. It goes without saying that when identical phospholipids are used these vesicles are more susceptible to complete disruption and leakage than multilamellar vesicles. Based on studies where unilamellar liposomes were targeted to hepatic macrophages much more efficiently than multilamellar vesicles (23) one can conclude that their increased volume is an advantage and that they also have distinct fusion behaviour.

Protocol 2. Unilamellar liposomes

Unilamellar liposomes can be prepared from multilamellar liposomes (*Protocol 1*, steps 1–6). Two methods are described: (A) sonification (for small unilamellar liposomes) and (B) extrusion through filters of different pore sizes (for unilamellar liposomes with a determined maximal size dependent on the sizes of the filters used).

Equipment and reagents

- Liposome suspension (1–4 ml)
- Sonicator equipped with a flat top disruptor tip
- Concentration cell
- Nitrogen cylinder
- Polycarbonate filters (example pore sizes 0.2 μm, 0.4 μm; Nucleopore Inc.)

A. Sonication (24)

1. Put the liposome suspension in melting ice.
2. Place the sonifer tip in the suspension. Take care not to touch the wall of the tube containing the liposomes.
3. Sonicate for 1 min at 50 W.

B. Extrusion

The amount of liposome suspension for a filter is dependent on the size of the concentration cell. The following is for a 10 ml capacity cell.

1. Place 5 ml of liposome suspension in the cell equipped with 0.4 μm polycarbonate filter.
2. Attach the apparatus to the nitrogen cylinder and apply a pressure of 44 p.s.i. (3 bar) and collect the liposomes in a tube. Repeat this procedure four times.

3. Disassemble the concentration cell and replace the 0.4 μm filter with a 0.2 μm filter.
4. Place the liposome suspension in the cell and apply a pressure of 80 p.s.i. (5.5 bar) and collect the liposomes in a tube. Repeat this procedure four times.

5. Size

To a large extent liposome size determines the actual half-life and biodistribution of liposomes (25), and the larger the liposome the more chance there is of it being taken up by macrophages (18). When macrophage processing is desired, e.g. in the case of intact pathogens, targeting to macrophages can be ensured by using relatively large liposomes, e.g. giant liposomes containing live or attenuated microbes (26) (see below). Size is mainly dependent on the preparation technique (27) but can be corrected when the liposomes are formed using filter extrusion (see above) and size-exclusion chromatography (in a heterogeneously sized liposome suspension) as described below.

Protocol 3. Size-exclusion chromatography

Equipment and reagents

- Chromatography column (r = 0.5 cm, height 25 cm)
- PBS (see *Protocol 1*)
- Bio-Gel A-1.5 m (Bio-Rad)

Method

1. Pack the column with the Bio-Gel.
2. Wash the column with five bed volumes (approx. 100 ml) PBS.
3. Apply 1 ml of a liposome suspension to the column.
4. Elute the liposomes (in the void volume) with PBS.
5. The non-entrapped material can be collected by futher elution of the column.

6. Content

Although, because of their particulate nature, liposomes are rapidly taken up by macrophages liposomal membranes made with 'natural' phospholipids are essentially immunologically inert. This contributes to the fact that substances entrapped within the aqueous phase of the liposomes are effectively shielded from degrading influences after *in vivo* administration. This can be an advantage in those cases where fragile antigens are used (28), and may possibly explain the beneficial effects of liposomes in some (29) but not in other (30,31) oral immunization studies. However, it is necessary to employ care when preparing liposomes with 'fragile' substances since the preparation technique might also degrade the compounds used. When making reverse-phase liposomes with organic solvents, as described above, one should make sure that the membrane compounds (i.e. proteins such as antigens, antibodies for targeting, receptors, ligands, etc.) are not degraded in such a way that they lose their function or immunespecificity. To prevent this it would be prudent to use a milder technique, without organic solvents (e.g. alcohol or chloroform), such as the detergent dialysis method.

Protocol 4. Detergent dialysis liposomes (32)

Equipment and reagents

- Cholesterol
- Phosphatidylserine
- Egg phosphatidylcholine
- 1 M octylglucoside
- 10 mM Hepes buffer pH 7.4, 1 mM EDTA, 150 mM NaCl
- Lyophilizer

Method

1. Dissolve 3 mg cholesterol, 6 mg phosphatidylcholine, and 6 mg phosphatidylserine in 2 ml chloroform.
2. Transfer the lipid solution to a glass tube and dry the lipids to a film using nitrogen gas.
3. Place the lipid film in a lyophilizer for 60 min.
4. Dissolve the material to be entrapped in 0.5 ml Hepes buffer and add to the dry lipids.
5. After 30 min add 0.24 ml octylglucoside to the mixture and shake vigorously.
6. Transfer the sample to dialysis tubing (M_r cut-off 3500), and dialyse against 100 ml Hepes buffer for 24 h at room temperature.
7. Separate the entrapped material from the free material by size-exclusion chromatography (see *Protocol 3*).

7. Giant liposomes

For entrapment of large and/or particulate antigens one can make use of giant liposomes. The composition of the liposome will influence, and alter, intrinsic *in vivo* distribution and uptake by target cells of the entrapped compound. Furthermore, the liposome may function as a protective layer shielding the entrapped compound from degrading influences.

Protocol 5. Giant liposomes (26)

Reagents

- Cholesterol (Chol)
- Egg phosphatidylcholine (PC)
- Phosphatidylglycerol (PG)
- Triolein (TO)
- 150 mM sucrose solution
- 200 mM sucrose solution
- Diethyl ether
- 5% glucose solution
- 100 mM sodium phosphate buffer pH 7.4, 150 mM NaCl

Method

1. Mix, by vortexing for 45 sec, 1 ml of a 150 mM sucrose solution containing the material to be entrapped with 1 ml of a chloroform solution containing PC, PG, Chol, and TO (4:4:2:1 molar ratio; 9 μmol total lipid).
2. Mix, by vortexing for 45 sec, 0.5 ml diethyl ether solution containing PC, PG, Chol, and TO (4:4:2:1 molar ratio; 4.5 μmol total lipid) with 2.5 ml of a 200 mM sucrose solution.
3. Mix, by vortexing for 15 sec, the water in chloroform emulsion of step 1 with the water in diethyl ether emulsion of step 2.
4. Transfer the emulsion in a 250 ml conical flask and evaporate the organic solvents with nitrogen at 37 °C while the sample is gently agitated in a shaking incubator.
5. Transfer 40 ml of a 5% glucose solution to a 50 ml centrifuge tube. Layer the liposomes on top of the glucose solution.
6. Centrifuge for 5 min at 600 *g* at room temperature. Collect the pellet and suspend it in 1 ml of the phosphate buffer. Repeat step 5 and 6 once.

Labile material can be entrapped in giant liposomes in the absence of organic solvents using the dehydration–hydration method (see *Protocol 8*).

8. Cytotoxic T cells

To induce an efficient MHC class I restricted immune response, involving the production of antigen-specific cytotoxic T cells (CTL), it is necessary to target the antigen to the cytoplasm (33,34) or induce processing by dedicated macrophages (4,35,36). It has been shown that both anionic and cationic (16) pH-sensitive liposomes are able to enter the class I restricted (endoplasmic reticulum/Golgi) pathway (4,36,37). The addition of Quil A to liposomes has been shown to efficiently enhance their capacity to induce $CD8^+$ CTL (34) and spectacular results have been observed with the induction of virus-specific CTL *in vivo* without antigen by entrapment of mRNA alone (38).

For the delivery of liposome-associated substances to antigen-presenting cells *in vitro* one can also make use of electroporation and commercially available liposomes (39).

Protocol 6. pH-sensitive liposomes (40)

Equipment and reagents

- Dioleoylphosphatidylethanolamine (DOPE) (Avanti Polar Lipids)
- 1,2-dioleoyl-*sn*-3-succinylglycerol (DOSG) (Avanti Polar Lipids)
- 5 mM Hepes buffer pH 8.5, 135 mM NaCl
- Waterbath sonicator

Method

1. Dissolve 2.5 μmol of DOPE and 2.5 μmol DOSG in 1 ml of chloroform.
2. Evaporate the chloroform by nitrogen gas.
3. Remove the residual chloroform by placing the tube containing the dried lipid film in a vacuum desiccator for 30 min.
4. Add 250 μl of Hepes buffer to the lipid film and adjust the pH with NaOH to 8.5.
5. Vortex the mixture for 1 min, and incubate the mixture for 60 min at room temperature.
6. Sonicate the mixture for 5 min in a water-bath sonicator, and incubate the small unilamellar liposomes for 48 h in order to hydrate the liposomes.
7. Sonicate the liposomes for 3 min in a water-bath sonicator and adjust the pH to 8.5.
8. In order to trap material, the freeze–thaw protocol is used (*Protocol 9*).

9. Stealth (PEG; SL) liposomes

The administration and sustained release of hydrophobic compounds has been described as one of the major advantages of liposomes (41). The *in vivo* half-life, depot function, and slow release of content can be drastically improved when stealth liposomes are used (42,43). These non-reactive liposomes, with reduced recognition and uptake by the immune system, are also called sterically stabilized liposomes (SLs) because of the fact that they are made with a protective layer of polyethylene glycol (44). Stealth liposomes can exhibit half-lives up to 100 times longer than conventional liposomes as a result of the inhibition of interactions with cell surface receptors (delaying non-specific uptake), and opsonins, and lipoproteins in the serum (42).

Protocol 7. Polyethylene glycol (PEG; stealth, SLs) liposomes (45)

Equipment and reagents

- 1,2-dioleoyl-*sn*-glycero-3-phosphoethanolamine-*N*-(poly(ethylene glycol)5000) (PEG–PE) (Avanti Polar Lipids)
- Cholesterol (Chol)
- Egg phosphatidylcholine (PC)
- 0.145 M NaCl
- Waterbath sonicator
- Polycarbonate filters (pore sizes 0.2 μm, 0.4 μm; Nucleopore Inc.)

Method

1. Dissolve 2.5 μmol of Chol, 2.5 μmol PC, and 0.375 μmol PEG–PE in 1 ml of chloroform/ethanol (1:1) in a round-bottom glass tube.
2. Evaporate the organic phase by nitrogen gas.
3. Remove the residual organic phase by placing the tube containing the dried lipid film in a vacuum desiccator for 2 h.
4. Add 2 ml of 0.145 M NaCl containing the material to be encapsulated to the dried llpld film and incubate for 1 h at room temperature.
5. Vortex the mixture for 2 min, and incubate the mixture for 60 min at room temperature.
6. Extrude the liposomes through polycarbonate filters (see *Protocol 2*).
7. Separate the free from the entrapped material by size-exclusion chromatography (see *Protocol 3*).

10. Enhanced entrapment

In the two protocols described below alternatives for liposome formation with relatively high entrapment efficiency are given. The advantage of the dehydration method lies in the fact that the freeze-dried material can be stored almost indefinitly, provided that the lipids cannot oxidize (store under vacuum or under nitrogen). The freeze–thaw liposomes are very simple to prepare and require no freeze-drying apparatus.

Protocol 8. Dehydration–hydration liposomes (26)

Equipment and reagents

- 1 ml liposome suspension (giant, unilamellar, multilamellar)
- Lyophilizer
- 1 ml of the material to entrap

Method

1. Mix 1 ml of liposomes with 1 ml of the material to be encapsulated.

Protocol 8. *Continued*

2. Freeze-dry the material in a lyophilizer overnight under vacuum (< 0.1 Torr).
3. Rehydrate the freeze-dried material initially by the addition of 0.1 ml distilled water at 20 °C.
4. Swirl the suspension vigorously and incubate for 30 min.
5. Repeat the process first by the addition of 0.1 ml PBS and 30 min later by the addition of 0.8 ml PBS.
6. The entrapped material is separated from the free material by centrifugation for the multilamellar liposomes or giant liposomes (see conditions for *Protocols 1* and *5*) or by size-exclusion chromatography (see *Protocol 3*) for the small unilamellar liposomes.

Protocol 9. Freeze–thaw liposomes (40)

Equipment and reagents

- 1 ml liposome suspension (giant, unilamellar, multilamellar)
- Liquid nitrogen
- 0.1 ml of the material to entrap

Method

1. Mix 1 ml of liposomes with 0.1 ml of the material to be encapsulated.
2. Freeze the mixture rapidly in liquid nitrogen.
3. Slowly thaw the mixture at 4 °C.
4. Repeat this procedure three times.
5. The entrapped material is separated from the free material by centrifugation for the multilamellar liposomes or giant liposomes (see the conditions for *Protocols 1* and *5*) or by size-exclusion chromatography (see *Protocol 3*) for the small unilamellar liposomes.

11. Carbocyanin labelling of liposomes

Carbocyanins are very lipophilic fluorescent dyes originally used for the membrane labelling of living neurons. They have low toxicity and integrate with high stability into plasma membranes and consequently have a long half-life *in vivo*. In contrast to fluorescent labels such as FITC (fluorescein isothiocyanate) and TRITC (tetramethyl rhodamine isothyocyanate), they do not interfere with surface membrane proteins, and consequently they do not interfere with receptor–ligand interactions. The fact that the liposomes can be labelled after they are formed can be particularly advantageous in those

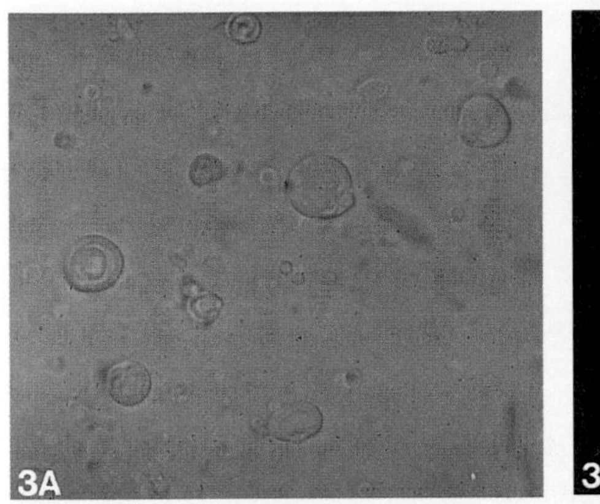

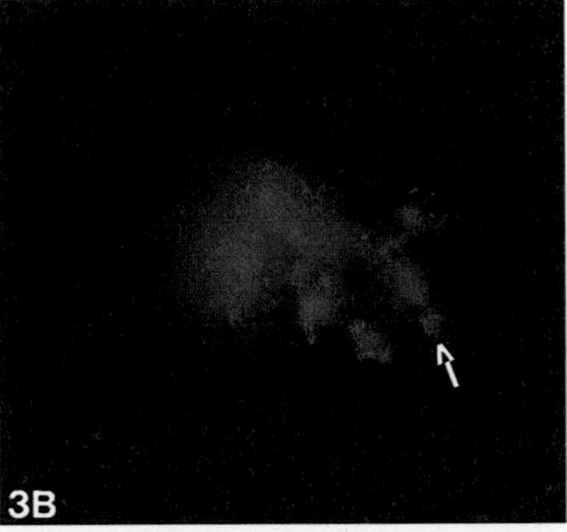

Figure 3. Multilamellar liposomes as viewed by phase-contrast light microscopy. When injected in mice and viewed *in situ* this would look like *Figure 2B*. Only after labelling with carbocyanins like DiI (yellow) and DiO (green, *arrow*) can the liposomes be visualized (with fluorescent light microscopy).

cases where liposomes have been used for *in vivo* studies (unlabelled as in *Figure 3A*) and are still available for *in vitro* labelling and subsequent localization studies. Furthermore, this method of labelling is preferred when the fluorochromes are quenched by (or interfere with) the contents (e.g. drug or enzyme) of the liposomes in the aqueous phase. Double staining (*Figure 3B*) by means of combination with 'routine' fluorescent labels such as FITC and TRITC is also possible but care should be taken to avoid quenching the label in the buffers or fixatives used (46). When using low amounts of dye relative to the amount of lipid all added dye will immediately be taken up by the liposomes. Only when very intense fluorescence is needed will one observe some extra liposomal crystal formation when labelling; these crystals can easily be removed by flotation gradient centrifugation (47).

By adding carbocyanins during preparation to the organic phase containing the (phospho) lipids, very efficient labelling can be obtained during liposome formation. The main advantage over post-formation labelling is the fact that all dye is taken up in the membrane, no crystals are formed, and no additional purification step is necessary. As shown in *Figure 4* liposomes given through the intravenous or intraperitoneal route will localize almost immediately in the marginal zone (macrophages) of the spleen and Kupffer cells of the liver (*Figure 6*). Almost no involvement of red pulp macrophages or dendritic cells is seen in the early uptake of these vesicles. As a secondary phenomenon, with time, a clear uptake by, or binding to, cells in the B cell follicles of the spleen can be observed (*Figure 5*). This latter aspect is probably involved with antigen presentation of liposomal constituents, whereas the uptake by marginal zone macrophages is mainly a non-immunological filter event (1). No liposomes are taken up by cells residing in the main T cell area (periarteriolar

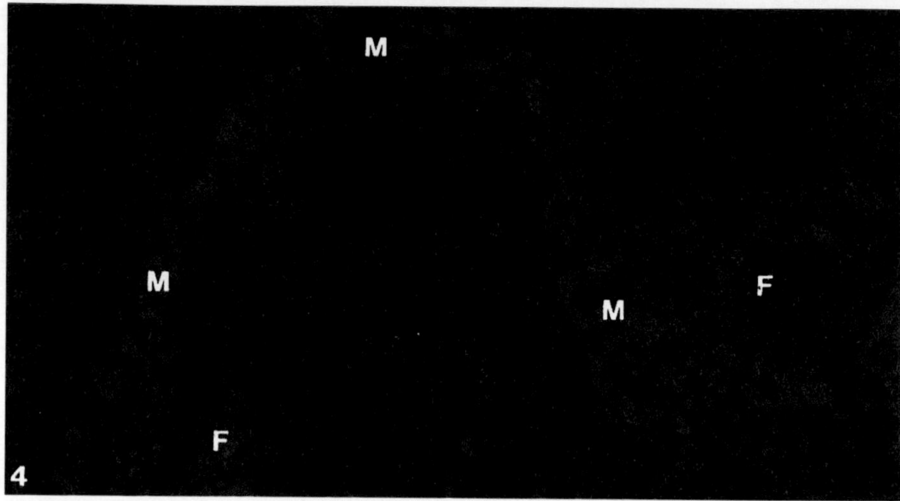

Figure 4. Fluorescent photomicrograph of carbocyanin (Dil) labelled liposomes, in a murine spleen, two hours after intravenous administration. Note that almost all liposomes are found in the marginal zone macrophages (M) and on follicular cells (F). Relatively few liposomes are taken up by the red pulp macrophages, and none by cells in the PALS (within the ring of the marginal zone).

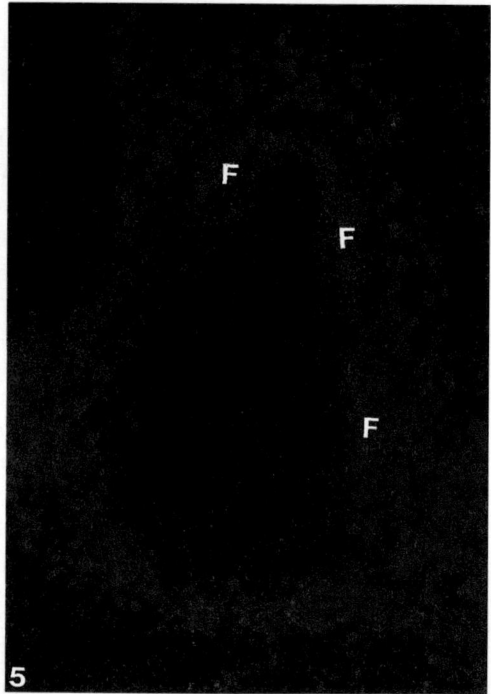

Figure 5. Animal treated as in *Figure 4* but viewed 24 hours after administration. Note the huge increase in follicular localization, with no material in the red pulp or PALS.

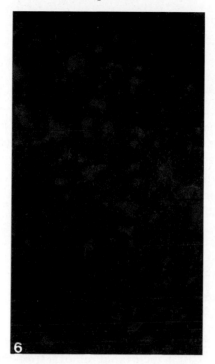

Figure 6. Fluorescent photomicrograph of carbocyanin (DiI) labelled liposomes, in Kupffer cells of murine liver, 24 hours after intravenous administration.

lymphocyte sheath PALS). Details of *in vivo* distribution of liposomes in lymph node and skin can be found elsewhere (compare ref. 1).

Protocol 10. Post-formation labelling of liposomes (47,48)

Equipment and reagents

- Liposomes to be labelled
- Vortex mixer
- Carbocyanin dye of choice (DiI, DiO, DiA from Molecular Probes, Eugene, USA or Europe Leiden The Netherlands)
- Large test-tube (30–50 ml)
- Ficoll, sucrose, or dextran of gradient quality
- Fluorescence microscope

Method

1. Dissolve 2.5 mg of carbocyanin dye in absolute ethanol (DiI) or DMSO (DiO; 2.5 mg/ml). The stock solution can be kept in the dark at room temperature for up to ten weeks.
2. Dilute the liposomal suspension to about 5 mg lipid per ml in suitable buffer (usually PBS but dependent on liposomes used) at room

Protocol 10. *Continued*

temperature, place tube on vortex mixer, and rigorously agitate the mixture.

3. Add the carbocyanin stock solution to the vortex in the liposomal suspension (DiI in the range of 5–20 μg/mg lipid and DiO 1–5 μg/mg lipid).
4. Mix for 2 min and check suspension under a microscope. Note structural integrity, or loss thereof, of liposomes and presence of brightly fluorescent carbocyanin crystals.
5. When necessary layer liposome suspension 1:1 (v/v) on Ficoll (Pharmacia) cushion and spin at low speed for separation of liposomes and crystals, or employ *Protocol 3*.

12. Conclusions

Liposomes can be formed in a number of different ways, some of which are extremely simple. The effective use of liposomes depends on a delicate balance between their function and the way in which the intact organism responds to them. Unfortunately, the very same factors that enhance their bioeffectiveness often assist in their rapid removal from the body. The advent of new synthetic lipids and a better knowledge of the innate and specific immune responses has resulted in a new generation of liposomes, with considerable promise in both vaccine research and drug targeting (1,49,50).

References

1. Claassen, E. (1996). In *Vesicles* (ed. M. Rosoff), p. 645. Surfactant Science Series, Marcel Dekker Inc., New York.
2. Alving, C. R. (1977). In *The antigens* (ed. M. Sela), p. 1. Academic Press, New York.
3. Heath, T. D., Edwards, D. C., and Ryman, B. E. (1976). *Biochem. Soc. Trans.*, **4**, 129.
4. Van Rooijen, N. (1995). In *Vaccines: new generation immunological adjuvants* (ed. G. Gregoriadis). Plenum Press, New York.
5. Ng, M. H., Ng, W. S., Ho, W. K. K., Fung, K. P., and Lamelin, J. P. (1978). *Exp. Cell. Res.*, **11**, 387.
6. Rivnay, B., Globerson, A., and Shinitsky, M. (1978). *Eur. J. Immunol.*, **8**, 185.
7. Schuster, B. G., Neidig, M., Alving, B. M., and Alving, C. R. (1979). *J. Immunol.*, **122**, 900.
8. Van Rooijen, N. and Van Nieuwmegen, R. (1980). *Immunol. Commun.*, **9**, 747.
9. Strejan, G. H., Essani, K., and Surlan, D. (1981). *J. Immunol.*, **127**, 160.
10. Alving, C. R. (1983). In *Liposome letters* (ed. A. D. Bangham), p. 269. Academic Press, New York.

11. Richards, R. L., Aronson, J., Schoenbechler, M., Diggs, C. L., and Alving, C. R. (1983). *J. Immunol.*, **130**, 1390.
12. Mayhew, E., Ito, M., and Lazo, R. (1987). *Exp. Cell Res.*, **171**, 195.
13. Claassen, E., Westerhof, Y., Versluis, B., Kors, N., Schellekens, M., and Van Rooijen, N. (1988). *Br. J. Exp. Pathol.*, **96**, 865.
14. Alving, C. R., Richards, R. L., Moss, J., Alving, L. I., Clements, J. D., Shiba, T., *et al.* (1986). *Vaccine*, **4**, 166.
15. Liu, D. X., Wada, A., and Huang, L. (1992). *Immunol. Lett.*, **31**, 177.
16. Wizel, B., Rogers, W. O., Houghten, R. A., Lanar, D. E., Tine, J. A., and Hoffman, S. L. (1994). *Eur. J. Immunol.*, **24**, 1487.
17. Claassen, E., Kors, N., and Van Rooijen, N. (1987). *Immunology*, **60**, 509.
18. Van Rooijen, N. (1995). In *Liposome mediated immunopotentiation and immunomodulation* (ed. G. Gregoriadis, *et al.*). Plenum Press, New York.
19. Van Rooijen, N. (1992). *Res. Immunol.*, **143**, 215.
20. Claassen, E. and Van Rooijen, N. (1986). *J. Microencapsulation*, **3**, 109.
21. Huitinga, I., Damoiseaux, J. G., Van Rooijen, N., Dopp, E. A., and Dijkstra, C. D. (1992). *Immunobiology*, **185**, 11.
22. Van Rooijen, N. and Sanders, A. (1994). *J. Immunol. Methods*, **174**, 83.
23. Camilleri, J. P., Williams, A. S., Amos, N., Douglas, A. G., Jones, D., Love, W. G., *et al.* (1995). *Clin. Exp. Immunol.*, **99**, 269.
24. Oosterlaken-Dijksterhuis, M. A., Haagsman, H. P., Van Golde, L. M. G., and Demel, R. A. (1991). *Biochemistry*, **30**, 8276.
25. Litzinger, D. C., Buiting, A. M. J., Van Rooijen, N., and Huang, L. (1994). *Biochim. Biophys. Acta*, **1190**, 99.
26. Antimisiaris, S. G., Jayasekera, P., and Gregoriadis, G. (1993). *J. Immunol. Methods*, **166**, 271.
27. Gregoriadis, G. (1994). *Immunomethods*, **4**, 210.
28. Mestecky, J., Moldoveanu, Z., Novak, M., and Compans, R. W. (1994). *Acta Paeditr. Japan*, **36**, 537.
29. Michalek, S. M., Childers, N. K., Katz, J., Dertzbaugh, M., Zhang, S., Russell, M. W., *et al.* (1992). *Adv. Exp. Med. Biol.*, **327**, 191.
30. Clarke, C. J. and Stokes, C. R. (1992). *Vet. Immunol. Immunopathol.*, **32**, 139.
31. Clarke, C. J. and Stokes, C. R. (1992). *Vet. Immunol. Immunopathol.*, **32**, 125.
32. Abraham, E. and Shah, S. (1992). *J. Immunol.*, **149**, 3719.
33. Huang, L., Reddy, R., Nair, S. K., Zhou, F., and Rouse, B. T. (1992). *Res. Immunol.*, **143**, 192.
34. Lipford, G. B., Wagner, H., and Heeg, K. (1994). *Vaccine*, **12**, 73.
35. Zhou, F., Rouse, B. T., and Huang, L. (1992). *J. Immunol.*, **149**, 1599.
36. Zhou, F. and Huang, L. (1994). *Immunomethods*, **4**, 229.
37. Martin, S., Niedermann, G., Leipner, C., Eichmann, K., and Weltzien, H. U. (1993). *Immunol. Lett.*, **37**, 97.
38. Martinon, F., Krishnan, S., Lenzen, G., Magne, R., Gomard, E., Guillet, J. G., *et al.* (1993). *Eur. J. Immunol.*, **23**, 1719.
39. Chen, W., Carbone, F. R., and McCluskey, J. (1993). *J. Immunol. Methods*, **160**, 49.
40. Zhou, F., Rouse, B. T., and Huang, L. (1991). *J. Immunol. Methods*, **145**, 143.
41. Weiner, A. L. (1994). *Immunomethods*, **4**, 201.
42. Lasic, D. D. and Papahadjopoulos, D. (1995). *Science*, **267**, 1275.

43. Kedar, E., Braun, E., Rutkowski, Y., Emanuel, N., and Barenholz, Y. (1994). *J. Immunother. Emphasis. Tumor. Immunol.*, **16**, 115.
44. Allen, T. M., Agrawal, A. K., Ahmad, I., Hansen, C. B., and Zalipsky, S. (1994). *J. Liposome Res.*, **4**, 1.
45. Klibanov, A. L., Maruyama, K., Beckerleg, A. M., Torchilin, V. P., and Huang, L. (1991). *Biochim. Biophys. Acta*, **1062**, 142.
46. Claassen, I. J. T. M., Osterhaus, A. D. M. E., and Claassen, E. (1995). *Eur. J. Immunol.*, **25**, 1446.
47. Claassen, E. (1992). *Res. Immunol.*, **143**, 235.
48. Claassen, E. (1992). *J. Immunol. Methods*, **147**, 231.
49. Van Rooijen, N. (1993). In *New generation vaccines* (ed. G. Gregoriadis), p. 11. Plenum Press, New York.
50. Buiting, A. M. J., Van Rooijen, N., and Claassen, E. (1992). *Res. Immunol.*, **143**, 541.

4

Immunofluorescence and immunoenzyme histochemistry

P. BRANDTZAEG, T. S. HALSTENSEN, H. S. HUITFELDT, and K. N. VALNES

1. Introduction

In 1941 Albert Coons and co-workers for the first time labelled the immunoglobulin (Ig) fraction of an antiserum with fluorescein to visualize the corresponding antigen in tissue sections by fluorescence microscopy (1,2). A new morphological discipline, based on probing for structural or functional markers, was thereby founded. The term immunohistochemistry should preferably be reserved for immunological probing in tissue sections, while immunocytochemistry usually refers to cell smears, cytospin preparations, and monolayer cultures. For simplicity, immunohistochemistry will be used as a general methodological term in this chapter.

Immunohistochemistry is widely used, both in biological research and in diagnostic histopathology and microbiology; it is applicable for transmitted light, fluorescence, and electron microscopy. The basic requirement is availability of a relevant antibody reagent that, when used as a specific probe on the test preparation, can be identified by direct or indirect labelling with a discernible signal. The reagent can be raised by polyclonal or monoclonal antibody technology against a variety of antigens ranging from single amino acids to large cellular glycoproteins. Major methodological advancements after the introduction of Coon's fluorescent antibody tracing are the development of antibody-conjugated enzyme labels (3,4), the introduction of unlabelled antibody bridge enzyme methods (5–7), and particularly the unlabelled peroxidase anti-peroxidase (PAP) method (8), as well as the alkaline phosphatase anti-alkaline phosphatase (APAAP) method (9).

Simultaneous visualization of more than one antigen by multicolour immunostaining is often desirable or even necessary, both for quantitative studies and to explore spatial relationships (topography) of functional significance. The introduction of rhodamine as an alternative fluorescent label (10), as well as narrow-band excitation and selective filtration of fluorescein (green) and rhodamine (red) emission (11), makes paired immunofluorescence a practically and scientifically acceptable probing method. Furthermore, immunoenzyme techniques can be adapted for multicolour staining either with the same enzyme and different substrates, as originally introduced by Nakane and Pierce (12), or with different enzymes and their substrates.

Altogether, numerous modifications of immunohistochemical staining methods have been introduced since the late 1960s. An outline of the most commonly employed antigen probing principles, with special emphasis on multicolour immunofluorescence and immunoenzyme staining, will be given below. The results obtained depend on many variables that are often interdependent, such as tissue substrate fixation, pre-treatment of tissue sections, incubation procedures, reagent specificity, sensitivity, efficiency, and reproducibility.

2. Immunostaining for fluorescence or light microscopy

2.1 Reagents

2.1.1 Fluorochromes and fluorescent antibodies

The IgG fraction of an antiserum, affinity purified polyclonal IgG antibody, monoclonal IgG antibody, and $F(ab')_2$ or Fab fragments of IgG can all be conjugated with fluorescent compounds called fluorochromes or fluorophores. The most common fluorochromes employed for immunohistochemical conjugates are fluorescein isothiocyanate (FITC), which emits apple-green fluorescence when excited by ultraviolet or preferentially blue light, and tetramethylrhodamine isothiocyanate (TRITC), which emits orange fluorescence when excited by ultraviolet or preferentially green light (13). Several other fluorochromes are currently used for commercially available conjugates, such as difluoroboradiazaindacene (BODIPY®) that emits green fluorescence, Lissamine® rhodamine B sulfonyl chloride (RB200SC) and its derivative Texas Red®, indocarbocyanine (Cy3®), or indodicarbocyanide (Cy5®) that all emit orange to red fluorescence (14), and Cascade Blue® as well as aminomethylcoumarin acetic acid (AMCA) that both emit blue fluorescence (15).

The approximate absorption and emission maxima for the most commonly used fluorochromes appear in *Table 1*; there is generally only a slight shift (1–10 nm) to a higher wavelength of maximal absorption (λ_{max}) after conjugation, depending on the degree of labelling (16). R-phycoerythrin (R-PE) is included for comparison because it is commonly applied in multicolour immunostaining for flow cytometry. This is one of several light-harvesting phycobiliproteins from cyanobacteria and eukaryotic algae exploited as fluorescent labels (17). R-PE conjugates have a broad absorption range for uptake of energy and may provide a signal five to ten times more intense than corresponding FITC conjugates. However, because of the large size and rapid fading of R-PE, it has only occasionally been applied in immunohistochemistry (18).

Table 1. Optical characteristics of some common fluorescent labels

Fluorescent label[a]	**Absorption maximum (nm)**[b]	**Emission maximum (nm)**
FITC	494 (blue)	520 (green)
TRITC	500, 550 (blue-green)[c]	575 (orange)
RB200SC	565 (green)	590 (orange)
Texas Red	593 (orange)	615 (orange-red)
Cy3	550 (green)	570 (yellow-orange)
Cy5	650 (red)	680 (dark red)
R-PE	480, 546, 565 (blue-green)	578 (orange)
AMCA	353 (ultraviolet)	448 (dark blue)

[a] Abbreviations are explained in the text.
[b] Also called λ_{max}; this maximum is often slightly higher after conjugation, depending on the degree of labelling (16).
[c] First λ_{max} depends on fluorochrome batch, its storage, and animal species of conjugated IgG (16).

Conjugation of IgG and $F(ab')_2$ fragments with fluorochromes such as FITC, TRITC, or RB200SC is simple and can be performed by different procedures in a reproducible manner (16,19). Several commercial companies have specialized in the production of fluorochromes and/or their conjugation to antibodies (Biological Detection Systems, DAKO, Jackson ImmunoResearch Laboratories, Molecular Probes, Sigma, Southern Biotechnology). Excess of free fluorochrome is easily removed by gel filtration, and thereafter the conjugate can be characterized. The optical density (OD) ratio ($OD_{280\ nm}$: $OD_{\lambda\ max}$), as proposed by Cebra and Goldstein (20), may be used as a simple and generally applicable estimate of the degree of labelling, where OD at 280 nm mainly reflects the protein (IgG) content of the conjugate. However, some producers prefer to give the reverse ratio—that is, $OD_{\lambda\ max}$: $OD_{280\ nm}$. When a pure standard of free fluorochrome is available, both types of estimate can conveniently be converted to the actual molar fluorochrome-to-protein (F:P) ratio (16).

The F:P ratio obtained after removal of free fluorochrome, is merely an average estimate as considerable heterogeneity exists for most conjugates. The negative charge introduced by bound fluorochrome will reflect the degree of labelling when a conjugate is subjected to anionic exchange chromatography (20). Such separation provides fractions with a relatively homogeneous F:P ratio (16) and has been adopted by several commercial companies to remove overlabelled as well as underlabelled IgG from fluorochrome conjugates.

Another essential feature of the conjugate is its actual concentration. Labelled protein can be satisfactorily estimated by OD with $E^{1\%,\ w/v}_{280\ nm,\ 1\ cm} = 14$ for IgG or $F(ab')_2$ when a correction factor is introduced, depending on the fluorescent label (16,20). Information about the protein concentration and the labelling degree should be available when the optimal working conditions of a conjugate are determined by performance testing, taking both its specific and non-specific staining properties into consideration (19,21). The immunohistochemical results obtained cannot be appropriately evaluated without knowledge about the various characteristics of the conjugate (see Section 5).

2.1.2 Microscopical separation of fluorescent colours

An ideal fluorochrome should have a high quantum yield, an absorption maximum close to a strong spectral line of the 100 W mercury arc lamp generally used on modern fluorescence microscopes, and a good separation between its λ_{max} (preferably used for excitation) and its emission peak (that is, a large Stokes shift). All of the fluorochromes listed in *Table 1* have such properties.

Modern fluorescence microscopes employ incident excitation light (epi-illumination) provided by a Ploem-type vertical beam splitter that contains several interchangeable dichroic mirrors (11). The combined excitation and barrier filter sets are constructed according to the Stokes shifts of the individual fluorochromes and are mounted in removable holders (Omega® Optical, Brattleboro, VT). Three and preferably more filter holders are placed in sliders or turrets, which allows rapid switching of the optical conditions; these can be selected with bandwidths that are more or less selective for the isolation of green, red, or blue emission colours. Thus, by changing the filter sets, each fluorescent signal from a morphological element can be observed one after the other (*Figure 1a,b*).

The first successful simultaneous recording of paired immunofluorescence staining (green and red) was achieved by Brandtzaeg in 1974 by double-exposing colour slides through a Ploem-type epi-illuminator while blocking the film transport (22).[1] Such rather cumbersome multicolour documentation

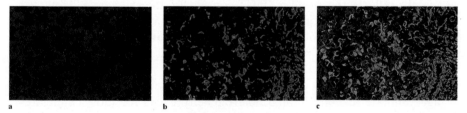

Figure 1. Two-colour immunofluorescence staining for cytokeratin with rabbit antiserum (red: swine IgG–TRITC conjugate, indirect staining) and for vimentin with murine mAb (green: FITC-labelled avidin–biotin sequence) in a section from an ethanol-fixed and paraffin-embedded specimen of nasopharyngeal carcinoma. (a) Selective filtration of red emission shows cytokeratin in cancer cells. (b) Selective filtration of green emission shows vimentin expression in mesenchymal cells and variable co-expression of this marker in many cancer cells. (c) Co-expression identified by yellow colour in double exposure of same field (fluorescence microscopy, × 112).

[1] Anecdotally it is interesting to note that this paper initially was not accepted for publication because the referee wanted "... the addition of ultraviolet excitation with a colourless barrier filter to ... have enhanced histological discrimination", and concluded that "The fluorescence microscopy employed is a limiting technical feature of the study". The appreciation of overlay procedures certainly changed profoundly over the next two decades.

(*Figure 1c*) has been used for several immunobiological and immunopathological studies in our laboratory over the last two decades (19) and has also been adopted by other laboratories. We have more recently applied the same principle to record triple-stained images either directly or by means of computerized image analysis (23,24).

Subsequent authors have called the photographic double-exposure method (*Figure 1c*) 'fluorescent overlay antigen mapping' (FOAM) and have defined several technical variables that may disturb the obtained images (25,26). These errors include the well-known problems with image shift differences (geometrical errors) and lack of colour fidelity. The main reason for the latter is 'bleed-through' of contrasting emission colours or autofluorescence, often caused by inappropriate filter set combination or photographic over-exposure. To avoid geometrical errors, it is crucial that the images are completely overlapping, and the emission colours should ideally reflect the true distribution of different antigens; these problems concern both photographic recording of multicolour staining and visual inspection by rapid filter switching. When three markers are analysed, the results are often best recorded and accurately superimposed by computerized image analysis (24,27) employing narrow bandpass filters (see Section 3.3).

Simultaneous visualization of different fluorescent colours by double- and triple-band filter sets (Omega® Optical) has recently made direct microscopical inspection of FOAM feasible. In theory, this outstanding advancement of practical immunofluorescence microscopy should eliminate the need for photographic double- or triple-exposures and thereby the problem with image shifting (25). However, inherent limitations of the interference coatings on the filters decrease to some extent the possibilities of producing satisfactory images within the visible spectrum. Therefore, the multiband filter sets provide lower emission intensities than the ideal single colour sets and hence faint or imbalanced colour mixing may be difficult to recognize. In fact, the single colour dichroic filter sets remain the 'gold standard' for verification of antigen co-localization and for ensuring lack of unwanted bleed-through of contrasting emission signals. Also, photographic documentation of FOAM may require fine-tuning of individual images by adapting the exposure times manually one after the other. Paired immunofluorescence staining can in fact often be well documented by parallel black-and-white illustrations of the separated fluorescent signals.

2.1.3 Preservation of fluorescent colour signals

Signal fading is an inherent problem of immunofluorescence methods, especially when FITC conjugates are used. Reduction of the colour intensity is particularly noticed during photographic recording because of relatively long exposure times. It was therefore of great interest when various compounds were introduced for the preservation of fluorescence (28). However, when we re-evaluated these chemicals with regard to their practical applicability, it became apparent that they reduced the initial emission intensity and thereby the staining efficiency (29). This important drawback has generally been neglected.

In our laboratory Tris-buffered polyvinyl alcohol (PVA) has always been used as a semi-solid mounting medium for immunofluorescence (30,31); it is practical, requires no sealing of the coverslips, and can be stored indefinitely at 4 °C in the dark, provided that weekly readjustment (1 M NaOH) to pH 8.5–9.0 is performed. Freshly prepared buffered (pH 8.7) PVA (Sigma) containing paraphenylendiamine (PPD), *n*-propyl gallate (NPG), or 1,4-diazobicyclo (2,2,2)-octane (DABCO), was compared with PVA alone or with buffered glycerol (pH 8.7) with respect to preservation of FITC immunofluorescence (29). At a concentration of 0.2–2.0 g/litre and 6 g/litre, respectively, PPD and NPG were shown to retard effectively fluorescence fading. To avoid a substantial decrease of the initial emission intensity, the modified PVA had to be rather fresh and the mounted preparations had to be examined within a few days. Although addition of DABCO (6 g/litre) afforded a mounting medium that tolerated storage reasonably well, both PPD and NPG were more advantageous in practice. For ordinary PVA and buffered glycerol, the relative degree of fading was comparable and most pronounced during the first 45 seconds, but the initial intensity was significantly lower with buffered glycerol than with PVA.

In our opinion, PPD at a concentration of approximately 1 g/litre is most useful when added to the PVA mounting medium. This addition is helpful for prolonged microscopy (for instance cell counting) at high magnifications, and for photographic documentation in special instances. However, remounting in ordinary PVA is necessary for prolonged storage of tissue sections (29). Even FITC-labelled preparations can be stored in PVA at 4 °C in the dark for several years without any notable decrease of the fluorescence intensity (unpublished observations). The storage properties of AMCA-labelled preparations are limited by the increase in bluish autofluorescence emitted by several tissue elements (see Section 5.5.1).

In practice, counting of fluorescent cells and double- or triple-exposures can usually be performed satisfactorily after mounting in ordinary buffered PVA, provided that adequate filter and microscopy conditions are available. One important requirement for photography is that 100% of the emission light reaches the film. Rhodamine fluorochromes, which in contrast to FITC do not have strongly pH-dependent characteristics, show relatively little fading, and single-stained preparations can be mounted in ordinary organic media. BODIPY® has been recommended as a pH-insensitive alternative to FITC (Molecular Probes).

2.1.4 Enzyme labelling systems

Various enzymes and their chromogens (*Table 2*) have been used as immunohistochemical labels since Avrameas and Uriel (3) and Nakane and Pierce

Table 2. Enzymes and corresponding chromogenic substrates most commonly used as immunohistochemical labels

Enzyme label	Substrate (chromogen)	Colour reaction
Horseradish peroxidase (Px)	Diaminobenzidine (DAB)	Brown
	3-Amino-9-ethylcarbazole (AEC)	Reddish
	Tetramethyl benzidine	Brownish-black
	Benzidine dihydrochloride (BDHC)	Blue
	4-Chloro-1-naphthol (CN)	Blue-black
	p-Phenylenediamine–HCl and pyrocatechol	Blue-black
Alkaline phosphatase (AP)	Fast Blue BB salt and naphthol AS-MX	Blue
	Fast Red salt	Red
	New Fuchsin	Red
Glucose oxidase	Nitro-blue tetrazolium	Blue-black
β-Galactosidase	5-Bromo-4-chloro-3 indolyl-β-D-galacto-pyranoside and ferri/ferrocyanide	Dark blue

(12) independently introduced horseradish peroxidase (Px) in 1966. The most commonly used substrate for Px is diaminobenzidine (DAB), which polymerizes upon oxidation with H_2O_2 and produces a brown colour that contrasts well with nuclear haematoxylin staining (*Figure 2*). The DAB reaction can be further enhanced by a variety of agents such as osmium (32), $CuSO_4$, $CoCl_2$, $NiCl_2$ (33), imidazole (34), thioglycolic acid–silver nitrate (35), or ferric ferricyanide (36). Such enhancers are also commercially available (Vector Labotatories).

An advantage of the benzidine-based compounds is their stability in organic solvents; a drawback is their potential carcinogenicity, although DAB is now considered less dangerous than previously (37). Several alternatives to DAB have been developed. Burstone (38) originally introduced 3-amino-9-ethylcarbazole (AEC) for the localization of cytochrome oxidase, and Graham *et al.* (39) extended its use to the detection of Px. Sections stained with AEC must be aqueously mounted because the reaction product dissolves in organic solutions. Tetramethyl benzidine has also been found to be a very sensitive chromogen, but crystallization on the tissue section may be a problem (40). Benzidine dihydrochloride (BDHC) produces a blue colour that contrasts well with the brown DAB reaction product (41). An alternative non-carcinogenic chromogen with a blue-black permanent end-product is *p*-phenylenediamine–HCl in combination with pyrocatechol (42). Also 4-chloro-1-naphthol (CN) that generates a similar colour may be useful for paired staining (4).

Endogenous Px is formalin-resistant and can therefore interfere with specific immunostaining even in routine paraffin sections. Such disturbing enzymatic activity may be blocked by methanol–H_2O_2 (43), phenylhydrazine (44), or periodate oxidation (45); but the possibility of destroying antigenic

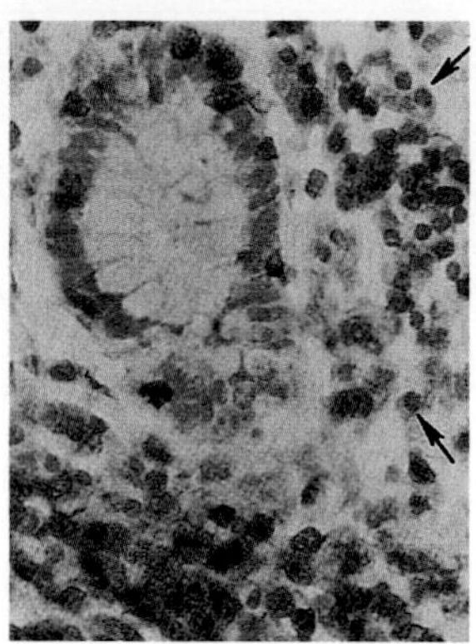

Figure 2. Immunoenzyme staining with mAb-based PAP in a trypsinized section from routinely formalin-fixed and paraffin-embedded specimen of human colonic mucosa. Brown colour shows surface membrane expression of leucocyte common antigen (CD45) on lymphocytes in lamina propria and crypt epithelium, whereas plasma cells (*arrows*) are mainly negative (haematoxylin counterstain, × 250).

epitopes by this pre-treatment must always be considered (46). If intense unwanted reactivity is present in the test preparation (e.g. eosinophils), another immunohistochemical method should be chosen.

Alkaline phosphatase (AP) has been increasingly used as an immunohistochemical label, particularly after the introduction of paired immunoenzyme staining techniques (47). AP was originally visualized with a substrate of Fast Blue BB salt and naphthol AS-MX, giving a blue reaction product that contrasts well with DAB in paired staining (*Figure 3*). Fast Red salt can also be used and provides excellent contrast with haematoxylin counterstain (*Figure 4a,b*) and sensitive detection of single membrane-positive cells in smears (*Figure 4c*). Aqueous mountants are required for both these AP chromogens. An alternative substrate is New Fuchsin (48) or Vector Red (Vector Labotatories) whose reaction products are resistant to organic solvents. Amplification of the red colour signal can be obtained under the fluorescence microscope, and the narrow emission spectrum offers potential for use in paired immunofluorescence methods (201).

Endogenous AP staining is generally abolished by routine formalin fixation and paraffin embedding, but isoenzyme activity often occurs in frozen or ethanol-fixed preparations of various tissues. Several blocking agents can be used, such as levamisole (49), acetic acid (50), and periodate oxidation (51), because they have little effect on AP from calf intestine (or from *Escherichia coli*) that is most frequently used as label. However, human intestinal AP is not blocked by levamisole; although the other agents may be useful (52), Px or fluorescence is often better on sections of gut mucosa, particularly for intraepithelial immunostaining.

Glucose oxidase from *Aspergillus niger* (53) has been subjected to con-

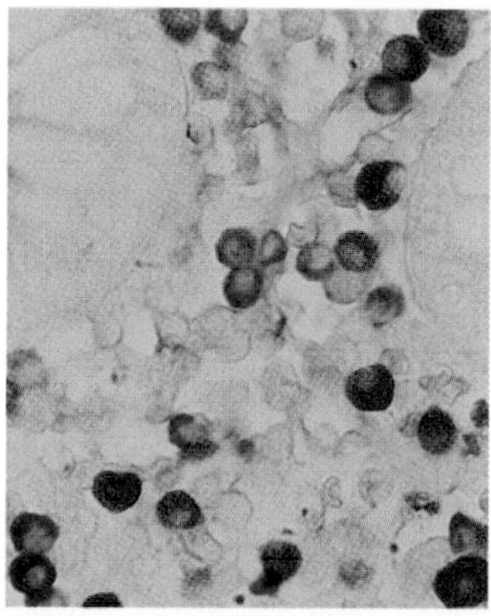

Figure 3. Two-colour immunoenzyme staining with unlabelled primary rabbit antibody reagents to different human Ig light chains in a section from paraffin-embedded specimen of colonic mucosa fixed with Susa fixative. Cells expressing κ chain are decorated brown and those with λ chain blue. The first sequence was based on PAP–DAB and the second on indirect AP–Fast Blue BB staining (no counterstain, × 262).

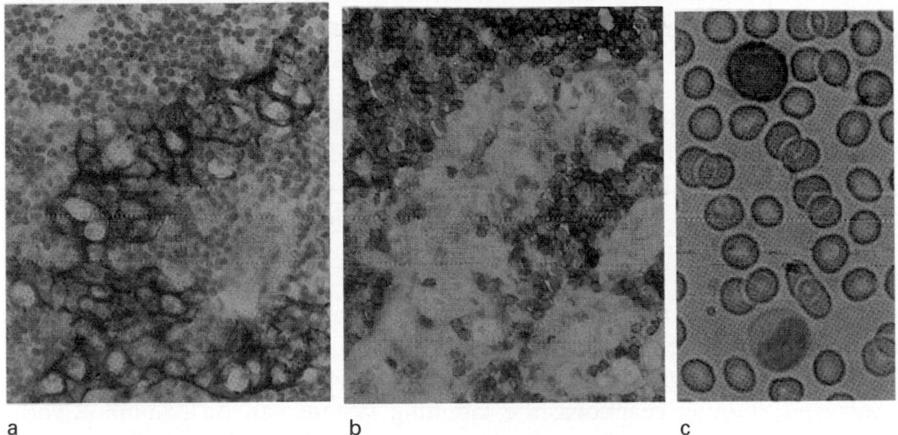

a b c

Figure 4. Immunoenzyme staining with mAb-based APAAP in (a, b) two trypsinized serial sections from routinely formalin-fixed and paraffin-embedded specimen of nasopharyngeal carcinoma, and in (c) formalin-methanol (1 : 9, v/v)-fixed (3 sec) smear of human peripheral blood. (a) Red colour shows cytokeratin in carcinoma cells. (b) Comparable field in adjacent section shows expression of leucocyte common antigen (CD45) on mononuclear cells surrounding and to some extent invading the carcinoma. (c) Red colour shows lymphocyte surface membrane expression of CD4, while another mononuclear cell as well as erythrocytes are negative (haematoxylin counterstain, a,b, × 282; c, × 450).

siderable interest as an antibody label because this enzyme does not exist in mammalian tissues and can be used for paired immunostaining as well (54). Mammalian tissues also lack β-galactosidase and this enzyme has been recommended as another useful antibody label (55). Nevertheless, Px and AP remain the two most popular enzymes.

Covalent conjugation of IgG or $F(ab')_2$ fragments with enzyme can be obtained either by employing glutaraldehyde or periodate (53,56). Improved conjugation procedures have minimized the risk of antibody and enzyme denaturation and reduced the presence of free enzyme or antibody in the final conjugate preparation (56,57). The problem of enzyme-to-enzyme or IgG-to-IgG conjugation can also be minimized (58). So-called EPOS ('enhanced polymer one-step staining') conjugates (Dako) are based on an inert backbone molecule to which several primary antibody and Px molecules are chemically linked. However, direct staining even with such enhanced conjugates cannot be expected to provide the same sensitivity as indirect multistep methods (59). An additional advantage of the unlabelled indirect methods based on immune complexes or avidin–biotin complexes is that chemical enzyme conjugation is totally avoided (see Section 2.2.1.*ii*).

2.1.5 Metallic labelling systems

The use of colloidal gold particles as labels in immunohistochemistry was originally developed for electron microscopy (60); this approach has become the most important subcellular immunohistochemical method (61). Colloidal gold particles can be seen under the light microscope as a reddish colour when highly concentrated conjugates are applied but such suspensions are quite unstable. This problem can be avoided by diluting the conjugate and enhancing the reaction by silver precipitation that produces a strong black colour (62). In addition to being a label for polyclonal and monoclonal antibody reagents, colloidal gold is often used in combination with protein A. Other methods have also been described, such as the 'antigen-coated colloidal gold granules' or the GLAD ('gold-labelled antigen detection') technique (63).

Immunogold–silver staining for light microscopy has the advantage of high sensitivity, particularly when viewed through an epipolarization filter (IGS, Nikon, Nippon Kogaku KK, Tokyo, Japan); the colour develops without subsequent staining reactions; the labelling system can be combined with counterstains (201); and the preparation of the gold conjugates is easy and economic (63). Nevertheless, the relatively poor penetration of the conjugates into fixed tissues is a disadvantage, and staining of cryosections often results in non-specific silver precipitation.

2.2 Immunohistochemical staining methods

The immunohistochemical label can principally be bound to the actual test antigen either by pure immunological methods (see Sections 2.2.1, 2.2.2, and 2.2.3) or by methods in which part of the staining sequence is non-immunological (see Sections 2.2.4 and 2.2.5). It is important in the planning of indirect methods that the staining sequences are carefully designed. Flow charts should be prepared in order to minimize the risk of introducing unwanted interspecies cross-reactivity with endogenous Ig in the test preparation, or between the different sequences in multicolour experiments. A variety of staining protocols have recently been published for immunoenzyme methods (48,59,63–65) and are also available from several commercial companies (DAKO; Jackson ImmunoResearch; Vector Laboratories). Protocols will be provided below for some recent multicolour principles applicable for immunofluorescence as well as for immunoenzyme staining.

2.2.1 Basic immunofluorescence and immunoenzyme principles

i. Labelled antibody methods

The label (fluorochrome or enzyme) can be conjugated to the primary or to the secondary antibody, referred to as direct and indirect labelled antibody methods, respectively. These are the simplest possible immunostaining principles, including direct (*Figure 5a*) and indirect (*Figure 5b*) immunofluorescence, as well as direct and indirect immunoenzyme techniques. The direct approach provides no immunological amplification of the colour signal relative to the number of antigenic sites in the preparation. This limitation is often a drawback, particularly for the detection of cell membrane antigens that usually occur in small amounts. It is also a drawback that every primary antibody reagent of a desired specificity must be directly conjugated. Enhancement of the staining intensity over that obtained by ordinary indirect immunofluorescence, has been achieved by combined direct–indirect staining (66), sequential indirect staining (67), indirect staining by repeated application of the first antibody layer (68), and two indirect steps including biotin–avidin (66).

ii. Unlabelled antibody bridge methods

In these techniques, various enzymes (primarily Px) have exclusively been used for labelling. A second-stage anti-Ig antibody acts as bridge between the first antibody and subsequent steps (6,7), which either include anti-enzyme antibody and the corresponding enzyme in four steps (*Figure 6a*), or complexes

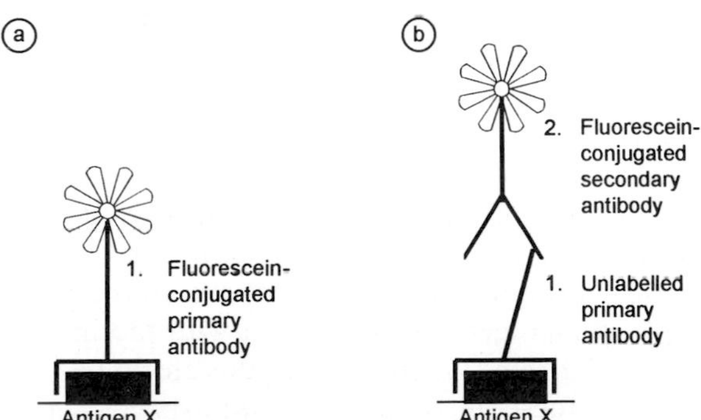

Figure 5. (a) Direct labelled antibody, and (b) indirect (two-step) labelled antibody (immunofluorescence) methods with fluorescein as labels.

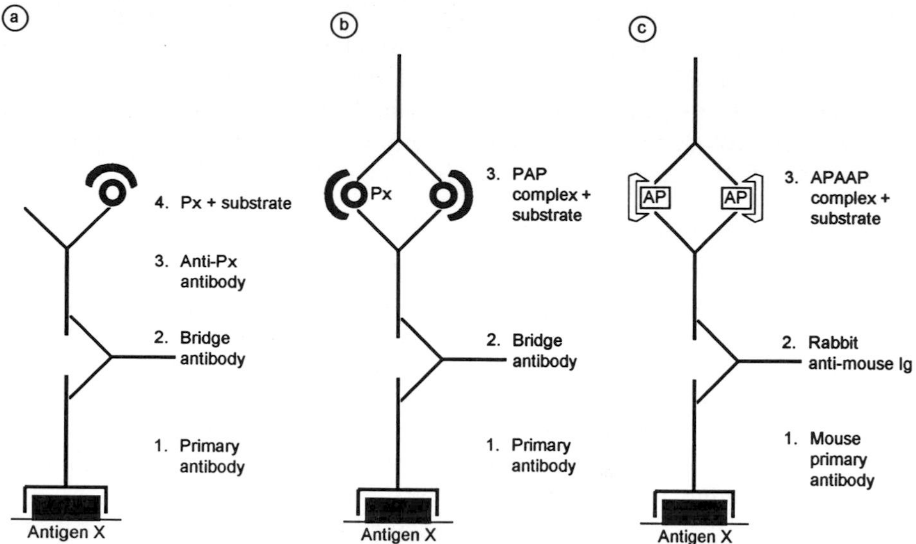

Figure 6. (a) Four-step unlabelled antibody immunoenzyme (peroxidase, Px) bridge method, (b) three-step Px anti-Px (PAP) complex method, and (c) three-step alkaline phosphatase (AP) anti-AP (APAAP) complex method.

of anti-enzyme antibody and the enzyme in three steps (*Figure 6b*). These two approaches are called the unlabelled antibody bridge method and the PAP method, respectively (8). They were originally designed for primary rabbit antibody but can easily be adapted for murine monoclonal antibody (mAb), the second method then being referred to as 'mouse PAP' or 'mono-PAP'. The three-step approach also includes the APAAP technique (9,69) originally developed for mAbs (*Figure 6c*) but subsequently extended to exploit primary rabbit antibody by the incorporation of a mAb specific for rabbit Ig (DAKO). The intensity of the Px or AP colour signal can be considerably enhanced by performing one or more repeats with the two last incubation steps (48).

With these methods, it is important to apply the bridge antibody in excess, thereby ensuring that one of its antibody combining sites is available to interact with the next step in the sequence (*Figure 6*). It follows that if the bridge antibody reacts specifically with the primary antibody, it will bind to the same antigenic site of the corresponding antibody in the PAP or APAAP complexes. In contrast, unwanted antibodies present in the bridging reagent that bind to non-Ig tissue antigens will not react with the immune complexes. A low degree of background staining can therefore be obtained with this approach provided there is absence of interspecies cross-reactivity with endogenous Ig in the test preparation. Moreover, the immune complexes are relatively stable and produce substantial signal amplification. The average

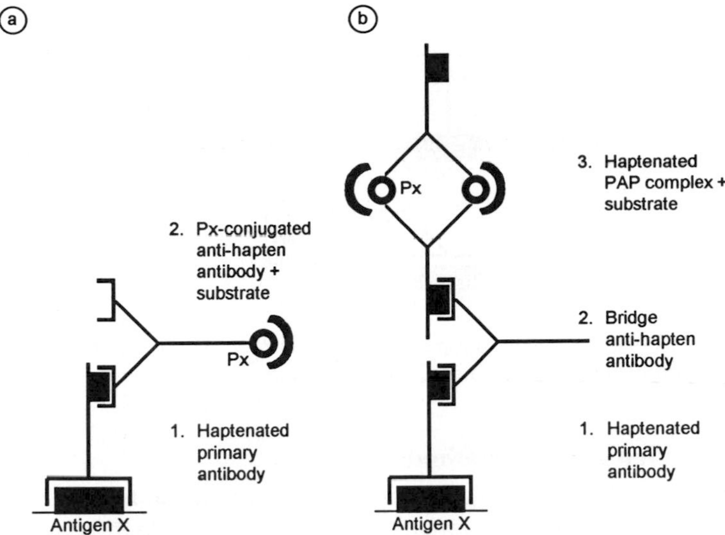

Figure 7. (a) Two-step hapten-labelled antibody immunoenzyme method based on secondary peroxidase (Px)-labelled antibody, and (b) three-step Px haptenated anti-Px (PAP) complex method with unlabelled anti-hapten antibody as bridge.

molecular ratio of Px to anti-Px antibody is 3:2 in the PAP complexes (70), whereas the enzyme ratio is 2:1 or 1:1 in the APAAP complexes (9,71).

2.2.2 Hapten-labelled antibody methods

Hapten-labelled antibodies were introduced by Cammisuli and Wofsy (72). A primary antibody can be labelled with many hapten groups, thereby providing considerable amplification. This approach can be used both for immunofluorescence (73) and immunoenzyme techniques (74,75). In the indirect method, the haptenated primary antibody is followed by a labelled antibody specific for the hapten (*Figure 7a*), analogous to the indirect immunofluorescence and immunoenzyme techniques. In a three-stage method (75), addition of excess anti-hapten bridge antibody is followed by haptenated PAP complexes (*Figure 7b*).

The main advantages of these methods are: minimal loss of antibody activity because of mild coupling procedures, for example by employing bifunctional amidinating reagents; greater amplification by introducing on average 20 hapten molecules per IgG molecule; and the possibility for multicolour staining by conjugating different primary antibodies from the same species with non-cross-reacting haptens, such as FITC, biotin, dinitrophenol, *p*-azobenzene arsonate, *p*-azobenzoyl glutamate, or *p*-azobenzoyl glycine (see Section 3.2.1.*iii*). Antibodies to haptens can also be used in various immunostaining approaches to intensify the colour signal, for example by applying polyclonal or monoclonal anti-FITC or anti-biotin as an enhancement step.

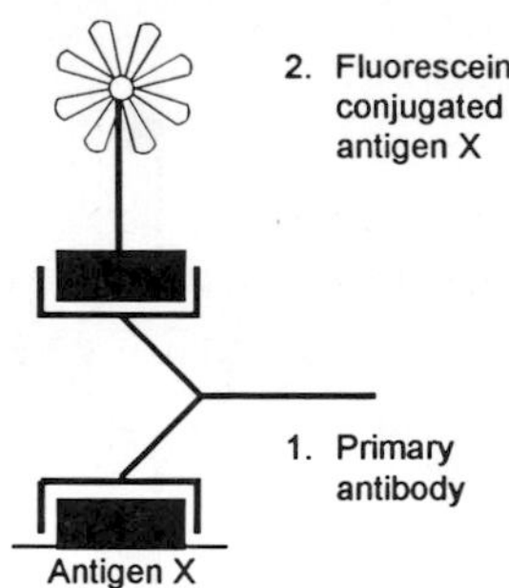

Figure 8. Two-step labelled antigen immunofluorescence method with unlabelled primary antibody and fluorescein-conjugated antigen.

2.2.3 Labelled antigen methods

In these methods (*Figure 8*), the unlabelled primary antibody is applied in excess followed by labelled antigen (76–78). This approach is highly specific but depends on relatively large amounts of available purified antigen for conjugation with fluorochrome or enzyme. Its applicability is therefore rather limited, although the same approach is important for direct detection of antibody-producing cells in tissue sections (see Section 3.2.1.*ii*).

2.2.4 Protein A methods

The specific binding of protein A from *Staphylococcus aureus* to the Fc portion of IgG from many animal species has been exploited in a variety of immunohistochemical methods. Protein A can be conjugated with fluorescein (79), Px (80), and AP (81), or be adsorbed to colloidal gold (61,62). Two-stage protein A methods employ unlabelled primary antibody followed by labelled protein A (*Figure 9a*); and with free protein A as bridge, a protein A–PAP complex method can be performed (*Figure 9b*).

Advantages of the protein A methods are: low background staining (provided binding to endogenous IgG in the tissue section is avoided); few limitations with respect to the animal species in which the primary antibody is raised; and the possibility of paired staining (82) as described later (see Section 3.2.3).

2.2.5 Avidin–biotin methods

The 68 kDa basic glycoprotein avidin from egg white has an extraordinarily high affinity ($K_a > 10^{15}$ M^{-1}) for the small coenzyme biotin (part of the vitamin B complex), and this property is exploited extensively in immunohistochemistry (83). One molecule of avidin will bind four molecules of biotin by a non-covalent interaction that is essentially irreversible because it is at least 10^6 times stronger than most antibody–antigen reactions. Both avidin and

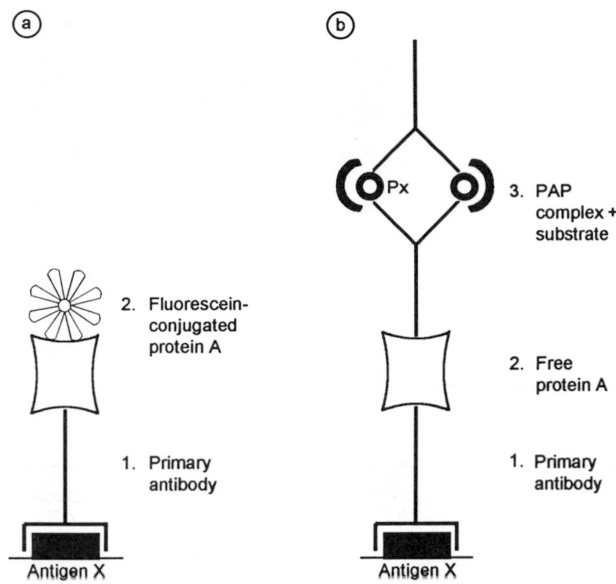

Figure 9. (a) Two-step protein A immunofluorescence method with unlabelled primary antibody and fluorescein-conjugated protein A, and (b) three-step peroxidase (Px) anti-Px (PAP) complex immunoenzyme method with free protein A as bridge.

biotin can be conjugated with fluorochromes (84) or enzymes (83) without interfering with the binding affinities.

Several immunofluorescence and immunoenzyme variants of the avidin–biotin system have been described (*Figure 10*). For immunoenzyme staining, the avidin–biotin complex (ABC) method proposed by Hsu *et al.* (85) has been popular; a biotinylated secondary antibody is used to bridge the unlabelled primary antibody and complexes of avidin and biotinylated Px (*Figure 10c*). This approach can be used for polyclonal as well as for monoclonal primary antibodies. Optimal staining is achieved by preparing the complexes at an avidin : Px ratio of 4:1, and the high sensitivity obtained is probably explained by amplification through the formation of a lattice with many biotinylated Px molecules (85). The ABC method can also be used with biotinylated primary antibody, an approach that can be advantageous in order to avoid possible cross-reactions between secondary antibody and endogenous Ig in the tissue section.

Endogenous biotin or biotin receptors in various tissues may make blocking procedures necessary (62,86,87). In addition, some avidin preparations bind non-specifically to certain cellular components, probably because of electrostatic interactions (83,86). Mast cells and macrophages are particularly prone to producing such non-specific staining, which may be prevented by applying the ABC solution at pH 9.4 (88). Moreover, commercial avidin–biotin blocking kits are available (DAKO, Vector Laboratories).

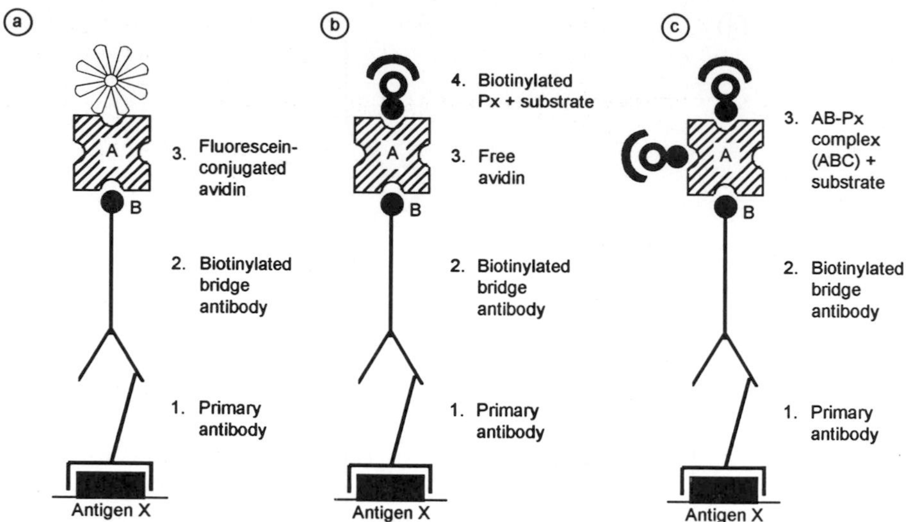

Figure 10. (a) Three-step fluorescein-labelled avidin (A)–biotin (B) immunofluorescence method, (b) four-step biotinylated peroxidase (Px) AB method, and (c) three-step AB–Px complex (ABC) immunoenzyme method.

The use of streptavidin is recommended to minimize spurious staining produced by avidin binding sites present in some tissues (89). This homotetramer from *Streptomyces avidinii* shows an affinity for biotin that is several orders of magnitude lower than that of egg white avidin, but its fairly neutral isoelectric point and unglycosylated state favour immunohistochemical performance.

A possible drawback of the ABC method may be steric hindrance because of the large size of the complexes, although this is advantageous in paired staining to reinforce the DAB blocking effect (see Section 3.2.3). Simplified and enhanced staining is obtained by the labelled streptavidin–biotin (LSAB) method based on sequential application of biotinylated bridge antibody and streptavidin conjugated with AP or Px. Such conjugates are available commercially (DAKO; Vector Laboratories; Ventana Medical Systems) and they have potentially more available binding sites for the bridge antibody than those provided by the ABC method. Similar conjugates of modified avidin (ExtrAvidin®) can also be purchased (Sigma).

3. Multicolour immunostaining and its evaluation

Simultaneous visualization of two or more antigens can be achieved by a variety of combinations of the different immunohistochemical methods and their modifications. Whether the immunoreagents are applied sequentially, in parallel, or partly simultaneously, avoidance of unwanted interactions between the different staining sequences is imperative. Several approaches may be successful to this end but many pitfalls exist (65), particularly when it comes to detecting three or more rather than two antigens in the same preparation. The technical problems are mainly related to the availability of relevant primary antibodies from only one animal species, which often turns out to be a limitation.

3.1 Primary antibodies from different species

By applying primary antibodies from different animal species (90,91), two indirect staining sequences can conveniently be combined based on immunofluorescence (*Figures 1* and *11a,b*) or immunoenzyme (*Figure 11c*) methods. This principle has been extended to three antigens employing FITC, TRITC, and AMCA as labels (92), but the availability of primary antibodies from different species limits its applicability. For paired immunoenzyme staining, Campbell and Bhatnagar (54) used glucose oxidase and Px, while Mason *et al.* (93) have reported detailed protocols for the use of Px–DAB and AP–Fast Blue BB. To ensure reliable co-localization of two antigens, it is important that all antibodies are applied before the sheltering effect of the coloured end-product is developed, particularly that of DAB (see Section 3.2.3). Several modifications have been explored, such as a direct–indirect immunofluorescence sandwich (66) combined with an avidin–biotin sequence (*Figure 11b*), two unlabelled antibody sequences (*Figure 11c*), and an ABC and unlabelled antibody bridge method (94).

It should be pointed out, however, that despite the use of primary antibodies from different animal species, troublesome interspecies reactions may occur (92). Interactions between the two staining sequences can be avoided by appropriate absorptions with IgG or normal serum from the species that shows unwanted binding, or preferably by using secondary antibodies from the same species. Precautions must also be taken to avoid cross-reactions of secondary antibodies with endogenous Ig present in the tissue section. We have, for example, observed that a commercial horse anti-mouse Ig reagent claimed to show less than 1% activity with human Ig by radioimmunoassay, nevertheless cross-reacted sufficiently to visualize distinctly Ig-producing plasma cells when applied on human tissue sections (unpublished observations). Omission of the primary antibodies, alternatively one or both, is an imperative control in indirect staining methods.

3.2 Primary antibodies from the same species

3.2.1 Cross-reactions avoided by choice of staining method

i. Direct labelled antibody methods

By combining two primary conjugates, either in direct immunofluorescence (*Figure 12*) or direct immunoenzyme staining, interaction between the reagents is usually no problem. The conjugates can therefore be applied

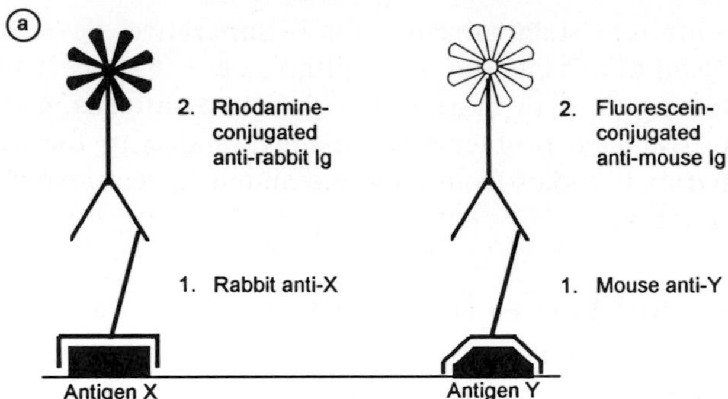
a
2. Rhodamine-conjugated anti-rabbit Ig
1. Rabbit anti-X
Antigen X
2. Fluorescein-conjugated anti-mouse Ig
1. Mouse anti-Y
Antigen Y

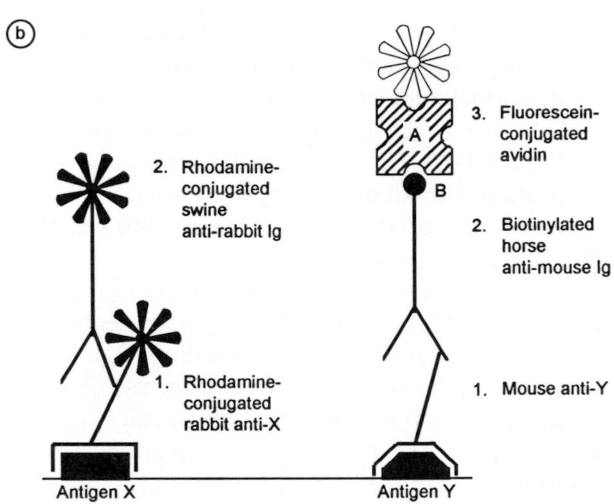
b
2. Rhodamine-conjugated swine anti-rabbit Ig
1. Rhodamine-conjugated rabbit anti-X
Antigen X
3. Fluorescein-conjugated avidin
A
B
2. Biotinylated horse anti-mouse Ig
1. Mouse anti-Y
Antigen Y

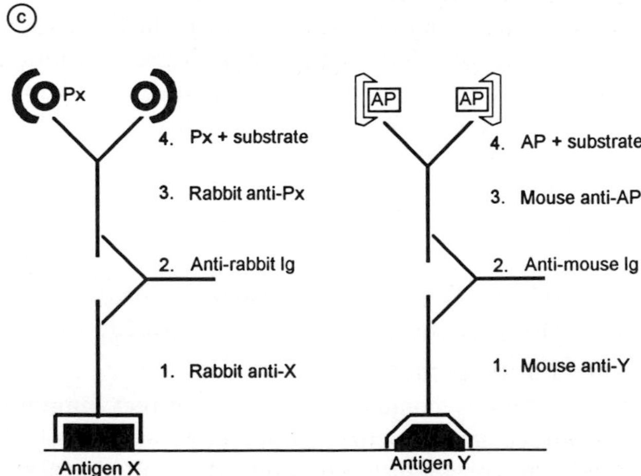
c
Px
4. Px + substrate
3. Rabbit anti-Px
2. Anti-rabbit Ig
1. Rabbit anti-X
Antigen X
AP
AP
4. AP + substrate
3. Mouse anti-AP
2. Anti-mouse Ig
1. Mouse anti-Y
Antigen Y

Figure 11. Two-colour immunohistochemistry with primary antibodies from different animal species. (a) Two indirect parallel two-step immunofluorescence sequences with unlabelled rabbit and mouse primary antibodies and rhodamine- and fluorescein-labelled secondary antibody conjugates, (b) modified direct–indirect immunofluorescence (rhodamine) two-step method combined with a parallel three-step avidin (A)–biotin (B) sequence with fluorescein as label, and (c) two parallel four-step unlabelled antibody immunoenzyme sequences applying peroxidase (Px) and alkaline phosphatase (AP) as labels developed with contrasting colours.

---

simultaneously, which is clearly the simplest and speediest approach for paired staining. However, if one or both of the reagents have been absorbed with soluble antigens, excess of this absorbent can exert unwanted blocking effects; the immunostaining then has to be performed by sequential incubations with intermediate rinsing. Conjugates from different species may also be mixed provided interspecies interactions are avoided by appropriate absorption (see Section 3.1). With mAbs such direct immunohistochemical staining is often not feasible because of faint colour signals (95).

ii. Direct or indirect labelled antigen methods

Labelled antigen methods have been used with bridge antibody for paired staining (96) by applying Px- and AP-conjugated antigens (*Figure 13*). Different fluorochromes can also be employed as labels, which is a simple method for multicolour staining although restricted by the limited availability of purified non-cross-reacting antigens. The same approach can be used in a direct manner to detect one or more specific antibody-producing cell populations in tissue sections. For this purpose, the number of different colours can be increased by mixed labelling of one or two antigens because a single plasma cell *a priori* will bind only one non-cross-reacting antigen (97). Antibody-producing cells, moreover, can be detected by an indirect (unlabelled antigen) method when the corresponding antibody specificity is available as a conjugate (22); with this approach paired staining for cytoplasmic Ig is necessary to exclude direct decoration of engulfed antigen in macrophages (98).

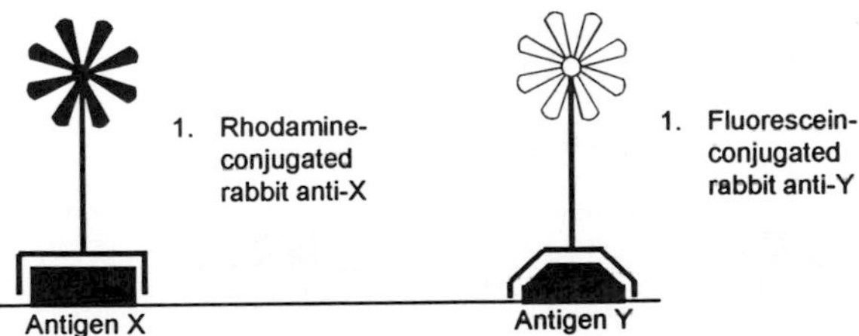

Figure 12. Two-colour direct immunofluorescence staining with rhodamine- and fluorescein-labelled rabbit antibody conjugates applied simultaneously in one step.

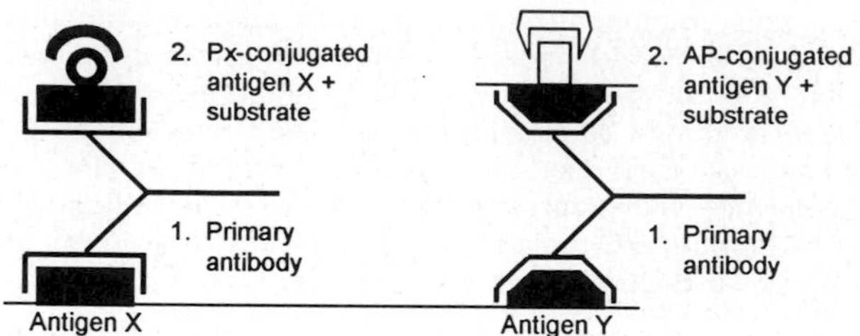

Figure 13. Two-colour immunoenzyme two-step staining with peroxidase (Px)- and alkaline phosphatase (AP)-labelled antigens applied in parallel sequences after the respective unlabelled primary antibodies.

iii. Hapten-labelled antibody methods

After conjugating primary antibodies from the same species with different haptens (see Section 2.2.2), paired immunofluorescence or immunoenzyme (*Figure 14*) staining can be performed by secondary non-cross-reacting antibodies, for instance to detect cell surface antigens (99). This principle has also often been used for hapten sandwich procedures such as haptenated PAP or APAAP methods with murine mAbs (75).

iv. Ig class- or subclass-specific secondary antibodies

By combining primary antibodies of different classes (for instance, murine IgG and IgM), light chains (murine κ and λ chains), or subclasses (murine IgG1, IgG2a, IgG2b, and IgG3) from the same species, multicolour staining can be performed provided truly isotype-specific polyclonal secondary antibodies are available (24,93). Because the number of unique isotype epitopes on the primary mAb may be very small, an amplifying avidin–biotin sequence sometimes has to be introduced to obtain a sufficiently strong colour signal (*Figure 15*, *Protocol 1*). This step can be further enhanced by

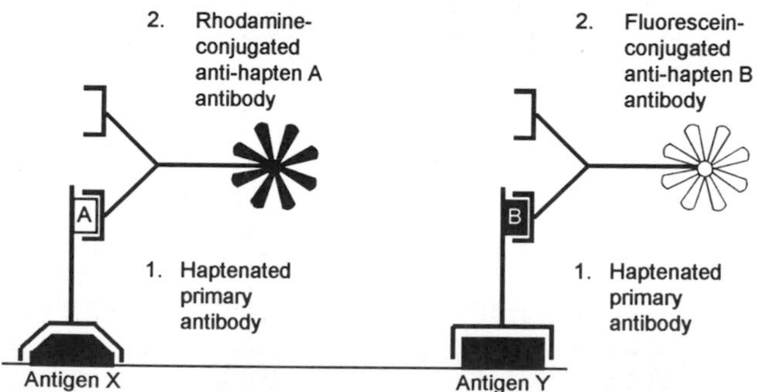

Figure 14. Two-colour immunofluorescence two-step staining with primary antibodies labelled with non-cross-reacting haptens (A and B), followed by corresponding secondary rhodamine- and fluorescein-labelled antibodies applied in parallel.

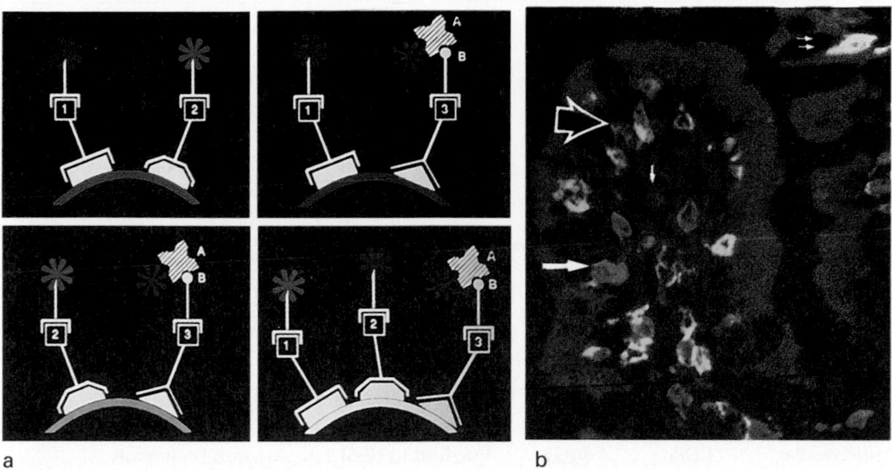

Figure 15. (a) Schematic illustration of results obtained in double- or triple-exposed photomicrographs of cell surface membranes decorated by multicolour immunofluorescence. Unlabelled primary mAbs of different murine IgG subclasses (1, 2, and 3) were applied in a mixture, followed by rhodamine-, fluorescein-, and biotin (B)-labelled goat anti-mouse IgG subclass-specific conjugates, and finally aminocoumarin-labelled streptavidin (A) as secondary reagents. Blending of red (rhodamine) and green (fluorescein) produces yellow; blending of red and dark blue (aminocoumarin) produces purple; blending of green and dark blue produces light blue; and blending of all three colours produces white. (b) Three-colour immunofluorescence staining for CD3 (green), CD4/8 (red), and CD45RB (blue) in a cryosection from the jejunal mucosa of a patient with treated coeliac disease. Note that light blue cells (large filled arrow) in the surface epithelium of a blunt villus are $CD3^{+}CD4/8^{-}$ with high RB expression ($CD45RB^{hi}$); dark blue cells are non-T cells ($CD3^{-}CD4/8^{-}$ and $CD45RB^{hi}$); pink cells are $CD3^{+}CD4/8^{+}$ with low RB expression ($CD45RB^{lo}$), but the latter cell type becomes white when $CD45RB^{hi}$ (double small arrows); yellow cells (open arrow) are $CD3^{+}CD4/8^{+}CD45RB^{-}$; and red lamina propria cells (small arrow) are $CD4^{+}$ macrophages (triple exposure based on computerized image analysis, × 1000).

adding biotinylated goat antibody to (strept)avidin (Vector Laboratories) followed by repeat incubation of the (strept)avidin–fluorochrome conjugate (Rugtveit and Brandtzaeg, unpublished observations).

Negative controls are obtained by replacing primary mAbs with irrelevant isotype- and concentration-matched mAbs (e.g. against KLH) and by totally omitting primary mAbs. Moreover, multicolour immunofluorescence provides inherent controls by displaying different staining patterns depending on the primary mAb.

For appropriate selection of mAb combinations, several clones must be subjected to immunohistochemical performance testing. Other limitations of this approach are the relatively high cost of the appropriate secondary antibodies and the fact that they occasionally show unwanted cross-reactions; this is best avoided when they are derived from the same animal species. In addition, most murine mAbs are of the IgG1 subclass, and murine IgM often

Table 3. Primary antibody reagents

Designation	Specificity	Isotype	Final working conc. (μg/ml or dilution)[a]	Source
Anti-Leu-4	CD3	IgG1	Purified Ig (2.5)	Becton Dickinson, Mountain View
BMA-180	CD3	IgG2a	Purified Ig (1/40)	Behringwerke, Marburg, Germany
RIV9	CD3	IgG3	Purified Ig (1/10)	Sanbio, Am Uden, The Netherlands
βF1	TcRα/β	IgG1	Purified Ig (1/40)	T-Cell Sciences, Cambridge, MA
TcRδ1	TcRγ/δ	IgG1	Purified Ig (1/20)	T-Cell Sciences
δTCS1	Vδ1/Jδ1	IgG1	Purified Ig (1/20)	T-Cell Sciences
Anti-Leu-3a & b	CD4	IgG1	Purified Ig (5.0)	Becton Dickinson
RIV6	CD4	IgG2a	Purified Ig (1/5)	Sanbio
Anti-Leu-2a	CD8α	IgG1	Purified Ig (2.5)	Becton Dickinson
BMA-081	CD8α	IgG2a	Purified Ig (1/40)	Behringwerke
Anti-Leu-2b	CD8α	IgG2a	Purified Ig (2.5)	Becton Dickinson
ACT-1	CD25	IgG1	Supernatant (1/10)	DAKO, Glostrup, Denmark
HD37	CD19	IgG1	Supernatant (1/10)	DAKO
L26	CD20	IgG2a	Supernatant (1/40)	DAKO
Anti-Leu-18	CD45RA	IgG1	Purified Ig (1/20)	Becton Dickinson
PD/7/16	CD45RB	IgG1	Supernatant (1/20)	DAKO
UCHL-1	CD45R0	IgG2a	Supernatant (1/10)	DAKO
FP 298A3	CD15	IgM	Purified Ig (1/20)	Biosys, Compiègne, France
L243	HLA-DR	IgG2a	Purified Ig (2.5)	Becton Dickinson
X39	KLH[b]	IgG1	Purified Ig (5.0)	Becton Dickinson
X40	KLH[b]	IgG2a	Purified Ig (5.0)	Becton Dickinson

[a] Diluted in phosphate-buffered (pH 7.5) isotonic saline (PBS) containing bovine serum albumin (12.5 mg/ml).
[b] Keyhole limpet haemocyanin.

performs poorly in immunohistochemistry. For three-colour staining it may therefore be practical to combine two murine mAbs with, for example, one primary rabbit antibody (24).

Protocol 1. Three-colour immunofluorescence *in situ* staining of human leucocyte markers

Equipment and reagents

- Clean glass slides coated with gelatin that is dissolved in water (10 g/litre) by heating and stabilized by mixing with an equal volume of potassium chromium sulfate (10 g/litre) before use—other adhesives may also be used (63) such as 2% 3-aminopropyltriethoxysilane (Sigma A-3648) in acetone or absolute ethanol (immerse slides for 2 min, rinse in two changes of distilled water, drain, and air dry)
- Fluorescence microscope equipped with a Ploem-type epi-illuminator containing filter sets for FITC, TRITC/Cy-3, Texas Red, and AMCA
- See *Tables 3* and *4*

Method

1. Orient the tissue sample immediately on a thin slice of carrot, embed in OCT (Tissue-Tek, Miles Laboratories, Elkhart, IN) and snap-freeze in liquid nitrogen.
2. Alternatively, place tissue sample in ice-chilled culture medium (RPMI 1640, Gibco) until freezing or fix immediately in ice-chilled periodate/lysine/0.5% paraformaldehyde (0.5% PLP) for 2–6 h and wash briefly in PBS before freezing.
3. Cut cryosections serially at 4 μm, place them on coated slides, dry overnight at ambient termperature, fix in acetone for 10 min, wrap in aluminium foil, and store at −20 °C until use.
4. Incubate with appropriate mixtures of primary mAbs of differing isotype in a moist chamber for 1 h at ambient temperature, followed by a 3 min rinse in PBS with slow agitation and one change.
5. After a brief rinse in ion-free water to remove salts, drain the sections and, without prolonged drying, incubate with appropriate secondary reagents for 1.5 h.
6. After rinsing as above, incubate with tertiary conjugates for 30 min, rinse, and then mount in PVA (see Section 2.1.3).

Table 4. Secondary antibody reagents and tertiary avidin conjugates

Binding specificity	Label or conjugate	Final working concentration (μg/ml)[a]	Species	Source
Mouse IgM	Biotin	20	Goat	Southern Biotechnology, Birmingham, AL
Mouse IgG1	Biotin	10	Goat	Southern Biotechnology
Mouse IgG1	Cy-3	2	Goat	Southern Biotechnology
Mouse IgG1	TRITC	50	Goat	Southern Biotechnology
Mouse IgG2a	FITC	50	Goat	Southern Biotechnology
Mouse IgG2a	TRITC	50	Goat	Southern Biotechnology
Mouse IgG3	FITC	50	Goat	Southern Biotechnology
Biotin	Streptavidin–Texas Red	3	*Streptomyces avidinii*	BRL, Gaithersburg, MD
Biotin	Streptavidin–AMCA	20	*Streptomyces avidinii*	Vector Laboratories, Burlingame, CA

[a]Appropriately diluted in PBS containing bovine serum albumin (125 mg/ml) and human IgG (0.8 mg/ml).

v. Various method combinations

Several possibilities exist for combining different staining methods when the bridging reagents do not cross-react, for example, indirect immunofluorescence combined with an avidin–biotin sequence (*Figures 11b* and *15a*, *Protocol 1*) or with a hapten sandwich method (100). Another less attractive possibility is to combine two staining principles with the primary antibody of the first sequence applied at a concentration well below that required for detection in the second sequence. This can be achieved when an indirect immunogold–silver technique (primary antiserum: 1/50 000) is followed by PAP staining (primary antiserum: 1/1000), or when PAP is combined with immunofluorescence (62,101).

3.2.2 Removal or denaturation of initial sequences

With the immunoenzyme methods, antibodies from the first sequence can be eluted from the tissue section without removing the coloured end-product; unwanted interactions may thereby be avoided when the next sequence is applied. Such stepwise staining was introduced by Nakane (4) when he reported simultaneous visualization of three antigens by consecutive immunoperoxidase sequences with different Px substrates (DAB = brown, α-naphthol = pink and CN = blue black); the section was incubated at low pH between each sequence.

Many methods have been reported for such elution, including glycine buffer and dimethylformamide (102), HCl (103), glycine buffer of low pH (104), $KMNO_4$–H_2SO_4 (105), and electrophoresis in acidic buffer or in the presence of dimethylformamide (106). When two sequences are used for immunofluorescence staining, the section has to be photographed before the elution step (107,108). Elution involves the risk of denaturing epitopes of antigen(s) to be subsequently visualized, and it is difficult to ensure complete removal of bound antibodies. Moreover, this approach is quite tedious.

An alternative method is to denature the antibodies applied in the first sequence. This was first achieved by the use of hot formaldehyde vapour (109) or plain heating at 130 °C for 4 min (110). More recently, heating tissue sections twice for 5 min in a microwave oven has been found to denature efficiently antibody reactivity as well as antigenicity and enzyme activity of immunoenzyme staining sequences (111). By employing intervening microwaving in sequential APAAP (blue) and PAP staining, the latter developed stepwise with different chromogens (AEC, red; DAB, brown; and DAB plus 1% nickel ammonium sulfate, black), the authors were able to decorate simultaneously three or four antigens located at separate sites (cell membrane, cytoplasm, nucleus, and basement membrane). Co-localization of two or more antigens was not attempted, however, and with cryosections the microwaving denatured not only the applied reagents but also cell membrane antigens that had not been decorated by the first staining sequence (111).

According to this principle, a sequential LSAB (Ventana) method has been developed in our laboratory for distinct visualization of three markers expressed by separate cells (*Figure 16*). Three murine mAbs can be used, disregarding their IgG subclasses, or a combination of polyclonal or monoclonal primary reagents. It is important to note that in addition to intervening microwaving, blocking of the avidin-binding activity (see Section 3.2.3) of every preceding biotin-based step is necessary to avoid disturbing colour mixing. The most robust marker should preferably be stained in the first sequence.

3.2.3 Blocking of active sites in first and second sequence

When the PAP method was first adapted for stepwise multicolour staining (70,112), it turned out that antibody elution could be rendered unnecessary because an extensively developed DAB product shields all reagents of the first sequence (*Figure 17*). This principle has been exploited for paired indirect immunoenzyme staining with Px–DAB and AP–Fast Blue BB (*Figure 3*) based on primary antibodies from the same species (113). DAB shielding can be further enhanced by heavy metal salts (see Section 2.1.4). Several modifications have been explored, including the use of murine mAbs as primary reagents (71,93,113). Nevertheless, co-localization of two antigens at the same site cannot be reliably achieved (112,114) unless one of the sequences is based on primary antibody from a non-cross-reacting species (113) as described in Section 3.1.

A similar shielding effect has been obtained with immunogold–silver staining in the first sequence (115). The same authors showed that sequential staining with this black colour product first, followed by Px–AEC and AP–Fast Blue BB in order of sensitivity, permitted decoration of three antigens at separate sites (115). However, the AEC colour product is in principle permeable and can facilitate co-localization of two antigens, provided that the next sequence does not cross-react and produces a balanced mixing of blue with red (115). Nevertheless, even an intense AEC precipitate has been shown to provide a shield for subsequent antibody reactions, although avidin–biotin interactions are less likely to be blocked because of their strength (116).

Feller *et al.* (117) introduced a fully AP-based paired staining technique with murine mAbs and two different chromogens. The methodological requisite was immunological blocking of all available antigenic determinants on the first mAb with a secondary rabbit anti-mouse IgG followed by saturation of the latter with goat anti-rabbit IgG (*Figure 18*). The same principle has been applied for two-colour immunofluorescence, and for two- or three-colour immunoenzyme staining in which final blocking of the first sequence (mAb and anti-mouse IgG) was performed by the addition of normal mouse serum (116,118,119).

In the avidin–biotin system, blocking can be performed with free biotin, for example after the first sequence of biotinylated mouse antibody and

FITC-labelled avidin (86). Commercial avidin–biotin blocking kits can be used for this purpose (DAKO, Vector Laboratories), preceded by microwaving when an immunoenzyme sequence is involved (see Section 3.2.2). In the protein A systems, the Fc receptors on protein A and the Fc portion of IgG must likewise be satisfactorily blocked in order to obtain distinct paired staining (82). However, some authors have experienced problems with such blocking (120,121), presumably due to binding of protein A to both the Fab and the Fc regions (122).

Several authors have reported that the blocking of a previous immunostaining sequence with antibody (*Figure 18*) or normal serum is not always reliable (65). To facilitate the use of two primary antibodies from the same species without intervening blocking, Wessel and McLay (123) employed sequential indirect immunofluorescence with secondary reagents consisting of FITC- and TRITC-labelled monovalent Fab fragments. Franzusoff *et al.* (124) subsequently used unlabelled Fab fragments in a three-step sequence of paired immunofluorescence staining. More recently, Carl *et al.* (125) extended this principle for indirect immunofluorescence by blocking the first conjugate (TRITC-labelled) with normal Ig corresponding to the primary antibody, followed by a second blocking with monovalent Fab fragments before application of the next sandwich (FITC conjugate). The necessary reagents are available commercially (Jackson ImmunoResearch), but both we (unpublished observations) and others (111) have not consistently obtained complete blocking even with this immunological approach.

Tuson *et al.* (126) first attempted blocking of antibody cross-reactivity in indirect immunostaining by performing soluble absorption before reagent application; normal human serum was added to a pre-incubated mixture of human mAb and Px-labelled anti-human Ig, thereby successfully abolishing unwanted binding of the conjugate to endogenous Ig present in human tissue sections. This principle was recently used for sequential paired indirect immunoenzyme staining to avoid cross-reactivity between the two sequences (127). The method was designed for an initial Px–AEC sandwich followed by an AP–Fast Blue BB biotin/avidin-enhanced sequence (*Figure 19*, *Protocol 2*).

Figure 16. (a) Three-colour sequential immunoenzyme nine-step labelled streptavidin–biotin (LSAB) method with primary antibodies from the same or different species. The first sequence employs streptavidin (SA) conjugated with peroxidase (Px) and developed with diaminobenzidine (brown), whereas the subsequent sequences are based on alkaline phosphatase (AP) conjugates developed with Fast Red (FR) and Fast Blue (FB), respectively. (b) Three-colour staining with the LSAB method (Ventana) combining polyclonal and monoclonal primary antibodies and a mixture of biotinylated second antibodies against rabbit and mouse Ig. Microwave-treated routine paraffin section of lymph node infiltrated with melanoma metastasis shows T cell zone (CD3, brown), B cell follicles (CD20, red), and islands of malignant melanoma (melanoma-associated antigen, dark blue). (c) Higher magnification shows distinct differentiation between the three cellular phenotypes with no apparent colour mixing. Courtesy: Hogne Røed Nilsen (faint haematoxylin counterstain, b, × 75; c, × 150).

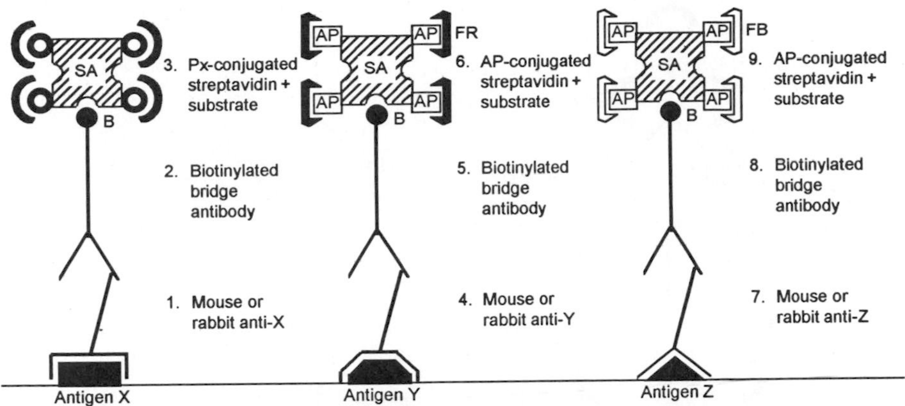
SA
B
3. Px-conjugated streptavidin + substrate
2. Biotinylated bridge antibody
1. Mouse or rabbit anti-X
Antigen X
AP
FR
6. AP-conjugated streptavidin + substrate
5. Biotinylated bridge antibody
4. Mouse or rabbit anti-Y
Antigen Y
FB
9. AP-conjugated streptavidin + substrate
8. Biotinylated bridge antibody
7. Mouse or rabbit anti-Z
Antigen Z

a

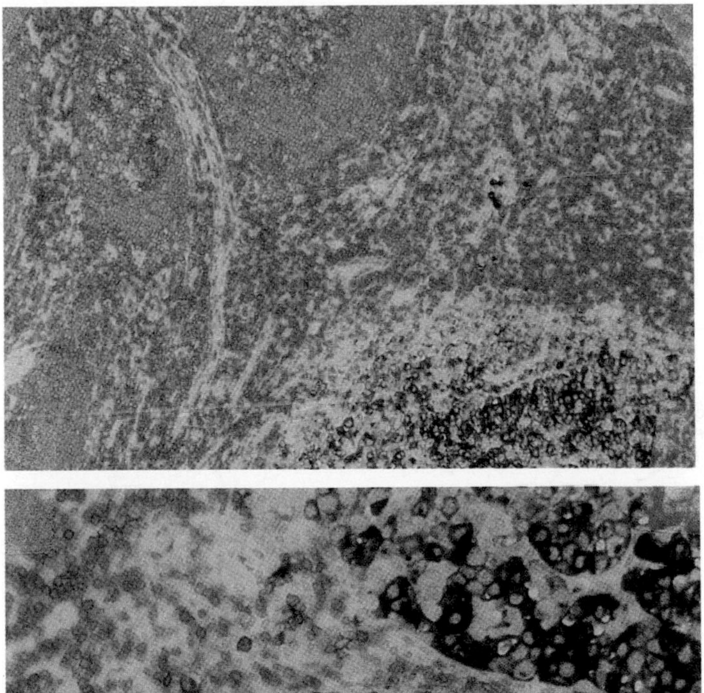

b

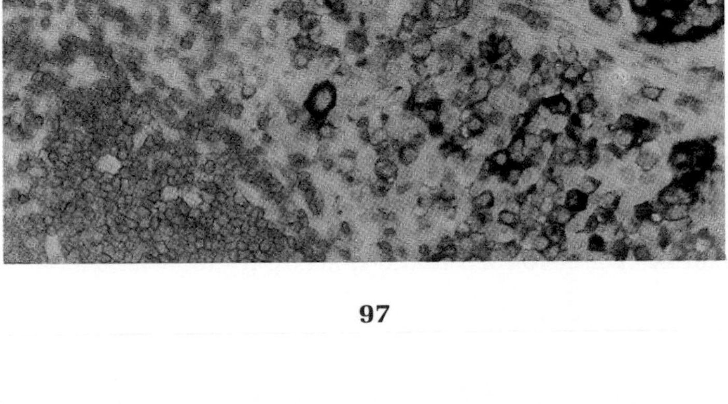

c

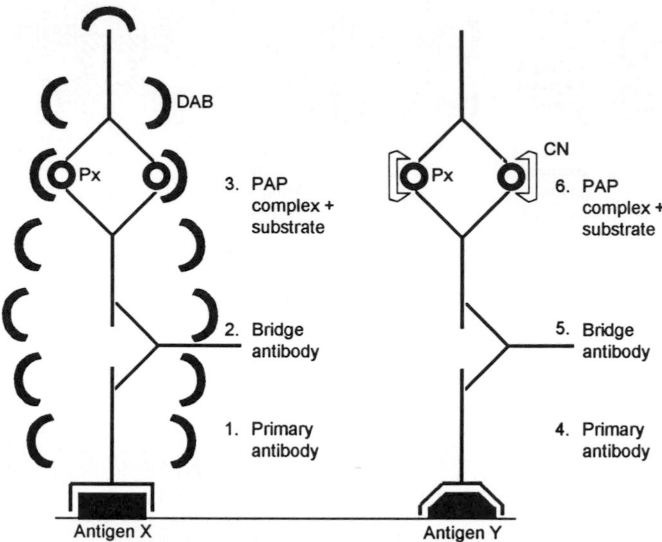

Figure 17. Two-colour sequential immunoenzyme staining with unlabelled primary antibodies from the same animal species including six steps, the first sequence based on the peroxidase (Px) anti-Px (PAP) complex method with extensively developed diaminobenzidine (DAB) as substrate, and then a second PAP sequence with 4-chloro-1-naphthol (CN) as substrate.

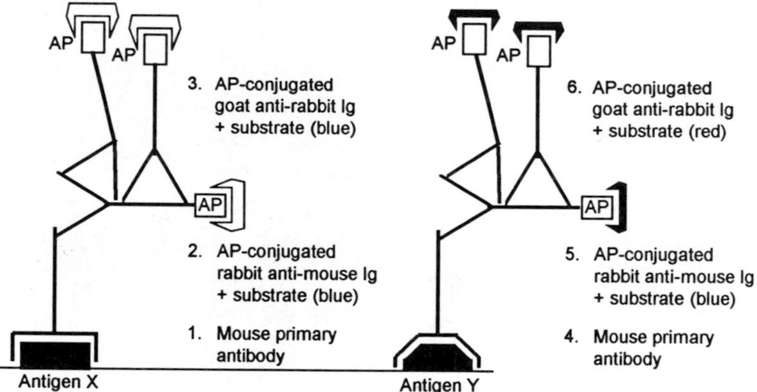

Figure 18. Two-colour sequential immunoenzyme six-step staining based on unlabelled primary murine mAbs and alkaline phosphatase (AP)-labelled secondary and tertiary antibodies in both sequences, the enzyme colours being developed with different substrates (blue, Fast Blue BB; red, New Fuchsin).

The authors documented pure colours for separate localization of the two antigens and colour mixing for balanced co-localization (127). We have applied this principle for paired indirect immunofluorescence staining with primary murine IgG mAbs and found it necessary to include a blocking step

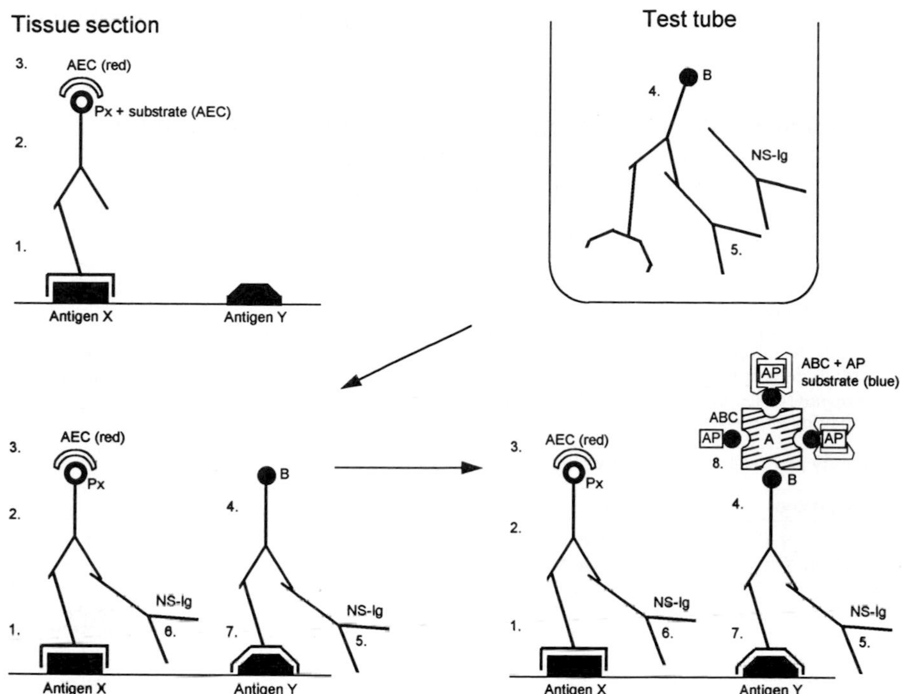

Figure 19. Two-colour sequential immunoenzyme staining with unlabelled primary antibodies from the same animal species. The various steps (1–8) are explained in *Protocol 2*. AEC, 3-amino-9-ethylcarbazole; AP, alkaline phosphatase; A, avidin; B, biotin; Ns-Ig, normal serum immunoglobulins.

with normal mouse serum after the first sandwich to obtain pure colours for separate antigen localization (J. Rugtveit and P. Brandtzaeg, unpublished observations). However, several mAbs apparently do not preserve their activity in immune complexes (127). In such cases, the reagents of the liquid pre-incubation step may be replaced by direct application of a biotinylated mAb after thorough blocking of the secondary reagent in the first sandwich (128).

3.2.4 Reversed sequential paired staining

The indirect methods described above for multicolour immunostaining with primary antibodies from the same species, are tedious and exhibit several restrictions in performance: elution or denaturation of the initial staining sequence is possible only when the remaining antigens of interest are rather robust or can be stabilized by cross-linking fixatives (111); various approaches to block available reactive sites of antibodies bound to the tissue section are not consistently reliable (111); and to block unwanted cross-reactivities by pre-absorption of immune complexes in solution is incompatible with some primary antibodies, and apparently applicable only with biotinylated secondaries (127).

Protocol 2. Paired sequential immunostaining with primary antibodies from the same species based on the blocking of secondary antibodies

Equipment and reagents

- Light microscope for immunoenzyme staining; fluorescence microscope equipped with a Ploem-type epi-illuminator and appropriate filter sets for contrasting colours of immunofluorescence staining
- Eppendorf test-tube coated with defatted dried-milk (1% (w/v), 1 h, 37°C)
- Clean glass slides coated with adhesive (see *Protocol 1*)
- Two primary antibodies of different non-cross-reacting specificities produced in the same animal species—example will be based on rat mAbs applied on murine cryosections (127)

Primary and secondary antibody reagents:

Designation	Specificity	Final dilution[a]	Source
RM 4–5 (rat IgG2a)	Mouse CD4	1/400	Dinova, Germany
ER-HR 52 (rat IgG2b)	Mouse MHC class II	1/100	Dinova
Px-labelled goat IgG	Rat Ig	1/75	Dinova
Biotinylated goat IgG	Rat Ig	1/50	Vector Laboratories

Method

1. Pre-incubate murine cryosections with 3% H_2O_2 for 5 min to block endogenous Px, and with 4% normal goat serum for 5 min to inhibit unwanted binding, before applying the first primary rat mAb for 45 min at ambient temperature, and rinsing for 3 min (one change) in TBS.
2. Apply the Px-labelled secondary antibody (anti-rat IgG) in 4% mouse serum (to inhibit cross-reactivity with endogenous mouse Ig) for 45 min, and rinse in TBS.
3. Develop the enzyme reaction for 15 min with AEC substrate made up as a 1% solution in dimethylformamide and diluted to 0.03% with 0.05 M sodium acetate buffer pH 5.2, containing 0.017% H_2O_2 as activator, followed by three 2 min rinses in TBS.
4. Concomitant with these steps, incubate the second primary rat mAb in a test-tube with biotinylated secondary antibody for 1 h at 37°C.
5. Add 4% normal rat serum for 1 h at 37°C to allow rat Ig to block available binding sites of the secondary reagent, together with 4% normal mouse serum to inhibit subsequent cross-reactivity with endogenous mouse Ig.
6. In parallel, incubate the tissue section with 4% normal rat serum at ambient temperature to block available binding sites for rat Ig in the first secondary reagent.

7. Apply the immune complex solution from the test-tube to the tissue section for 1 h at ambient temperature, and rinse three times in TBS.
8. Prepare complexes of biotinylated alkaline phosphatase and avidin (ABC–AP) as recommended by the manufacturer (Vector).
9. Apply APC–AP on the tissue section for 30 min at ambient temperature and develop the enzyme for approx. 10 min with the naphthol AS–MX substrate (made up as a 1% solution in dimethylformamide and diluted to 0.03% in 0.05 M Tris–HCl buffer pH 8.8, containing 0.025% levamisole to block endogenous AP) and Fast Blue BB salt (0.04%) as chromogen.

[a]Diluted in 0.05 M Tris–HCl buffer pH 7.6, containing 0.15 M NaCl (TBS) and 1% normal bovine serum.

Reversed sequential paired staining circumvents all these problems; it should therefore be considered as an alternative method to obtain information about co-localization or separate localization of two cell type-specific antigens in three different subsets (129). This approach may be particularly useful when two mAbs of the desired specificities are available only in the same murine IgG subclass. By recording the fraction of single-stained (TRITC-positive) cells in two adjacent tissue sections, it can be concluded that subset B contains only antigen Y (*Figure 20a*), whereas subset A contains only antigen X (*Figure 20b*). The difference between the percentage of FITC-positive cells (double-stained by various types of cross-reactivity) in the first section and those stained only by TRITC in the second, represents subset C that expresses both markers. This percentage for co-localization can be confirmed by reversing the calculation—that is, by subtracting the fraction of purely TRITC-stained cells in the first section from the double-stained population in the second.

We have successfully applied variants of this paired immunofluorescence method to determine phenotypic subsets of T cells (130) and eosinophils (131). Because the second mAb in each sequence is used to identify only the subset that exclusively expresses the corresponding marker (*Figure 20*), the same approach should be applicable for sequential immunoenzyme staining as well (129), regardless of whether successful colour mixing is obtained or not (see Section 3.2.3).

3.3 Computerized image analysis of multicolour fluorescence

Computerized image analysis has several potential uses in fluorescence microscopy:

(a) Overlay of several images representing different fluorescent markers.

(b) Improvement of image quality, particularly reduction of out-of-focus glare.

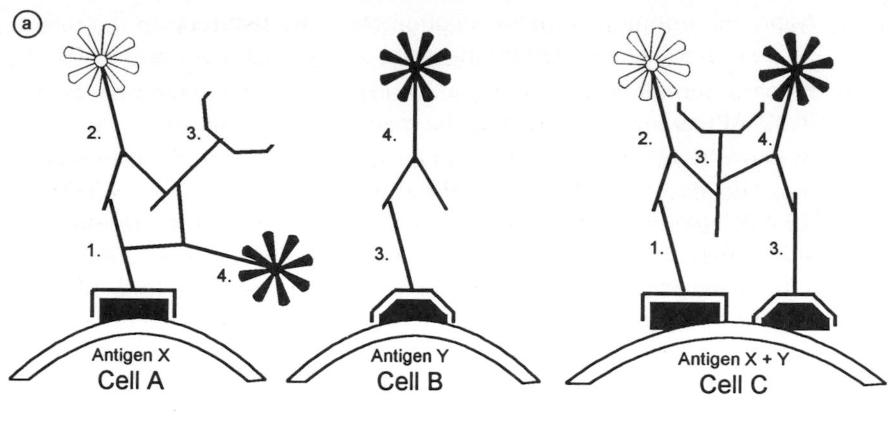

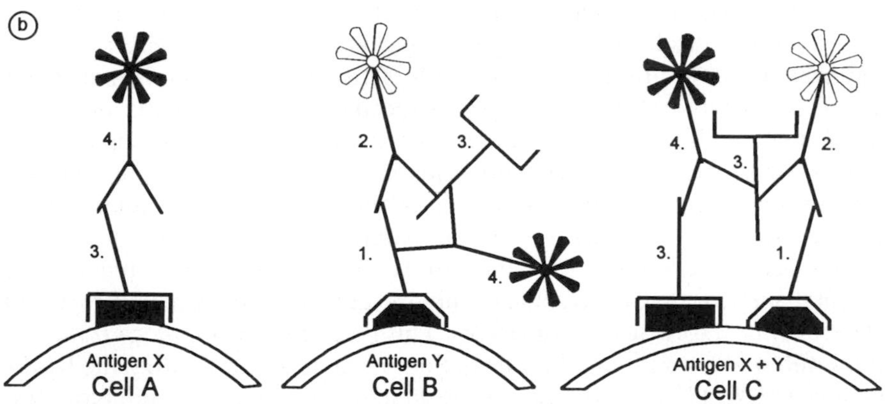

Figure 20. Reversed sequential indirect immunofluorescence staining with primary antibodies (1 and 3) from the same animal species applied to two serial sections. (a) On the first section, the secondary fluorescein conjugate (2) is incubated before the next primary antibody (3) and the subseqent secondary rhodamine conjugate (4). (b) On the second section, the whole sequence is reversed. Interpretation of the staining results for the three cell subsets indicated (A, B, and C), are explained in the text.

(c) Fluorometric quantitations, including cell enumerations, as well as measurements of staining intensities and positive areas (that is, morphometry).

Furthermore, image analysis is an important adjunct of confocal laser scanning microscopy (see Section 3.4 and Chapter 5).

The reader is referred to more extensive texts (132) for a general discussion of image analysis. Here we will focus on quantitative fluorescence methods as applied in our laboratory (27,133). It is possible to analyse three or even more labels simultaneously (27,134) and bright-field microscopy can be included as well. Therefore, these techniques are more versatile (although somewhat more complex) than image analysis of immunoenzyme staining. When the latter is used for multicolour analyses, the chromogens must be carefully selected to make clear colour separation feasible. Immunofluorescence is better for identification and quantification of two or more co-localized markers because separation of the fluorochrome emissions is objectively obtained with the Ploem-type epi-illuminator equipped with appropriate selective filter sets (see Section 2.1.2). Commercial image analysis systems are available for certain selected bright-field or fluorescence applications (Becton Dickinson), and more general systems can be adapted for various analytical purposes. Most modern set-ups are based on Windows® (Microsoft, Armonk, NY) or OS/2® (IBM, Redmond, WA) operating systems.

3.3.1 Video camera

High-sensitivity monochrome video cameras that detect very low light levels, in the range of 10^{-4} to 10^{-5} lux ('moon light'), are well suited for computerized image analysis of immunofluorescence. They employ silicone-intensified tubes and are therefore referred to as SIT cameras. Geometrical distortion and uneven sensitivity in different areas of the field is often a problem that, however, can be compensated for by shade correction. Such procedures involve storage of a reference image in the computer memory and must be based on proportional adjustments (not merely background subtractions) if quantitative data are required. It should be noted that correction routines reduce the effective dynamic range of the image.

Although 'charge coupled device' (CCD) cameras are geometrically correct with even sensitivity, the same problem as above occurs when an SIT intensifier is added. In our experience it is easier to control the uneven sensitivity of an SIT-intensified CCD camera but the resolution is not as good as with a tube camera. Cooled CCD cameras with 'image integration' have recently been introduced; in these the 'black current' (random electrical impulses) are reduced, thereby lowering the 'noise' and providing enhanced sensitivity by accumulation of images. At low sensitivities, these cameras are very slow due to long accumulation times, which renders focusing and orientation in the tissue section difficult. Standardization of the sensitivity for quantitative analyses, as well as fading of fluorescence, may also be a problem. Cooled CCD colour cameras are also available; these can be used to record immunofluorescence emissions separated through double- or triple-band filter sets (see Section 2.1.2).

Images to be analysed must be measured at the same camera sensitivity. It is therefore necessary to replace the automatic 'gain control' and 'black offset' with a manual control. The black level should be set to zero to give a pixel value of O for a completely dark image; the sensitivity (gain) should be as high as possible without inducing distortion of the image. Some SIT cameras rotate or move the image slightly when the sensitivity is altered; this may cause problems with the image overlay.

SIT cameras should be moved as little as possible, and horizontal mounting is often needed to prevent dust from damaging the tube. It is noteworthy that these cameras are more sensitive to infrared light than the human eye and therefore 'see' relatively much red background fluorescence. A cut-off filter absorbing light above about 700–750 nm may substantially improve the image quality.

3.3.2 Computer and software

Although a 6-bit digitizer (64 grey levels) may be sufficient for most applications, the image analyser should contain an 8-bit digitizer (256 grey levels) to provide improved quantitative resolution. The images should be at least 512 × 512 pixels, and the image memory must be big enough (4–8 megabytes) for six to eight images (three or four primary images, one or several reference images, some transformed images, and some binary images).

If an overlay of several images is required, the computer's capacity for colour display must be carefully considered. In our experience, at least 64 grey levels are needed for each colour; this means a 6-bit display for grey images. When colour images are used, 64 × 3 colours are needed (there are three primary colours: red, green, and blue), which means an 18-bit display. A normal VGA monitor can only show 256 different colours (8-bit display) simultaneously, although these can be chosen from a larger colour palette. Many commercial image analysers use 12-bit displays (16 grey levels per colour), but this is not satisfactory. Modern operating systems can handle 24-bit displays, but many commercial image analysis programmes do not exploit this capacity. Some image analysers compensate by calculating the 'most significant' (that is, the most frequent) colours and display these. However, such routines do not perform satisfactorily because in immunostained images, the most frequent colours are often the background fluorescence.

General image analysis programmes usually provide the opportunity to create 'macros' or 'task lists' that repeat standard procedures for image capturing and modification, segmentation, and subsequent measurements. In this way several fields may be measured in a standardized manner, which favours speed and objective data. Because procedures may be required that are not included in the standard design, some computer systems provide programming libraries and support for tailored applications.

Most image analysis programmes include integrated optical density (IOD) as a measurement option; some also include the opportunity to measure IOD for the same object in several images, e.g. in each of the three overlaid images that constitute a multicoloured image (red, green, and blue: RGB mode). IOD can be used for quantitations in transmitted light microscopy, in which the colour product is measured by absorbance. This involves logarithmic transformation of the actual grey levels in the image. Epifluorescence microscopy measurements are accomplished with integrated fluorescence that is a linear function of the actual grey levels. It is critical to recognize that although the OD of one pixel may be transformed back to the original grey level value, IOD cannot be converted to integrated fluorescence values (unless the values of all individual data points contributing to the IOD are known). Because most analysing systems do not offer fluorescence (or intensity) values as a measurement option, it is necessary to programme this feature and integrate it into the provided programme. This modulation should allow assessment of grey levels in at least three overlaid images (or in every component of an RBG image), so that each integrated fluorescence value can be determined. Vendors should be able to offer support for such programming.

3.3.3 Standardization and applications

Because several grey images that represent different tissue structures in the same section area are analysed, one fluorescent marker is often used to define the region of interest, while another identifies a specific cell type or a structural feature in this region (*Protocol 3*). Areas to be measured are defined as objects in a binary overlay (*Figure 21a*). It is often necessary to use two different binary images, one representing the actual region, the other a particular feature, as a basis for assessment of 'objects within objects' (also called 'nested objects'). Thus, the programme should recognize each object in the first binary image, and look inside it in the second binary image for cell counts (*Figure 21b*) and measurements of objects (*Figure 21c*). The database software must distinguish between these levels and provide access to data of one level through the inclusion criteria from the other. Because some analytical problems are very custom-specific, it is often necessary to export data from the image analysis programme to a general format (i.e. ASCII files, popular spreadsheet, or database programme formats).

A fluorescent standard (available from vendors) must be used for quality controls of quantitative data. First, one should check if measurements improve by averaging several grey images. Also, the standard should be repeatedly analysed at intervals to control for variations or drift in lamp intensity or camera sensitivity. The stability of both the camera and the fluorescence lamp may benefit from the use of a current stabilizer. The standard should furthermore be measured in different positions of the field to record geometric distortion and sensitivity variations. In this way, the quality of the shade correction routine can be controlled. In addition, the standard should be measured at different light intensities to examine whether the 'standard curve' of emission versus measured integrated fluorescence is linear. Different emissions are obtained by inserting grey filters that block defined percentages of the passing light between the lamp and excitation filter. Finally, the standard is useful for calibration of camera sensitivity before each work session; this ensures that data from different examinations can be compared.

Strict routines to avoid unnecessary light exposure before and during photo-

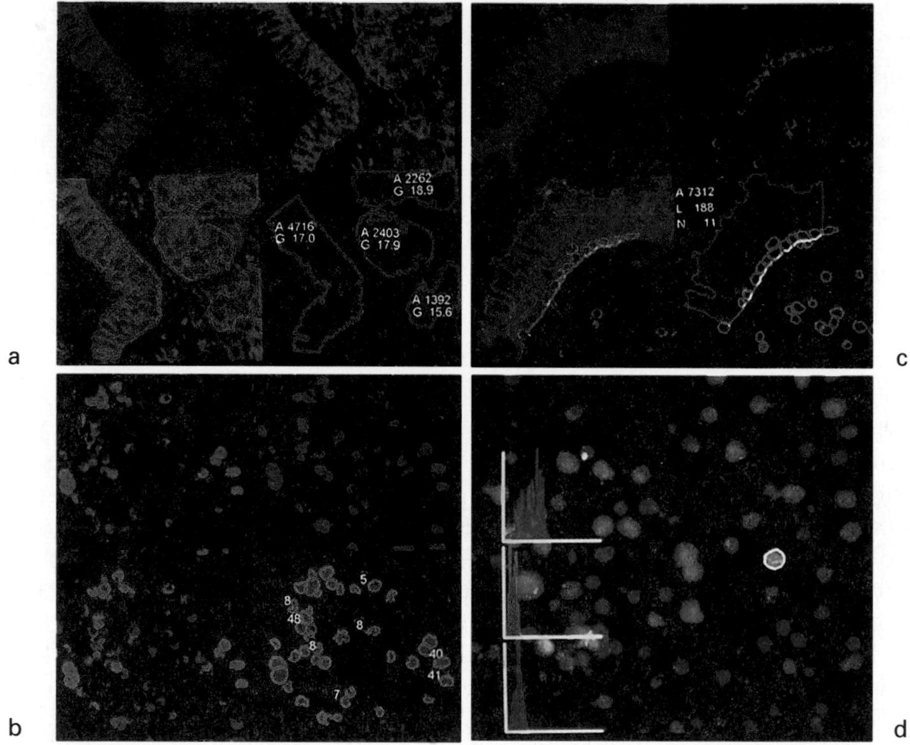

graphy should be implemented, and 100% of the emitted light should reach the video camera. For the identification of areas to be measured, one can often use transmitted light with phase-contrast or a fluorescent marker not included in the quantitations. Images should be captured immediately after exposure to the excitation light; the digitized image is then available for further evaluation. With strict routines, exposure times for each fluorochrome are less than one second. This methodological basis makes it possible to obtain quantitative data in a relative manner, thereby allowing comparisons of fluorescent markers for different cell populations or other tissue elements. If truly quantitative data are required, biological standards with predetermined marker quantities need to be included.

When several fluorochrome labels are analysed in the same tissue area, image overlaying is essential. Grey images that represent each colour are sequentially captured by the monochrome SIT camera and subsequently stored in the memory. For convenience, each digitized image can be assigned a pseudocolour according to the actual fluorochrome. If a colour image analysis system is used, these three colours can be projected simultaneously on the screen, making direct visual evaluation of multicolour staining possible. This is often the simplest way to record triple staining when a photounit is available (*Figures 15b* and *21c*).

Figure 21. Image analysis of two-colour immunofluorescence staining performed on (a-c) sections from ethanol-fixed and paraffin-embedded human gastric mucosa, and on (d) cryosection from rat liver. The experiments are detailed in *Protocol 3*. (a) Section was stained for cytokeratin (TRITC) and HLA-DR (FITC). Red (upper left panel) and green (upper right panel) emissions were sequentially captured with a monochrome SIT camera and designated the correct colours by the image analyser. These images were overlaid (lower left panel) and red was used to create a binary overlay (red outline) defining the objects. Areas of object (A, μm^2) and their mean green fluorescence intensities (G) were determined by the image analyser and are displayed for each object (lower right panel). (b) Section was stained for cytokeratin (TRITC, upper left panel) and CD3 (FITC, upper right panel) to identify epithelium and T cells. These images were overlaid (lower left panel) and binary overlays defining the epithelium (red outline), the T cells (green outline), and the basement membrane (purple) were created by combining grey value threshold settings and interactive editing. The image analyser calculated the epithelial area (A, μm^2), the length of the basement membrane (L, μm), and the number of T cells (N) within the defined epithelial area. (c) Section was stained for cytoplasmic IgA (FITC, upper left panel) and J-chain (TRITC, upper right panel) in lamina propria plasma cells. Computer-created overlay (lower left panel) demonstrated IgA-positive cells with (yellow) or without (green) J-chain, as well as IgA-negative cells with J-chain alone (red). IgA-positive cells were defined by a binary overlay created from the green image (yellow outline, lower right panel), and the relative J-chain concentration in IgA-positive cells was determined as exemplified by the displayed numbers. (d) Liver section from rat fed the carcinogen AAF and injected with BrdUrd, were triple-stained for nuclear DNA (Hoechst dye), AF–DNA adducts (FITC), and BrdUrd (Texas Red). Blue, green, and red emissions were sequentially captured, and a colour overlay was created as described above. Histograms representing fluorescence intensities (horizontal axes) versus pixel frequencies (vertical axes) within a defined replicating nucleus (encircled) are displayed. This illustrates the possibility of quantifying intensities in three different overlays.

Fluorescent markers can be measured in tissue sections as well as in cell cultures and smears. The total cellular number can be counted when nuclear DNA is stained with Hoechst dye or propidium iodide, and total DNA per cell can be quantified and used for ploidy determinations in single cell populations (135). In tissue sections, only relative concentration data (fluorescence intensities) can be obtained (*Figure 21d*, *Protocol 3*), because most structures of interest are larger than the section thickness and the sectioning causes nuclear capping. When structures (cell, nuclei, etc.) are enumerated in a tissue section, stereological considerations should be applied to avoid overcounting of large objects.

Standardization of measurements and of staining procedures is a requisite for good analytical results. Only tissue sections stained in the same batch should be compared. Weak signals provide poor reproducibility, and when only part of an object is positive, this signal is 'averaged' for the whole object. Even a strong signal (in a small area) may then be difficult to distinguish from the background. Consequently, cell membrane staining and cytoplasmic staining of cells with a small cytoplasm-to-nucleus ratio are difficult to measure.

Protocol 3. Computerized image analysis for immunological marker distribution within a defined tissue area, compartmentalized cell counting, and relative cellular concentrations of cytoplasmic or nuclear components within selected cell populations

Equipment

- Nikon Microphot microscope equipped with an epi-illuminator attachment (HMX-HBO 100 W lamphouse)
- Current stabilizer (Type GMS 350, Noratel, Oslo, Norway) to ensure consistent illumination
- The excitation light intensities applied for the different fluorochrome labels are adjusted to the sensitivity range of the video camera by a cassette of grey filters: a B2E filter block (450–490 excitation filter, 515 dichroic mirror, and a 520–560 barrier filter) is used for FITC, a G2E filter block (510–560 excitation filter, 580 dichroic mirror, 610 barrier filter) for TRITC/Texas Red, and a modified V filter block (330–380 excitation filter, 400 dichroic mirror, 450–490 barrier filter) for Hoechst dye
- The microscope is equipped with a high sensitivity monochrome SIT video camera (JAI 733, SIT, JAI, Copenhagen, Denmark), modified to allow manual setting of the gain and black offset
- The camera is connected to a Magiscan image analysis sytem (Joyce-Loebl, Gateshead, UK) that employes the Genias general image analysis programme
- Images (512 × 512 pixels, 6-bits) are digitized
- The programme is modified with the supplied Genial general image analysis library and a Pascal compiler to include measurements of mean grey intensities of the same object in three overlaid grey images

A. *Standardization of fluorescence intensity measurements*

1. Carry out performance testing with a fluorescence standard (Leitz 621 059 fluorescence standard, Leica, Wetzlar, Germany) to ensure reproducibility of quantitative intensity determinations. Start out with different capture routines (averaging, accumulation) and shade correction routines. Quantify the emission from the standard at several (e.g. 9–16) different locations within the view field, and select a suitable routine based on the data dispersion of these measurements.
2. Use the selected capture and shade correction routines, and measure the fluorescence standard at least ten times at 100%, 50%, and 25% lamp intensity by inserting grey filters between the lamp and the epi-illuminator. Control that the measurements are linear and proportional by plotting the lamp intensities against the measured emission values. Ensure that the data dispersions at different lamp intensities are acceptable.
3. Before subsequent measurements, calibrate the video camera by adjusting the black offset to zero and the gain (camera sensitivity) to a predetermined mean grey intensity of the fluorescence standard.

B. *Quantification of epithelial HLA-DR expression and T cell numbers in human gastric mucosa*

1. Perform paired immunostaining in parallel tissue sections (6 μm) for cytokeratin (TRITC) and HLA-DR (FITC), or for cytokeratin (TRITC) and

CD3 (FITC), with a combined indirect and avidin/biotin-enhanced immunofluorescence method (133).

2. Capture and digitize the cytokeratin and HLA-DR immunofluorescence, either as two different grey images or as the red and green component of an RGB colour image.
3. Define the epithelium by its cytokeratin staining, and create a binary overlay from this red component by a 'sharpen' operator (to reduce the halo effect of fluorescent objects) followed by grey-level threshold setting and interactive editing.
4. Determine with this overlay the relative area and mean fluorescence intensity of epithelial HLA-DR expression from the relevant grey image (or green component).
5. In the adjacent section, create a binary overlay representing CD3-positive T cells in addition to an overlay representing cytokeratin-positive epithelium as above.
6. Let the computer measure epithelial areas and count the number of T cells within each area (objects within objects).

C. *Quantification of cytoplasmic J-chain expression by IgA-producing human mucosal immunocytes*

1. Perform paired immunostaining in gastrointestinal tissue section (6 μm) for IgA (FITC) and J-chain (TRITC) with direct immunofluorescence (136).
2. Capture sequentially the corresponding grey images and digitize them. Use the green component to define a binary overlay according to the procedure outlined above (part B, step 3).
3. Store in memory also the original unprocessed image and use it for later intensity measurements.
4. Define each IgA-positive cell (green) as an 'object' in a binary image and delete those smaller than 4 mm^2. For each object, measure area as well as green and red mean fluorescence intensities. Express cytoplasmic J-chain content of each cell either as relative concentration (mean red fluorescence intensity) or as J-chain : IgA ratio (mean red : green fluorescence intensities).

D. *Quantification of DNA, DNA damage, and DNA synthesis in nuclei of rat hepatocytes*

1. Immunostain liver sections from animals fed a carcinogen (2-acetylaminofluorene) and injected with the DNA synthesis marker bromodeoxyuridine (BrdUrd) with appropriate antibodies (27) to damaged DNA (adducts) and BrdUrd (FITC and Texas Red, respectively). Add fluorescent Hoechst dye (bisbenzimide H 33254 fluorochrome, 0.05 μg/

Protocol 3. *Continued*

ml; Calbiochem-Behring, La Jolla, CA) to the final washing solution to stain nuclear DNA blue for 10 min.

2. Capture sequentially green, red, and blue emissions. Capture each grey image either as components of an RGB colour image, or as separate colour images that are compiled into one image containing the three original images.
3. Create a binary overlay as described above (part B, step 3) representing each nucleus from the blue (Hoechst dye) component. Measure the area and the mean red, green, and blue fluorescence intensities in each object. Use measurements from rats fed a control diet to define a threshold for DNA adduct detection. Mean DNA adduct immunofluorescence intensities plus 2 SD of control nuclei defines a satisfactory threshold.

3.4 Confocal microscopy

Confocal microscopy is designed for epi-illumination and provides increased resolution combined with reduced out-of-focus glare in fluorescence microscopy. Geometrically correct images of high resolution and even sensitivity are obtained when planar objectives are used. Optimally designed microscopes are well suited for two- or three-colour staining and produce accurate image overlays.

Confocal laser scanning microscopy is based on digitized images and is excellent for image analysis of immunofluorescence. It can be applied for detailed intracellular marker studies (137–139), but attention must be paid to the combination of laser and fluorochromes. Ideally, only one laser with several excitation lines suitable for appropriate fluorochromes should be used to overcome common problems such as overlay shifts and filter 'bleed-through'. Krypton–argon lasers provide three strong excitation lines (488 nm, 568 nm, and 543 nm), compatible with FITC, Texas Red, and Cy5. Confocal microscopy is considered in greater detail in Chapter 5.

4. Methodological considerations

4.1 Tissue preparation methods

4.1.1 A field of compromises

Tissue preparation is one of the cornerstones in immunohistochemistry but remains a subject of much antiquity and ambiguity. Nevertheless, the final result will significantly depend on the handling of the tissue specimen, regardless of the quality of the applied immunostaining method.

Any selection of tissue preparation method is a compromise between the limitations in obtaining morphology identical to that existing *in vivo*, and the desire to demonstrate *in situ* the antigens under study with the best possible signal-to-noise ratio and in correct proportions. Regrettably, it is a rather unrealistic hope to develop a standard procedure that at the same time can immobilize all types of antigens, preserve adequately and equally their antigenic epitopes, provide optimal access of the applied antibodies, and retain satisfactorily the structural integrity of tissues and cells.

Immobilization of antigens and optimal preservation of morphology generally requires immediate fixation of the tissue specimen, although satisfactory and sometimes superior immunohistochemical results may be obtained with cryostat sections, particularly for membrane constituents that are not subjected to diffusion. However, cryostat temperatures favour the formation of ice crystal artefacts and membrane damage, and frozen tissue blocks are neither permanent nor easily handled, especially when sections need to be cut from the same specimen on repeated occasions. It is therefore important that a sufficiently large number of cryosections are prepared in each series and stored at –20 °C after drying and acetone fixation (*Protocol 1*).

The use of fixed and permanently embedded tissue (e.g. paraffin blocks) offers the advantage of relatively good morphological preservation together with convenient handling and storage of the specimens. Although alternative methods such as freeze-drying and freeze-substitution may be used to obtain permanent blocks (63), fixation is a much simpler and often an adequate preparation method. Nevertheless, statements made about generalized applicability of certain fixatives are likely to be false. It seems that many antigens require tailored tissue preparation for optimal immunoreactivity and precise localization. From a morphological point of view, cross-linking fixatives are often preferable but they induce variable degrees of antigenic masking (140,141). Although antigen retrieval is possible (see Section 4.1.3), optimal preservation of both antigenicity and morphology is not always compatible with this approach.

In conclusion, it is important when entering the field of immunohistochemistry to be aware of the fact that success is not a matter of mere stain technology in terms of antigen probing. The primary and crucial target for all *in situ* immune reactions is the antigenicity that has been preserved and rendered accessible in the tissue section. In addition comes the goal of adequate morphology. The choice of tissue preparation method (*Table 5*) must be guided by the purpose of the investigation.

4.1.2 Practical approaches

Antigens are generally surprisingly robust, particularly small peptides and carbohydrates that often tolerate cross-linking fixatives quite well. Large glycoproteins, cytoskeletal elements, and cell membrane components constituents are usually better preserved by precipitating fixatives. The result obtained with cross-linking fixatives is often unpredictable, both for cell surface

Table 5. Variables in the preservation of antigens for immunohistochemistry

Handling and transport of tissue sample
Properties of antigen and its location
Fixation conditions:
- precipitating (coagulative)
  - acetone
  - ethanol
  - methanol
- cross-linking
  - aldehyde-based agents
  - carbodiimide
  - parabenzoquinone
  - periodate–lysine–paraformaldehyde (PLP)

Fixation time, temperature, pH
Embedding conditions:
- wax, plastic, freeze-drying

Treatment of fixed or frozen sections:
- permeabilization with detergent
- antigen retrieval procedure
- blocking of endogenous enzymes

molecules (142,143) and other cellular markers, including the intermediary filaments (144). Limited reactivity is especially encountered with mAbs, which often function satisfactorily only on cryosections. However, the availability of mAbs reactive with robust epitopes increases steadily, thereby expanding the possibilities for probing on sections of routinely formalin-fixed and paraffin-embedded tissue, particularly after antigen retrieval procedures (see Section 4.1.3).

Space does not permit a full account of fixation principles and the reader is referred to extensive texts on tissue preparation methods (63,145). Fixatives providing satisfactory morphology combined with superior preservation of cell membrane-bound as well as diffusible cytoplasmic antigens (such as cytokines) have been reported (146–148), but they often involve quite specialized procedures and have restricted applications. Tailored tissue preparation is likewise required for reliable detection of Ig markers expressed on or in B cells. Such localization often poses interpretative problems not encountered with antigens occurring at only low concentrations in interstitial fluid. Lymphoid cells are generally surrounded by very high levels of diffusible Ig components that are retained in directly fixed specimens (*Figure 22*). Therefore, many tissues (especially skin and mucosa) subjected to precipitating fixative, show strong background staining which interferes with the visualization of Ig-expressing cells and immune deposits (22). With aldehyde-based fixatives, antigenic masking is extensive where the microenvironmental concentration of bystander proteins is high (66,140). As a con-

Intravascular compartment	Extravascular compartment	Immunohisto-chemical detection of cell surface Ig after removal of diffusible Ig
Ig ~15 g/l Ig-κ Ig-λ	Ig ~7 g/l B B	B B

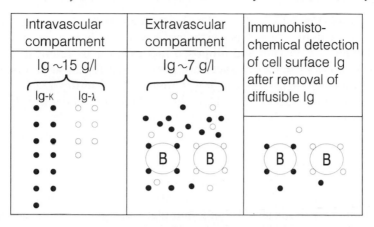

Figure 22. Schematic illustration of the intravascular and extravascular distribution of serum immunoglobulin (Ig) with κ or λ light chains. B lymphocytes (B) expressing monotypic Ig (κ or λ light chains) are visualized immunohistochemically against a relatively negative background after removal of diffusible extracellular Ig (right panel).

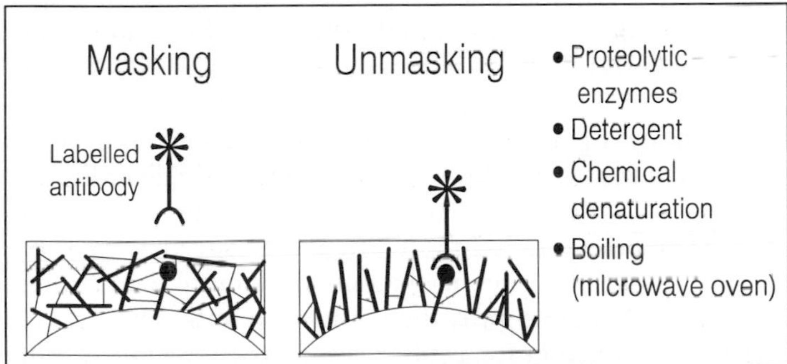

Figure 23. Putative scheme suggesting how aldehyde-based fixatives produce immunohistochemical masking of antigenic epitopes (●) on a cell surface by hindering access of antibody through the formation of numerous bridges (—) that cross-link antigen with extracellular protein molecules (——) abundantly present in the ground substance. Unmasking of epitope can be achieved by various enzymatic or denaturing procedures that break up the protein meshwork. This is usually more readily achieved for intracellular antigens (not shown).

sequence, Ig present on lymphoid cells (either expressed as surface membrane protein or adsorbed from interstitial fluid) becomes unreactive due to cross-linking with a variety of extracellular proteins, both serum-derived and part of the ground substance (*Figure 23*). Antigen retrieval methods will lead to antigenic unmasking and thereby again increase the Ig background staining, including both the κ and λ light chains (19,66,145).

Monotypic (either κ or λ) light chain staining is the best immunohistochemical criterion for monoclonality of B cell lymphomas (66,149). Studies of such expression may be performed with cryosections from which diffusible Ig has, to some extent, leached. Nevertheless, several authors have observed too much bitypic background and proposed methods for its removal (150–152). In our laboratory, thin tissue slices are pre-washed for 24–48 hours, fixed in cold ethanol, and embedded in low temperature paraffin (22,66,145). For most Ig-expressing cases of B cell lymphoma, this method permits determination of monoclonality by two-colour immunofluorescence detection of κ and λ chains. Moreover, this approach provides an internal control for every cell with regard to bitypic (κ plus λ) staining caused by *in vivo* or *in vitro* uptake of Ig from interstitial fluid (66,145). Immune deposits can also be clearly demonstrated after such tissue preparation (145,153). However, washing of unfixed tissue will to some extent destroy structural details. Therefore, reliable localization of cell surface Ig and immune deposits presents an inherent dilemma that should not be neglected (154).

4.1.3 Antigen retrieval

Sections of formalin-fixed and paraffin-embedded tissue specimens are increasingly used for immunohistochemical staining as an important and often decisive adjunct in diagnostic pathology. As discussed above, antigenic masking is a problem after use of aldehyde-based fixatives (140), which nevertheless remain the 'gold standard' of morphological tissue preservation. Loss of immunoreactivity is particularly common when formalin-fixed sections are probed with mAbs which by definition detect only a single antigenic epitope.

Antigen retrieval with various proteolytic enzymes (pronase, trypsin, or pepsin) has been practiced for more than two decades on formalin-fixed tissue sections. The striking beneficial result apparently reflects breakdown of protein cross-linking, thereby providing enhanced antibody access to relevant epitopes as well as freedom for protein antigens to assume a more reactive conformation (*Figure 23*). However, such digestion is a relatively unpredictable procedure because the degree of cross-linking depends on variables that are often uncontrolled, including the concentration of formaldehyde reaching the centre of large tissue specimens, fixation temperature and pH, time of exposure to fixative, and partial reversal of methylene bridges by rinsing before paraffin embedding. Moreover, a balance has to be found between proteolytic antigen retrieval and loss of sensitive epitopes as well as deterioration of the tissue structure (19,63,66,140,144,145).

The same limitations afflict other methods used for antigen retrieval, such as detergents combined with denaturing agents (155) and heating by microwaving. The latter approach has become increasingly popular since it was proposed by Shi *et al.* in 1991 (156). Nevertheless, the method is somewhat cumbersome and difficult to standardize, with hot and cold spots in the oven (157). Moreover, because of violent boiling with extensive evaporation of the buffer in which the sections are immersed, monitoring of the procedure and repeated bursts (usually two times 5 min) are generally required.

Plain boiling at 120°C by autoclaving in plastic Coplin jars filled with citrate buffer (pH 6.0) for 5–10 min (158), or boiling in a pressure cooker for 2–5 min (159), has been proposed as a simpler method with larger capacity, and apparently provides better preservation of morphology and enhanced retrieval of some epitopes. Microwaving has usually been carried out in the same buffer, sometimes combined with urea or heavy metals, but Tris–HCl or sodium acetate buffer at pH 8–9 may improve the reactivity of most antigens (160). We apply ordinary boiling under pressure (116°C) in this buffer as a convenient method to unmask certain membrane antigens. However, the choice of retrieval method should be based on performance testing; tailoring a combination of heating and short proteolytic digestion may sometimes be useful.

Although some epitopes seem to tolerate proteolytic enzymes better than heating (161), microwaving has turned out to have a remarkably wide applicability for antigen retrieval in diagnostic immunohistochemistry (162). To increase the detection signals even further, immunoenzyme staining with particularly designed enhancement sequences has been recommended (163). Furthermore, prolonged incubation of primary antibodies or application at raised temperature (37°C–40°C) facilitates their reactivity, especially with partially denatured epitopes (149).

4.2 Choice of immunostaining method

The practical methodological performance and the desired immunohistochemical information are both decisive for the choice of staining technique. The scarce supply or high cost of many primary antibody reagents, combined with applicability for light microscopy, makes immunoenzyme staining particularly attractive in diagnostic pathology laboratories (*Table 6*). Because the coloured product of most enzyme chromogens contrasts well with nuclear counterstain, immunological and morphological evaluation can be performed simultaneously, and potentially problematic autofluorescence is avoided (see Section 5.5.1). By new developments, immunoenzyme methods are made simpler with good sensitivity, such as the enhanced polymer one-step staining (EPOS) approach. The EPOS conjugates consist of an inert polymer backbone molecule to which several molecules of primary antibody and Px are chemically linked. Several useful specificities are commercially available (Dako) for this rapid and reproducible method.

As stated before by others (164), there is no reason to expect some mysterious difference between immunoenzyme and immunofluorescence performance, regardless of the method employed for tissue preparation (165). In fact, good contrast against a dark background may render optimally performed immunofluorescence advantageous for detection of cell surface markers (66,149,164). Nuclear staining obtained by a final brief rinse of the section in PBS containing the fluorescent (blue) Hoechst dye (*Protocol 3D*), provides

Table 6. Comparison of immunofluorescence and immunoenzyme staining methods

Immunofluorescence	**Immunoenzyme**
Specialized microscope	Ordinary light microscope
Reagents used at relatively high concentrations; most economic in manual applications	Reagents often extensively diluted, well suited for staining machines
Technically simple and often less time-consuming	Includes additional steps and often technically more complex
Staining result may be disturbed by autofluorescence	Staining result may be disturbed by endogenous enzymes
Easy to adapt for multicolour staining with two or three fluorochromes	Multicolour staining not always reliable when different antigens are co-localized at same site
Sometimes difficult morphological orientation	Staining signals can be related to morphology
Difficult to discuss without photography or image analysis	Easy to demonstrate and discuss with colleagues
Preparations not permanent	Preparations better suited for storage

morphological orientation and facilitates precise cell counting. Topographic mapping of intraepithelial lymphocytes or immunolocalization in relation to subepithelial structures can be further visualized by the inclusion of antibody to cytokeratin, laminin, β4 integrin, or various types of collagen in two- or three-colour staining (23,24,166,167). Moreover, immunofluorescence circumvents background noise from endogenous enzymes that sometimes disturbs the evaluation of immunoenzyme staining. Finally, certain multicolour analyses based on enzyme labels present inherent technical problems that are difficult to overcome (65).

The methodological basis for several sequential multicolour immunoenzyme staining protocols (70,112) with primary antibodies from the same or different species, has been the shielding effect exerted by dense DAB deposits (*Figure 17*). In combination with immunofluorescence, the quenching effect of DAB on emission colours must also be considered (101). DAB shielding is apparently enhanced in combination with the ABC method, presumably because the complexes provide additional steric hindrance (71,168). Although we have shown that PAP–CN staining followed by PAP–DAB can result in a mixed bluish-brown colour (112), other authors have reported that with sequential ABC staining, even the colour product of CN may block the active sites of the primary reagent sequence (169). The same has been claimed for a well-developed AEC end-product (116). Therefore, the penetrability of the chromogen precipitates is always an important variable to be considered in multicolour immunoenzyme staining.

In our experience, a reliable result of multicolour immunoenzyme staining can best be obtained when the actual antigens are known *a priori* to occur at different sites (112,114)—that is, disparate marker expression by separate cells or non-overlapping cellular phenotypes (*Figures 3* and *16*), as well as concomitant localization of nuclear and surface membrane or cytoplasmic antigens in the same cell (170). Other authors have likewise expressed this opinion (41,63,171,172). Certain immunological blocking methods may facilitate sequential multicolour immunoenzyme staining with primary antibody from the same species (see Section 3.2.3), but antigens present at disproportionate concentrations in the same location are not reliably revealed (65). The same problem applies even to immunoenzyme staining methods based on primary antibodies from different species (see Section 3.1). Despite enthusiastic statements in the literature, the interpretation of mixed colours is often very difficult in the light microscope. Although methods exist to enhance the detection sensitivity for antigens expressed at low levels, technical modulation to obtain balanced colour mixing is cumbersome and cannot always be trusted. Therefore, several prominent experts on immunoenzyme staining (63,65,93) seem to support our view that co-localization of two or more antigens occurring at differing concentrations, is best evaluated by multicolour immunofluorescence either directly in the microscopy, by FOAM in double- or triple-exposed colour slides (see Section 2.1.2), or after computerized image analysis (see Section 3.3) that may include confocal laser scanning microscopy (see Section 3.4).

5. Immunohistochemical reliability criteria

For comparison and evaluation of immunohistochemical staining methods, it is important to consider the following reliability criteria: specificity, accuracy, precision, sensitivity, and efficiency (173).

5.1 Specificity criteria

5.1.1 Immunological specificity

The antibody specificity of immunostaining can only be ensured by performance studies with known antigens present in a relevant preparation. For immunohistochemical applications, the antibody reagents must be tested on tissue sections, even when the specificity has been established by other methods such as radioimmunoassay. A specific radioimmunoassay relies merely on the competitive interaction between radiolabelled and unlabelled purified antigen, whereas a specific immunohistochemical signal depends on restricted binding of antibody to the corresponding tissue antigen and may be severely jeopardized by unknown antibody–antigen interactions (173). Flow cytometric analysis of cell surface antigens is likewise insufficient for immunohistochemical specificity testing because the sectioning may disclose previously undetected cross-reacting antigens (174). Therefore, even the application of primary mAbs to tissue sections can produce quite surprising results (175).

Immunohistochemical performance testing over a wide range of antibody dilutions on both positive and negative tissue preparations is necessary to ensure that unwanted antibodies or cross-reacting specificities are absent from the primary reagent. Although vendors generally indicate appropriate working concentrations of commercial reagents, serial dilutions should be made for every new batch to establish its actual immunohistochemical performance. Absorption of polyclonal reagents with defined purified antigen (not the immunogen itself!) is an additional desirable control which, however, does not necessarily establish immunological specificity and anyhow often cannot be performed due to lack of appropriate antigen (63). Moreover, this control is of little value in terms of absolute antigen specificity of mAbs which by definition react only with a single epitope. Therefore, it is not possible to remove cross-reactivity of mAbs without neutralizing all antibody activity, and isotype- as well as concentration-matched control mAbs should be included in every staining experiment (*Protocol 1*).

Despite appropriate testing for immunological specificity, cross-reactions may occur due to shared amino acid sequences of antigens. Little information is available about possible cross-reacting epitopes made accessible to the primary antibodies following tissue processing methods such as proteolytic digestion or heating of sections (63,176). However, species cross-reactivity of secondary anti-Ig reagents, for instance sharing of epitopes between mouse, rat, and human IgG (177), is a well-known and important problem in all types of indirect staining techniques (see Section 3, *Figure 19*, *Protocol 2*). It may rather be considered a problem of method specificity when the secondary antibodies react with endogenous Ig in the tissue (see Section 3.1). Immunological specificity is, in fact, linked to both method specificity (see Section 5.5.3) and detection efficiency (see Section 5.5.2); all these performance characteristics are significantly improved when the primary antibody reagents can be used at low concentrations. By extensive dilution, high-affinity antibodies are selected for binding to the relevant antigen, thus decreasing the possibility that unwanted or cross-reacting antibodies produce detectable colour signals.

5.1.2 Method specificity

Method specificity requires that all staining signals reflect immunological reactions caused by the primary antibodies, including the unwanted and cross-reacting ones. False positive signals appearing either as a diffuse background or as decoration of irrelevant cells or other tissue elements, can be caused by a variety of molecular interactions such as non-specific (electrostatic) binding of unconjugated or conjugated Ig (21), reaction of IgG with Fc receptors (63,178), direct binding of the enzyme label (179) or the avidin–biotin complexes (88), intrinsic enzyme activity being revealed in immunoenzyme staining, and reaction of endogenous biotin or biotin receptors when avidin–biotin sequences are used (see Section 2.2.5).

Problems of method specificity in immunohistochemistry are most often explained by non-specific Ig binding. Such affinity to cells and tissues may to some extent be caused by interactions with reactive groups preserved or produced by certain fixatives and are most pronounced for positively charged (acidophilic) tissue elements (e.g. necrotic areas). In liver tissue, unfixed Mallory bodies can absorb PAP complexes (180), and Ig can bind to cells containing pituitary ACTH (181). Other reports describe complement-mediated Ig binding (particularly involving C1q) to various endocrine cells (182), Ig binding to gastrin cells via non-specific ionic interactions (183), fixation-dependent Ig binding to polymorphonuclear leucocytes and macrophages (184), and binding of fluorochrome conjugates to eosinophils (21,185) and various epithelial cells, including goblet cells (21). Bergroth *et al.* (184) reported that PAP complexes produce non-specific staining of granulocytes, but it is difficult to exclude the possibility that incomplete inhibition of endogenous Px may induce slight positivity in such cells.

With the various immunoenzyme methods, in which the primary reagents are usually extensively diluted, non-specific staining is most often caused by the bridging antibodies (184) or the immune complexes (186,187). Pre-treatment with normal animal serum (for which there must be no wanted antibody activity in the staining sequence!), or dilution of the reagents with normal serum or another protein-rich solution (e.g. bovine serum albumin), may reduce the non-specific interactions but does not always abolish them. Progressive dilution of the primary reagent until the colour signal is omitted, is an important preliminary control for method specificity in all types of indirect immunostaining.

When mucous membranes are studied by immunofluorescence, several tissue elements such as eosinophils, squamous epithelium, goblet cells, and columnar epithelium, are prone to show non-specific staining, usually in that order (19,21). It may be quite difficult to distinguish between specifically fluorescent lymphoid cells and non-specific granulocyte staining. For example, eosinophils can interfere with the detection of Ig-producing plasma cells, particularly when highly-labelled FITC conjugates are used (185). There are several methods to block or identify such non-specific staining. For example, the tissue sections can be pre-treated with benzidine reagents and H_2O_2 (188) or with Lendrum's phenol chromotrope 2-R stain (189) and staining with FITC-labelled bovine serum albumin, that selectively binds to the eosinophils, can be paired with a specific rhodamine conjugate (188).

Such procedures to avoid non-specific fluorescence staining should be used only when absolutely necessary. Optimally labelled fluorochrome conjugates of good quality (see Section 2.1.1) do not cause problems when they can be applied at a low protein concentration—that is, when their end-point titre for the specific colour signal is low. The interval between the specific and the non-specific staining end-point is termed the specificity interval, defined by the specificity interval factor, SIF (*Figure 24*); this is an important performance characteristic of a fluorochrome conjugate (19,21).

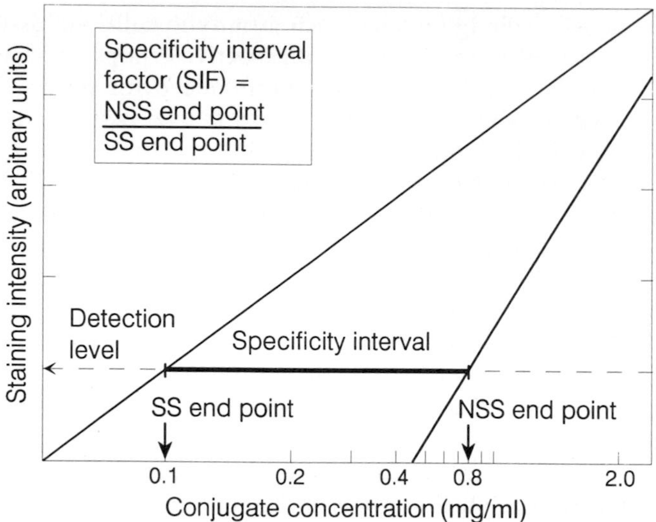

Figure 24. Specific binding of fluorochrome conjugate depends on the magnitude of its specificity interval factor (SIF). The specificity interval represents the range of concentrations that can be expected to produce only detectable immunological reactions with the actual test preparation. NSS, non-specific staining; SS, specific staining.

It cannot be over-emphasized that the best precaution against non-specific fluorescence staining is to use fractionated and well-characterized fluorochrome conjugates at the lowest applicable working concentration (see Section 2.1.1). Moderately labelled antibodies (F : P ratio = 1.5–3.0) usually cause few non-specific problems. Commercial conjugates, on the other hand, are often highly labelled (F : P ratios = 3.0–8.0) to produce strong colour signals; although such reagents generally perform well when applied on living cells (e.g. in flow cytometry), they are quite likely to cause non-specific staining in tissue sections (21). Indeed, it is sometimes difficult to obtain a strong and specific immunohistochemical signal combined with a satisfactory SIF because the conjugate does not work at a sufficiently low concentration; this problem may be circumvented by affinity purification of the antibody or by a new round of hyperimmunization to produce a reagent of higher affinity. These two measures are also useful for improving SIF in immunoenzyme staining.

5.2 Detection accuracy

In quantitative assays, accuracy describes how near a measurement is to the true value (190). In terms of immunohistochemistry, the definition relates to accuracy of antigen localization or microscopical resolution of the specific signal. With ordinary light microscopy, resolution has a lower limit of about 0.25 μm; it is probably somewhat poorer with fluorescence microscopy because of the scatter of emission light. Thus, blurring causes overlapping of fluorescent signals from juxtaposed tissue elements, thereby prohibiting separate analysis of the same marker in aggregated cells, for example co-expression of CD3 and HLA-DR on activated T cells lying adjacent to macrophages that are strongly positive for the latter marker (191). Although some authors claim that such co-expression can be examined by paired immunofluorescence staining (192), the documentation provided is in our opinion not convincing. However, the resolution can be improved by confocal lasar scanning microscopy (see Section 3.4 and Chapter 5).

The size of a single Px molecule, and even a PAP complex, is well below the limit of light microscopical resolution (8). Detectable Px staining can only be obtained by a certain degree of overstaining that produces a visible reaction precipitate. The resolution of immunoperoxidase procedures has been shown to be affected by diffusion and reabsorption of the DAB end-product, which is also of relevance for electron microscopical application of Px (193,194). Diffusion artefacts sometimes reduce even more the accuracy obtained with the water soluble coloured end-products (see Section 2.1.4).

5.3 Detection precision

Precision refers to the consistency of repeated measurements, and has relevance for immunohistochemical (morphological) antigen localization, enumeration reproducibility for positively stained cells, and consistency of specific signal intensity. Immunohistochemical methods performed with satisfactory specificity generally provide remarkably reproducible results for the localization of various tissue antigens such as hormones, neuropeptides, enzymes, and oncodevelopmental tumour markers (173). Reproducibility of cell counting has also been found to be highly satisfactory both with PAP staining (165) and immunofluorescence for cytoplasmic antigens (195,196), as well as with immunofluorescence for cell membrane markers (197). A relatively high reproducibility has also been obtained for quantitative estimation of fluorescence intensity (198,199).

5.4 Detection sensitivity

Staining sensitivity should preferably be defined as the lowest amount of detectable antigen (63,200) and can only be truly evaluated in a system with a range of known antigen concentrations (198,199). However, the lowest applicable working dilution of the primary antibody is often incorrectly taken to indicate sensitivity. This confusion between reagent economy and detection capacity explains to a large extent the prevailing opinion that the sensitivity of immunoenzyme staining is much higher than that of immunofluorescence.

Several variables influence immunohistochemical detection sensitivity, such as the affinity of the primary antibodies, the penetration of the reagents, the tissue preparation methods, the microscopy conditions and, to a lesser extent, prolonged incubation times, and raised primary antibody concentrations (199). Only minor differences in detection sensitivity have been documented when immunofluorescence has been directly compared with immunoenzyme staining methods (199). Nevertheless, the possibilities for staining enhancement are more extensive in some of the immunoenzyme methods, thus facilitating improved colour signal intensities.

5.5 Detection efficiency

Efficiency is defined as the 'signal-to-noise' ratio; it may be expressed as specific staining intensity minus unwanted background staining divided by the latter. Because of the influence of background staining, it is obviously important to apply the primary reagent at the highest possible dilution without sacrificing any specific staining signal. The efficiency will therefore depend on the reagent's SIF (*Figure 24*). However, particular problems such as self-masking and bystander protein masking of antigens subjected to cross-linking fixatives, are also important (19,145). Under such conditions, raised primary antibody concentration, and especially prolonged incubation, may improve the efficiency and lead to more intense staining, particularly when polyclonal reagents are applied (63,149,199).

5.5.1 Disturbing autofluorescence

The efficiency of immunofluorescence staining may be reduced by the fact that certain tissue elements emit primary fluorescence, mainly blue or blue-green. Such autofluorescence generally shows a broad emission spectrum combined with a short Stokes shift (see Section 2.1.2). Thus, it can often be distinguished from fluorochrome emission because of 'bleed-through' with several filter sets, and it can be reduced if fluorochromes and filter sets are adapted for a large Stokes shift. Cross-linking fixatives, particularly glutaraldehyde, tend to increase the bluish autofluorescence induced by ultraviolet excitation of proteins in general, and this phenomenon often becomes worse during storage of the tissue preparations. AMCA-stained sections should therefore be studied and recorded as soon as possible. Especially organized collagen and elastic fibres may produce very strong autofluorescence, rendering immunofluorescence studies of arterial walls, dermis, and certain tumours difficult. In addition, eosinophils, hepatocytes, carotenoids, vitamin A, and lipofuscin are autofluorescent. Lipofuscin granules with strong yellow emission are common in hepatocytes, glandular ducts, and certain macrophages. Autofluorescence may be exploited for morphological orientation, and the primary fluorescence of certain counterstains has also been used to this end. However, the latter approach is not recommended because immunoreactivity may be masked (63), except for the application of nuclear Hoechst dye (*Protocol 3D*) when needed (Section 4.2).

6. General conclusions

Comparison of immunofluorescence and immunoenzyme methods based on various reliability criteria, shows that the two staining approaches are interchangeable for most but not all purposes. Fluorescent colour signals exhibit a relatively consistent relationship to the actual antigen concentration in the test preparation and are better suited for quantitative computerized image analysis than light microscopic observations of immunoenzyme staining. Moreover, direct or indirect immunofluorescence is the most powerful and reliable immunohistochemical method for multicolour staining to evaluate co-localization of two or more antigens. Multicolour immunoenzyme staining provides an easily obtainable and reliable result only when the antigens are known *a priori* to be separately located. On the other hand, immunoenzyme methods are more economical in terms of reagent consumption and are therefore better suited for semi-automatic staining machines. Avoidance of autofluorescence can also be an advantage in certain tissues, particularly in old routinely fixed paraffin blocks. In addition, the superior morphological correlate provided by these methods, makes them more attractive for most purposes in diagnostic pathology laboratories.

Acknowledgements

Hege E. Svendsen is thanked for excellent secretarial assistance and Erik Kulø Hagen for the drawings. Studies in the authors' laboratory have been supported by the Norwegian Cancer Society, the Research Council of Norway, and Anders Jahre's Fund.

References

1. Coons, A. H., Creech, H. J., and Jones, R. N. (1941). *Proc. Soc. Exp. Biol. Med.*, **47**, 200.
2. Coons, A. H., Creech, H. J., Jones, R. N., and Berliner, E. (1942). *J. Immunol.*, **45**, 159.
3. Avrameas, S. and Uriel, J. (1966). *C. R. Acad. Sci. Paris*, **262**, 2543.
4. Nakane, P. (1968). *J. Histochem. Cytochem.*, **16**, 557.
5. Avrameas, S. (1969). *Immunohistochemistry*, **6**, 825.
6. Mason, T. E., Phifer, R. F., Spicer, S. S., Swallow, R. S., and Dreskin, R. D. (1969). *J. Histochem. Cytochem.*, **17**, 190.
7. Sternberger, L. A. and Cuculis, J. J. (1969). *J. Histochem. Cytochem.*, **17**, 190.
8. Sternberger, L. A., Hardy, P. H., Cuculis, J. J., and Meyer, H. G. (1970). *J. Histochem. Cytochem.*, **18**, 315.
9. Cordell, J. L., Falini, B., Erber, W. N., Ghosh, A. K., Abdulaziz, Z., Macdonald, S., *et al.* (1984). *J. Histochem. Cytochem.*, **2**, 219.
10. Silverstein, A. M. (1957). *J. Histochem. Cytochem.*, **5**, 94.

11. Ploem, J. S. (1967). *Z. Wissensch. Mikr.*, **68**, 129.
12. Nakane, P. K. and Pierce, G. B. (1966). *J. Histochem. Cytochem.*, **14**, 929.
13. Riggs, J. L., Seiwald, R. J., Burckhalter, J. H., Downs, C. M., and Metcalf, T. G. (1958). *Am. J. Pathol.*, **34**, 1081.
14. Titus, J. A., Haugland, R., Sharrow, S. O., and Segal, D. M. (1982). *J. Immunol. Methods*, **50**, 193.
15. Khalfan, H., Abuknesha, R., Rand-Weaver, M., Price, R. G., and Robinson, D. (1986). *Histochem. J.*, **18**, 497.
16. Brandtzaeg, P. (1973). *Scand. J. Immunol.*, **2**, 273.
17. Oi, V. T., Glazer, A. N., and Stryer, L. (1982). *J. Cell. Biol.*, **93**, 981.
18. Pizzolo, G. and Chilosi, M. (1984). *Am. J. Clin. Pathol.*, **82**, 44.
19. Brandtzaeg, P. (1982). In *Immunofluorescence technology. Selected theoretical and clinical aspects* (ed. G. Wick, K. N. Traill, and K. Schauenstein), p. 167. Elsevier Biomedical Press, Amsterdam, New York, Oxford.
20. Cebra, J. J. and Goldstein, G. (1965). *J. Immunol.*, **95**, 230.
21. Brandtzaeg, P. (1973). *Scand. J. Immunol.*, **2**, 333.
22. Brandtzaeg, P. (1974). *Immunology*, **26**, 1101.
23. Halstensen, T. S., Scott, H., and Brandtzaeg, P. (1990). *Eur. J. Immunol.*, **20**, 1825.
24. Halstensen, T. S., Scott, H., Farstad, I. N., Michaelsen, T. E., and Brandtzaeg, P. (1992). *Prog. Histochem. Cytochem.*, **26**, 201.
25. Bruins, S., de Jong, M. C. J. M., Heeres, K., Wilkinson, M. H. F., Jonkman, M. F., and van der Meer, J. B. (1994). *J. Histochem. Cytochem.*, **42**, 555.
26. Bruins, S., de Jong, M. C. J. M., Heeres, K., Wilkinson, M. H. F., Jonkman, M. F., and van der Meer, J. B. (1995). *J. Histochem. Cytochem.*, **43**, 715.
27. Huitfeldt, H. S., Brandtzaeg, P., and Poirier, M. C. (1991). *Lab. Invest.*, **64**, 207.
28. Johnson, G. D. and de C. Nogueira Araujo, G. M. (1981). *J. Immunol. Methods*, **43**, 349.
29. Valnes, K. and Brandtzaeg, P. (1985). *J. Histochem. Cytochem.*, **33**, 755.
30. Rodriguez, J. and Deinhardt, F. (1960). *Virology*, **12**, 316.
31. Lennette, D. A. (1978). *Am. J. Pathol.*, **69**, 647.
32. Busachi, C. A., Ray, M. B., and Desmet, V. J. (1978). *J. Histochem. Cytochem.*, **19**, 95.
33. Hsu, S.-M. and Soban, E. (1982). *J. Histochem. Cytochem.*, **30**, 1079.
34. Straus, W. (1982). *J. Histochem. Cytochem.*, **30**, 491.
35. Gallyas, F., Görcs, T., and Merchenthaler, I. (1982). *J. Histochem. Cytochem.*, **30**, 183.
36. Nemes, Z. (1987). *Histochemistry*, **86**, 415.
37. Weisburger, E. K., Russfield, A. B., Homburger, F., Weisburger, J. H., Boger, E., van Dongen, G. C., *et al.* (1978). *J. Environ. Pathol. Toxicol.*, **2**, 325.
38. Burstone, M. S. (1960). *J. Histochem. Cytochem.*, **8**, 67.
39. Graham, R. C., Lundholm, U., and Karnovsky, M. J. (1965). *J. Histochem. Cytochem.*, **13**, 150.
40. Mesulam, M.-M. (1978). *J. Histochem. Cytochem.*, **26**, 106.
41. Levey, A. I., Bolam, J. P., Rye, D. B., Hallanger, A. E., Demuth, R. M., Mesulam, M.-M., *et al.* (1986). *J. Histochem. Cytochem.*, **34**, 1449.
42. Hanker, J. S., Yates, P. E., Metz, C. B., and Rustioni, A. (1977). *Histochem. J.*, **9**, 789.

43. Streefkerk, J. G. (1972). *J. Histochem. Cytochem.*, **20**, 829.
44. Straus, W. (1972). *J. Histochem. Cytochem.*, **20**, 949.
45. Heyderman, E. and Neville, A. M. (1977). *J. Clin. Pathol.*, **30**, 138.
46. Fink, B., Loepfe, E., and Wyler, R. (1979). *J. Histochem. Cytochem.*, **27**, 1299.
47. Mason, D. Y. and Sammons, R. (1978). *J. Clin. Pathol.*, **31**, 454.
48. Mason, D. Y. (1985). In *Techniques in immunocytochemistry* (ed. G. R. Bulloch and P. Petrusz), Vol. 3, p. 25. Academic Press, London.
49. Borgers, M. (1973). *J. Histochem. Cytochem.*, **21**, 812.
50. Dearnaley, D. P., Sloane, J. P., Ormerod, M. G., Steele, K., Coombes, R. C., Clink, H. Mc.D., *et al.* (1981). *Br. J. Cancer*, **44**, 85.
51. Bulman, A. S. and Heyderman, E. (1981). *J. Clin. Pathol.*, **34**, 1349.
52. Van Noorden, S. (1986). In *Immunocytochemistry. Modern methods and applications* (ed. J. M. Polak and S. van Noorden), 2nd edn, p. 26. Wright, Bristol.
53. Avrameas, S. (1969). *Immunochemistry*, **6**, 43.
54. Campbell, G. T. and Bhatnagar, A. S. (1976). *J. Histochem. Cytochem.*, **24**, 448.
55. Bondi, A., Chieregatti, G., Eusebi, V., Fulcheri, E., and Bussolati, G. (1982). *Histochemistry*, **76**, 153.
56. Boorsma, D. M. (1983). In *Immunohistochemistry* (ed. A. C. Cuello), p. 87. John Wiley & Sons, Chichester, UK.
57. O'Sullivan, M. J., Gnemmi, E., Morris, D., Chieregatti, G., Simmonds, A. D., Simmons, M., *et al.* (1979). *Anal. Biochem.*, **100**, 100.
58. Nilsson, P., Bergquist, N. R., and Grundy, M. S. (1981). *J. Immunol. Methods*, **41**, 81.
59. Plenat, F., Martinet, Y., Martinet, N., and Vignaud, J.-M. (1994). *J. Immunol. Methods*, **174**, 133.
60. Faulk, W. P. and Taylor, G. M. (1971). *Immunochemistry*, **8**, 1081.
61. Roth, J. (1982). In *Techniques in immunocytochemistry* (ed. G. R. Bullock and P. Petrusz), Vol. 1, Chapter 11, p. 107. Academic Press, London.
62. Holgate, C. S., Jackson, P., Cowen, P. N., and Bird, C. C. (1983). *J. Histochem. Cytochem.*, **31**, 938.
63. Larsson, L.-I. (ed.) (1988). *Immunocytochemistry: theory and practice.* p. 272. CRC Press, Boca Raton, Florida.
64. Falini, B., Abdulaziz, Z., Gerdes, J., Canino, S., Ciani, C., Cordell, J. L., *et al.* (1986). *J. Immunol. Methods*, **93**, 265.
65. van der Loos, C. M., Becker, A. E., and van den Oord, J. J. (1993). *Histochem. J.*, **25**, 1.
66. Brandtzaeg, P. and Rognum, T. O. (1983). *Histochem. J.*, **15**, 655.
67. Jankovic, B. D. (1959). *Acta Haematol.*, **22**, 278.
68. Gu, J., Islam, K. N., and Polak, J. M. (1983). *Histochem. J.*, **15**, 475.
69. Falini, B., Martelli, M. F., Tarallo, F., Moir, D. J., Cordell, J. L., Gatter, K. C., *et al.* (1984). *Br. J. Haematol.*, **56**, 365.
70. Sternberger, L. A. and Joseph, S. A. (1979). *J. Histochem. Cytochem.*, **27**, 1424.
71. Hohmann, A., Hodgson, A. J., Di, W., Skinner, J. M., Bradley, J., and Zola, H. (1988). *J. Histochem. Cytochem.*, **36**, 137.
72. Cammisuli, S. and, Wofsy, L. (1976). *J. Immunol.*, **117**, 695.
73. Cammisuli, S. (1981). In *Immunological methods* (ed. J. Lefkovits), Vol. II, p. 139. Academic Press Inc., New York.
74. Farr, A. G. and Nakane, P. K. (1981). *J. Immunol. Methods*, **47**, 129.

75. Jasani, B., Wynford Thomas, D., and Williams, E. D. (1981). *J. Clin. Pathol.*, **34**, 1000.
76. Beutner, E. H., Holborow, E. J., and Johnson, G. D. (1965). *Nature*, **208**, 353.
77. Larsson, L.-I. (1979). *Nature*, **282**, 743.
78. Mason, D. Y. and Sammons, R. E. (1979). *J. Histochem. Cytochem.*, **27**, 832.
79. Biberfeld, P., Ghetie, V., and Sjöquist, J. (1975). *J. Immunol. Methods*, **6**, 249.
80. Dubois-Dalcq, M., Mcfarland, H., and Mcfarlin, D. (1977). *J. Histochem. Cytochem.*, **25**, 1201.
81. Engvall, E. (1978). *Scand. J. Immunol.*, **8**, 25.
82. Notani, G. W., Parsons, J. A., and Erlandsen, S. L. (1979). *J. Histochem. Cytochem.*, **27**, 1438.
83. Guesdon, J.-L., Ternynck, T., and Avrameas, S. (1979). *J. Histochem. Cytochem.*, **27**, 1131.
84. Berman, J. W. and Basch, R. S. (1980). *J. Immunol. Methods*, **36**, 335.
85. Hsu, S.-M., Raine, L., and Fanger, H. (1981). *J. Histochem. Cytochem.*, **29**, 577.
86. Wood, G. S. and Warnke, R. (1981). *J. Histochem. Cytochem.*, **29**, 1196.
87. Jones, C. J. P., Mosley, S. M., Jeffrey, I. J. M., and Stoddart, R. W. (1987). *Histochem. J.*, **19**, 264.
88. Bussolati, G. and Gugliotta, P. (1983). *J. Histochem. Cytochem.*, **31**, 1419.
89. Buckland, R. M. (1986). *Nature*, **320**, 557.
90. Erichsen, J. T., Reiner, A., and Karten, H. J. (1982). *Nature*, **295**, 407.
91. Wessendorf, M. W. and Elde, R. P. (1985). *J. Histochem. Cytochem.*, **33**, 984.
92. Staines, W. A., Meister, B., Melander, T., Nagy, J. I., and Hökfelt, T. (1988). *J. Histochem. Cytochem.*, **36**, 145.
93. Mason, D. Y., Abdulaziz, Z., Falini, B., and Stein, H. (1983). In *Immunocytochemistry. Practical applications in pathology and biology* (ed. J. M. Polak and S. van Noorden), p. 113. Wright & Sons Ltd., Bristol, London, Boston.
94. Klareskog, L., Forsum, U., Wigren, A., and Wigzell, H. (1982). *Scand. J. Immunol.*, **15**, 501.
95. Goding, J. W. (1980). *J. Immunol. Methods*, **39**, 285.
96. Falini, B., De Solas, I., Halverson, C., Parker, J. W., and Taylor, C. R. (1982). *J. Histochem. Cytochem.*, **30**, 21.
97. Claassen, E., Boorsma, D. M., Kors, N., and van Rooijen, N. (1986). *J. Histochem. Cytochem.*, **34**, 423.
98. Brandtzaeg, P. and Tolo, K. (1977). In *The borderline between caries and periodontal disease* (ed. T. Lehner), p. 145. Academic Press, London.
99. Wallace, E. F. and Wofsy, L. (1979). *J. Immunol. Methods*, **25**, 283.
100. Caligaris-Cappio, F., Gobbi, M., Bofill, M., and Janossy, G. (1982). *J. Exp. Med.*, **155**, 623.
101. Valnes, K. and Brandtzaeg, P. (1981). *J. Histochem. Cytochem.*, **29**, 703.
102. Vandesande, F. and Dierickx, K. (1975). *Cell Tissue Res.*, **164**, 153.
103. Erlandsen, S. L., Hegre, O. D., Parsons, J. A., McEvoy, R. C., and Elde, R. P. (1976). *J. Histochem. Cytochem.*, **24**, 883.
104. Martin-Comin, J. and Robyn, C. (1976). *J. Histochem. Cytochem.*, **24**, 1012.
105. Tramu, G., Pillez, A., and Leonardelli, J. (1978). *J. Histochem. Cytochem.*, **26**, 322.
106. Vandesande, F. and Dierickx, K. (1976). *Cell Tissue Res.*, **175**, 289.
107. Hökfelt, T., Skirboll, L., Rehfeld, J. F., Goldstein, M., Markey, K., and Dann, O. (1980). *Neuroscience*, **5**, 2093.

108. Bologna, M., Allen, R., and Dulbecco, R. (1986). *J. Immunol. Methods*, **86**, 151.
109. Wang, B.-L. and Larsson, L.-I. (1985). *Histochemistry*, **83**, 47.
110. Kolodziejczyk, E. and Baertschi, A. J. (1986). *J. Histochem. Cytochem.*, **34**, 1725.
111. Lan, H. Y., Mu, W., Nikolic-Paterson, D. J., and Atkins, R. C. (1995). *J. Histochem. Cytochem.*, **43**, 97.
112. Valnes, K. and Brandtzaeg, P. (1982). *J. Histochem. Cytochem.*, **30**, 518.
113. Van Noorden, S., Stuart, M. C., Cheung, A., Adams, E. F., and Polak, J. M. (1986). *J. Histochem. Cytochem.*, **34**, 287.
114. Valnes, K. and Brandtzaeg, P. (1984). *Histochem. J.*, **16**, 477.
115. Krenács, T., Krenács, L., Bozóky, B., Adams, E. F., and Ivány, B. (1990). *Histochem. J.*, **22**, 530.
116. Van der Heijden, F. (1987). *Acta Histochem.*, **82**, 59.
117. Feller, A. C., Parwaresch, M. R., Wacker, H.-H., Radzun, H.-J., and Lennert, K. (1983). *Histochem. J.*, **15**, 557.
118. Van der Loos, C. M., Das, P. K., and Houthoff, H.-J. (1987). *J. Histochem. Cytochem.*, **35**, 1199.
119. Van der Loos, C. M., van den Oord, J. J., Das, P. K., and Houthoff, H. J. (1988). *Histochem. J.*, **20**, 409.
120. Bendayan, M. and Stephens, H. (1984). In *Immunolabelling for electron microscopy* (ed. J. M. Polak and I. M. Varndell), p. 143. Elsevier Science Publications BV, Amsterdam, New York, Oxford.
121. Varndell, I. M. and Polak, J. M. (1984). In *Immunolabelling for electron microscopy* (ed. J. M. Polak and I. M. Varndell), p. 155. Elsevier Science Publishers BV, Amsterdam, New York, Oxford.
122. Young, W. W., Tamura, Y., Wolock, D. M., and Fox, J. W. (1984). *J. Immunol.*, **133**, 3163.
123. Wessel, G. M. and McClay, D. R. (1986). *J. Histochem. Cytochem.*, **34**, 703.
124. Franzusoff, A., Redding, K., Crosby, J., Fuller, R. S., and Schekman, R. (1991). *J. Cell Biol.*, **112**, 27.
125. Carl, S. A. L., Gillete-Ferguson, I., and Ferguson, D. G. (1993). *J. Histochem. Cytochem.*, **41**, 1273.
126. Tuson, J. R., Pascoe, E. W., and Jacob, D. A. (1990). *J. Histochem. Cytochem.*, **38**, 923.
127. Eichmüller, S., Stevenson, P. A., and Paus, R. (1996). *J. Immunol. Methods*, **190**, 255.
128. Würden, S. and Homberg, U. (1993). *J. Histochem. Cytochem.*, **41**, 627.
129. Johnson, G. D. and Walker, L. (1986). *J. Immunol. Methods*, **95**, 149.
130. Halstensen, T. S., Scott, H., and Brandtzaeg, P. (1989). *Scand. J. Immunol.*, **30**, 665.
131. Jahnsen, F. L., Brandtzaeg, P., and Halstensen, T. S. (1994). *J. Immunol. Methods*, **175**, 23.
132. Joyce-Loebl©. (1985). *Image analysis: principles and practice*, p. 250. Vickers, Gateshead, Tyne and Wear, England.
133. Valnes, K., Huitfeldt, H. S., and Brandtzaeg, P. (1990). *Gut*, **31**, 647.
134. Huitfeldt, H. S., Brandtzaeg, P., and Poirer, M. C. (1990). *Proc. Natl. Acad. Sci. USA*, **87**, 5955.
135. Gerlyng, P., Stokke, T., Huitfeldt, H. S., Stenersen, T., Danielsen, H. E., Grotmol, T., *et al.* (1992). *Cytometry*, **13**, 404.

136. Brandtzaeg, P. (1983). *Mol. Immunol.*, **20**, 941.
137. Larsen, T. H., Huitfeldt, H. S., Myking, O., and Sætersdal, T. (1993). *Cell Tissue Kinetics*, **272**, 201.
138. Skålhegg, B. S., Taskén, K., Hansson, V., Huitfeldt, H. S., Jahnsen, T., and Lea, T. (1994). *Science*, **263**, 84.
139. Huitfeldt, H. S., Skarpen, E., Lindeman, B., Becher, R., Thrane, E. V., and Schwarze, P. E. (1996). *J. Histochem. Cytochem.*, **44**, 227.
140. Brandtzaeg, P. and Rognum, T. O. (1984). *Pathol. Res. Pract.*, **179**, 250.
141. Brandtzaeg, P. and Rognum, T. O. (1984). *Histochemistry*, **81**, 213.
142. Pollard, K., Lunny, D., Holgate, C. S., Jackson, P., and Bird, C. C. (1987). *J. Histochem. Cytochem.*, **35**, 1329.
143. Warnke, R. A. and Rouse, R. V. (1985). *Hum. Pathol.*, **16**, 326.
144. Battifora, H. and Kopinski, M. (1986). *J. Histochem. Cytochem.*, **34**, 1095.
145. Brandtzaeg, P. (1982). In *Techniques in immunocytochemistry* (ed. G. R. Bullock and P. Petrusz), Vol. 1, p. 1. Academic Press, London.
146. Hall, P. A., Stearn, P. M., Butler, M. G., and D'Ardenne, A. J. (1987). *Histopathology*, **11**, 93.
147. Bradding, P., Feather, I. H., Wilson, S., Bardin, P. G., Heusser, C. H., Holgate, S. T., *et al.* (1993). *J. Immunol.*, **151**, 3853.
148. Anderson, J., Abrams, J., Björk, L., Funa, K., Litton, M., and Ågren, K. (1994). *Immunology*, **83**, 16.
149. Brandtzaeg, P. (1981). *J. Histochem. Cytochem.*, **29**, 1302.
150. Wood, G. W. and Travers, H. (1982). *J. Histochem. Cytochem.*, **30**, 1015.
151. Warnke, R. A., Bindl, J., and Doggett, R. (1983). *Histochem. J.*, **15**, 637.
152. Pankow, M. L., Davism, L. E., Becker, S. P., Ossoff, R. H., and Anderson, B. E. (1984). *J. Histochem. Cytochem.*, **32**, 771.
153. Halstensen, T. S., Mollnes, T. E., Garred, P., Fausa, O., and Brandtzaeg, P. (1990). *Gastroenterology*, **98**, 1264.
154. Brandtzaeg, P. (1995). *J. Pathol.*, **177**, 439.
155. Peränen, J., Rikkonen, M., and Kääriäinen, L. (1993). *J. Histochem. Cytochem.*, **41**, 447.
156. Shi, S.-R., Key, M. E., and Kalra, K. L. (1991). *J. Histochem. Cytochem.*, **39**, 741.
157. Boon, M. E. and Kok, L. P. (1989). *Microwave cookbook of pathology. The art of microscopic visualization*, 2nd edn. Leiden: Coulomb Press Leyden.
158. Bankfalvi, A., Navabi, H., Bier, B., Böcker, W., Jasani, B., and Schmid, K. W. (1994). *J. Pathol.*, **174**, 223.
159. Miller, K., Auld, J., Jessup, E., Rhodes, A., and Ashton-Key, M. (1995). *Adv. Anat. Pathol.*, **2**, 60.
160. Shi, S., Imam, S. A., Young, L., Cote, R. J., and Taylor, C. R. (1995). *J. Histochem. Cytochem.*, **43**, 193.
161. Cattoretti, G., Pileri, S., Parravicini, C., Becker, M. H. G., Poggi, S., Bifulco, C., *et al.* (1993). *J. Pathol.*, **171**, 83.
162. Brown, R. W. and Chirala, R. (1995). *Modern Pathol.*, **8**, 515.
163. Merz, H., Malisius, R., Mannweiler, S., Zhou, R., Hartmann, W., Orscheschek, K., *et al.* (1995). *Lab. Invest.*, **73**, 149.
164. Curran, R. C. and Gregory, J. (1978). *J. Clin. Pathol.*, **31**, 974.

165. Valnes, K., Brandtzaeg, P., Hanssen, L. E., Stave, R., Larsen, S., and Londong, W. (1983). *Histochem. J.*, **15**, 1011.
166. Jahnsen, F. L., Farstad, I. N., Aanesen, J. P., and Brandtzaeg, P. (1997). *Am. J. Respir. Crit. Care Med.* (In Press).
167. Bruins, S., De Jong, M. C., Heeres, K., Wilkingson, M. H., Jonkman, M. F., and Van der Meer, J. B. (1995). *J. Histochem. Cytochem.*, **43**, 649.
168. Mullik, H., Henzen-Logmans, S. C., Alons-van Kordelaar, J. J. M., Tadema, T. M., and Meijer, C. J. L. M. (1986). *Cell. Pathol.*, **52**, 55.
169. Butterworth, B. H., Khong, T. Y., Loke, Y. W., and Robertson, W. B. (1985). *J. Histochem. Cytochem.*, **33**, 977.
170. Gerdes, J., Schwarting, R., and Stein, H. (1986). *J. Clin. Pathol.*, **39**, 993.
171. Falini, B., Abdulaziz, Z., Gerdes, J., Canino, S., Ciani, C., Cordell, J. L., *et al.* (1986). *J. Immunol. Meth*ods, **93**, 265.
172. Gown, A. M., Garcia, R., Ferguson, M., Yamanaka, E., and Tippens, D. (1986). *J. Histochem. Cytochem.*, **34**, 403.
173. Petrusz, P., Ordronneau, P., and Finley, J. C. W. (1980). *Histochem. J.*, **12**, 333.
174. Ghosh, S. and Campbell, A. M. (1986). *Immunol. Today*, **7**, 217.
175. Zola, H. (1985). *Pathology*, **17**, 53.
176. Heyderman, E. (1979). *J. Clin. Pathol.*, **32**, 971.
177. Houser, C. R., Barber, R. P., Crawford, G. D., Matthews, D. A., Phelps, P. E., Salvaterra, P. M., *et al.* (1984). *J. Histochem. Cytochem.*, **32**, 395.
178. Itoh, G., Miura, S., and Suzuki, I. (1977). *J. Histochem. Cytochem.*, **25**, 252.
179. Omata, M., Liew, C.-T., Ashcavai, M., and Peters, R. L. (1980). *Am. J. Clin. Pathol.*, **73**, 626.
180. Sim, J. S. and French, S. W. (1976). *Arch. Pathol. Lab. Med.*, **100**, 550.
181. Pouplard, A., Bottazzo, G.-F., Doniach, D., and Roitt, I. M. (1976). *Nature*, **261**, 142.
182. Buffa, R., Crivelli, O., Fiocca, R., Fontana, P., and Solcia, E. (1979). *Histochemistry*, **63**, 15.
183. Grube, D. (1980). *Histochemistry*, **66**, 149.
184. Bergroth, V., Reitamo, S., Konttinen, Y. T., and Tolvanen, E. (1982). *Histochemistry*, **73**, 509.
185. Brandtzaeg, P. and Baklien, K. (1976). *Lancet*, **i**, 1297.
186. Childs, G. and Unabia, G. (1982). *J. Histochem. Cytochem.*, **30**, 713.
187. Hsu, S.-M., Cossman, J., and Jaffe, E. S. (1983). *Am. J. Clin. Pathol.*, **80**, 429.
188. Valnes, K. and Brandtzaeg, P. (1981). *J. Histochem. Cytochem.*, **29**, 595.
189. Johnston, N. W. and Bienenstock, J. (1974). *J. Immunol. Methods*, **4**, 189.
190. Loraine, J. A. and Bell, E. T. (1976). *Hormone assays and their clinical applications.* Churchill Livingstone, Edinburgh, London, and New York.
191. Halstensen, T. S., Scott, H., Fausa, O., and Brandtzaeg, P. (1993). *Scand. J. Immunol.*, **38**, 581.
192. Nagata, S., Yamashiro, Y., Maeda, M., Ohtsuka, Y., and Yabuta, K. (1993). *Pediatr. Res.*, **33**, 557.
193. Seligman, A. M., Shannon, W. A., Hoshino, Y., and Plapinger, R. E. (1973). *J. Histochem. Cytochem.*, **21**, 756.
194. Courtoy, P. J., Picton, D. H., and Farquhar, M. G. (1983). *J. Histochem. Cytochem.*, **31**, 945.

195. Kett, K., Brandtzaeg, P., Radl, J., and Haaijman, J. J. (1986). *J. Immunol.*, **136**, 3631.
196. Nilssen, D. E., Söderström, R., Brandtzaeg, P., Kett, K., Helgeland, L., Karlsson, G., *et al.* (1991). *Clin. Exp. Immunol.*, **83**, 17.
197. Halstensen, T. S., Farstad, I. N., Scott, H., Fausa, O., and Brandtzaeg, P. (1990). *Immunology*, **71**, 460.
198. Brandtzaeg, P. (1972). *Immunology*, **22**, 177.
199. Valnes, K., Brandtzaeg, P., and Rognum, T. O. (1984). *Histochemistry*, **81**, 313.
200. Borth, R. (1957). In *Vitamins and hormones. Advances in research and application* (ed. R. S. Harris, G. F. Marrian, and K. V. Thimann), Vol. 15. Academic Press Inc., Publishers, New York.
201. Van der Loos, C. M. and Becker, A. E. (1994). *J. Histochem. Cytochem.*, **42**, 289.

5

Confocal laser scanning microscopy

G. D. JOHNSON

1. Introduction

The development of confocal laser scanning microscopy (CLSM) has considerably enhanced the study of biological specimens stained by immunofluorescence (IF) which continues to be the preferred method of immunolabelling in a wide range of applications. These include rapid diagnosis of infection, autoantibody screening, and cell surface (FACS) analysis of leukaemic cells, in addition to the applications in the research field where the unique properties of the method are highly valued. The increasing availability of potent alternative fluorochromes having characteristic spectral features (1) enables different structures to be recognized and analysed for co-localization at appropriate excitation/emission wavelengths—a property not available by other methods of immunostaining, e.g. immunoenzyme staining where minor staining may be masked by coincident strong reactivity. Further extension of the use of IF has been encouraged following advances in the methodology resulting in:

(a) Retardation of fading—long considered to be a major disadvantage (2).
(b) Identification of background structures by counterstaining.
(c) Long-term storage.

The advent of digital imaging eliminated the need for fluorescence microscopy to be essentially a dark-room activity—and also the problem of mentally relating the specific localization of staining obtained with different fluorochromes as observed by the use of alternate filter combinations. CLSM has further improved the potential for analysis by introducing new features to fluorescence microscopy that have considerably enhanced the value of the method as first described in 1950 (3). These include improved definition and 3D analysis in addition to the extensive analytical processes available through a computerized operating system. It should be noted that the basic images that are obtained are on a grey scale: all coloration is achieved by manipulation of the video display to produce pseudo-colour. The aim of this chapter is to document the general features of confocal microscopy—especially in the context of immunology—and to present a practical approach to the methodology in order to enable the reader who is not familiar with the instrumentation to exploit the system to maximum advantage, possibly even in the absence of a dedicated operator. Since the field of confocal microscopy is currently undergoing intensive commercial development in respect of the hardware available—and especially the accompanying software—it is not intended to be a review of the comparative features of the many systems available; nor would it be feasible to cover the many variables in the operating procedures required for different products.

1.1 Principle

In confocal microscopy both illumination and detection are limited to a single point in the specimen by the insertion of pin-hole apertures in the excitation and fluorescence emission light-paths: in-focus light emitted by the fluorochrome therefore passes to the detector but most light from planes above and below the focal plane is excluded and does not contribute to the image. The depth of focus is directly proportional to the diameter of the aperture: in practice this is adjusted to the minimum size commensurate with the fluorescence intensity of the analyte. Sequential scanning of the microscope field then produces a complete image of the field in view. This process results in images that have improved resolution—up to 30% higher lateral resolution—and show a marked reduction in out-of-focus flare. The latter property also has the effect of shortening the apparent depth of the field that is in focus so that it is possible to collect a series of 'optical *xy* sections' in the vertical *z* axis—and from them construct a three-dimensional view of the field, or, by combining the images in a 'projection', view the expression of the analyte throughout the full depth of the structure. Collection of serial optical sections at a fixed increment is facilitated by a motorized control attached to the focusing mechanism of the microscope. The rejection of out-of-focus signals is in contrast with conventional fluorescence microscopy where signal from adjacent structures has a marked effect on the quality of the image obtained. A full description of the technical considerations in the development of the scanning confocal microscope since the principle was first described in 1961 will be found in ref. 4. Lasers having emission wavelength(s) appropriate to the fluorochrome(s) in use provide the high-intensity illumination required for rapid scanning. Alignment of the point of illumination and signal detection is accomplished by the use of epi-illumination microscopy where the objective lens also serves as the condenser for transmitting the fluorescent emission signal to the detector system. The separate images collected from material stained by multiple labelling may be merged to enable precise analysis of coincident/non-coincident expression—a considerable advantage over viewing the preparation by conventional fluorescence microscopy with alternate filter sets. In addition to the possibility of analysing the expression of as many as three independent fluorescent signals with appropriate laser excitation, merged images can be produced to combine fluorescent analysis with reflection, e.g. gold labelling, or with transmitted (non-confocal) phase-contrast imaging. Commercial development of these principles has resulted in the availability of confocal operating systems differing in electromechanical design, comparative details of which would not be appropriate for discussion in this chapter.

2. Practical considerations relating to the equipment

The basic set-up, in addition to the laser light source and confocal scanning mechanism, includes a fluorescence microscope, focusing motor, VDU monitor for viewing the image produced, a second VDU for monitoring the computer operation, and other items listed below.

2.1 Microscope specification

A standard fluorescence microscope—upright or inverted configuration depending on the types of application proposed—may be incorporated in a confocal laser scanning system subject to the following requirements:-

(a) Incident (epi-)illumination.

(b) Incorporation of a 100% switch-over mechanism separating the viewing eye-piece assembly from the laser pathway—essential in order to prevent accidental laser entry to the visual field.

(c) Rotating stage—useful for orientating the field at the optimum angle for the object of interest to match the screen format.

(d) Independent coarse and fine focusing controls.

(e) Objective lenses having high numerical apertures, e.g. × 40 numerical aperture 0.9; × 16 numerical aperture 0.4—the enhanced light transmission enables the confocal aperture to be minimized, thus reducing the effective depth of focus—and spatial resolution is increased, with consequent improvement in image quality, while maintaining an adequate signal level.

2.2 Supplementary equipment

The following items should be included in a complete CLSM operating system:-

(a) Camera—reproduction of the images in colour may be obtained by on-line transfer systems to:- an instant printer: output from this is generally adequate for note-book records; a high-definition screen linked to a standard-format 35 mm camera. Colour transparency film provides the best quality hard-copy for projection and print enlargements—which are actually better in appearance than the original screen image.

(b) Image archive—the total digital information contained in a single full-screen image file occupies a substantial amount of computer memory, e.g. 384 Kbytes, which is considerably increased if multiple images are collected, say a *z*-series comprising 10–20 images. Long-term storage of images is essential for subsequent processing, photographic recording, and direct comparison with new findings, and a suitable archiving system may be incorporated either as an internal or external option. High density removable cartridge drives installed in early equipment have now been superseded by high capacity rewritable optical disk drives capable of using up to 230 Mb media.

(c) Data printer—the large amount of quantitative data generated by the image analysis software may be accessed by means of the 'Print Screen' facility connected to a standard external printer.

2.3 Operating adjustments

Different commercial CLSM systems will obviously vary in detail regarding their operational procedure. The following list includes common adjustments and settings that are standard requirements for routine imaging and should be carried out prior to every imaging session. Although standard test slides are available, e.g. comprising fluorochrome-stained tissue paper, in practice the best settings are obtained on a sample slide from the current test series that shows (preferably) moderate positivity.

(a) Selection of filter set(s) appropriate to the fluorochrome(s) and the laser employed (v.infra).

(b) Laser aperture pin-hole size—minimized as described above.

(c) Neutral density filter—maximized to reduce the damaging effect of the laser on the sample.

(d) Axial alignment of the laser—this should be checked at each session and any variation in the correspondence of fields obtained with different filter set-ups should always be corrected.

(e) Adjustment of photomultiplier gain and background settings. These are especially important when a comparison of relative intensity is to be made between different samples imaged under the same conditions. The optimum settings are determined on test samples showing maximum positivity and negative control background. This is facilitated by use of a colour-banding 'look-up table' (lut) where peak intensity, i.e. maximum staining is adjusted to 100% (computer value = 255) in one colour, and the negative background is set at 10–20% of maximum in a second colour.

(f) Zoom control. The possibility of increasing the effective microscope magnification by a variable factor up to10 × enables the object of interest to be accommodated optimally in the image field by use of a low power objective lens. It should be noted that the image obtained in this way contains maximum information—in contrast with application of the zoom command to a pre-existing image which produces 'empty' magnification. It will be apparent that with a high power immersion objective lens the possible final magnification is outside the range of conventional light microscopy. However, the dramatic fading of fluorescence (even in the presence of anti-fading agent) that results from focusing the laser energy on a very small area of the specimen imposes a practical limit on the zoom factor.

(g) Incremental step adjustment of focus control. When collecting a series of *xy* images in the *z* axis by use of the motorized focus control the increment is determined by the thickness of the specimen and the number of images required. Thus ten images to encompass the full thickness of a single cell 5 μm thick would be collected at 0.5 μm increments. The actual path-length is determined by trial-and-error adjustment of the incremental factor prior to setting-up the *z*-series command. It should be noted that the type of sample preparation employed has a significant effect on the perceived depth of objects: thus cells stained in suspension and attached to adherent slides without drying may appear as spherical 'balls' and appropriate for three-dimensional analysis—in contrast with cytocentrifuge preparations in which the cells are transformed into flattened discs, thus compressing the information available in the vertical axis.

(h) Scanning rate setting. This variable will generally be determined by the configuration of the individual system, with a default setting for the image collection mode. However when setting-up the system on a specimen it is convenient to select a high scanning rate in order to see the effect of small adjustments to the various settings on the image observed.

(i) Selection of electronic noise filter and number of scans. Various methods are available for eliminating irrelevant background interference attributable to electronic noise in the system. A very satisfactory result is obtainable with the Kalman-type filter which accumulates coincident (i.e. relevant) signals present in consecutive scans and discards non-coincident random noise. The minimum number of scans required is determined by the intensity of the staining in the specimen and the efficiency of the laser in exciting fluorescence—which together determine the photomultiplier gain setting. Test imaging generally establishes that five to ten scans are optimal: excessive scanning should be avoided because of the high risk of bleaching, especially at high magnification.

(j) Image format. The standard video full screen format may not be appropriate for a particular subject and a useful alternative may be to collect the image in a (smaller) horizontal, vertical, or square format. This provides further advantages: scanning time is shortened so that multiple serial images (as in a long z-series) are captured more quickly, and less computer disk space is required for storage. Precise image centration in the selected format may be accomplished by 'panning' the image with built-in controls: this is preferable to attempting slight adjustment of the slide location by means of the microscope stage controls.

(k) Microscope objective magnification. Although not an essential adjustment *per se* it is useful to record the lens magnification factor with the image data at the time of collection. This ensures that subsequent computerized image analysis based on linear/area measurements will be calculated with the appropriate scale factor.

3. Application of CLSM in immunological studies

The confocal microscope provides many advantages over conventional microscopy for the study of biological specimens stained by immunofluorescence.

3.1 Improved definition

The loss of out-of-focus flare and enhanced lateral space resolution facilitate the identification of sites of immunoreactivity in complex tissue sections, and especially in single cell analysis enable discrete areas of staining to be identified and related to adjoining structures. Thus immunological features of cell aggregates which develop in *in vitro* culture experiments, identifiable by their reactivity with specific antibody, can be studied in detail—especially the molecules associated with cell–cell recognition/interaction, e.g. adhesion molecules on leucocytes in relation to adjacent endothelial cells. The thinness of the optical section comprising a single image permits precise localization of the site of immunoreactivity on or in an individual cell by focusing on the point of interest, fluorescence emissions excited by the illuminating light in adjacent optical planes being effectively de-focused and excluded. Image quality is further enhanced by the significant improvement of around 30% in lateral resolution (5) and, as described above, a selected area of the overall image—which may have been collected with a zoom factor up to 10 ×—may be further magnified. This is particularly informative when fluorescence intensity is colour-banded as described below. At low power microscope magnification—× 10/16 objective and minimum zoom—a relatively large area, e.g. comprising a complete germinal centre in a tonsil section, may be imaged for quantitative analysis as described below (6): it is then essential to ensure that the centration of the excitation light is optimized in order to obtain even illumination. At high objective magnification as used for analysis at the single cell level (× 40 or higher) the use of a water—or non-fluorescent oil—immersion lens produces an impressive enhancement of image quality.

3.2 Image intensity enhancement

Immunofluorescent staining that is demonstrable by conventional fluorescence microscopy without difficulty produces the best results by CLSM which should not be expected to compensate for inadequately stained preparations. However it is possible to image lower levels of staining by enlargement of the laser aperture pin-hole, reduction of the density of the neutral filter, and increase in the photomultiplier gain. It should be noted that these adjustments will require appropriate compensation of the background setting in order to optimize the image. In some systems a fast photon-counting mode is available that produces higher quality images at low levels of staining than are obtainable in the normal operating mode. The identification of low intensity staining in the recorded image may be achieved by adjustment of the 'ramp parameters' so that peak intensity is set at a lower value than the computer standard of 255: in this way the apparent intensity may be enhanced up to tenfold but the threshold setting will require compensation to obtain a satisfactory background level. An ingenious method of viewing the image in order to visualize minimal levels of staining is the application of a 'look-up table' in which different levels of staining at the bottom of the intensity scale are identified in different colours. Such computerized manipulation of the video display by pseudo-colour plays an important role in obtaining maximum information from the grey-scale images produced by CLSM, and is further discussed below.

3.3 Optical sectioning and 3D reconstruction

The effective short depth-of-focus combined with loss of out-of-focus flare enables multiple optical sections in the *xy* plane of a complex tissue or even a single cell to be collected in the *z* axis. The focusing may either be performed manually, or by means of a computer-operated motorized attachment to the microscope focus control set at a predetermined increment which may be as small as 0.1 μm. Such analysis in the third dimension is a major factor in distinguishing CLSM from other image-analysis systems that are based on conventional fluorescence microscopy. The collection of images comprising the *z*-series may be processed in several ways:-

(a) Individual optical sections may be separately analysed in order to assess the staining at different levels in the vertical axis.

(b) Sequential display reveals the characteristic distribution of surface-associated antigen—e.g. IgG on the surface of a small lymphocyte—which is easily distinguishable from the appearance of intracellular antigen—e.g. CD21 in a follicular dendritic cell (*Figure 1*).

(c) A combination of all the images, retaining the maximum signal of each image without any offset, produces a 'projection' that is useful for

a

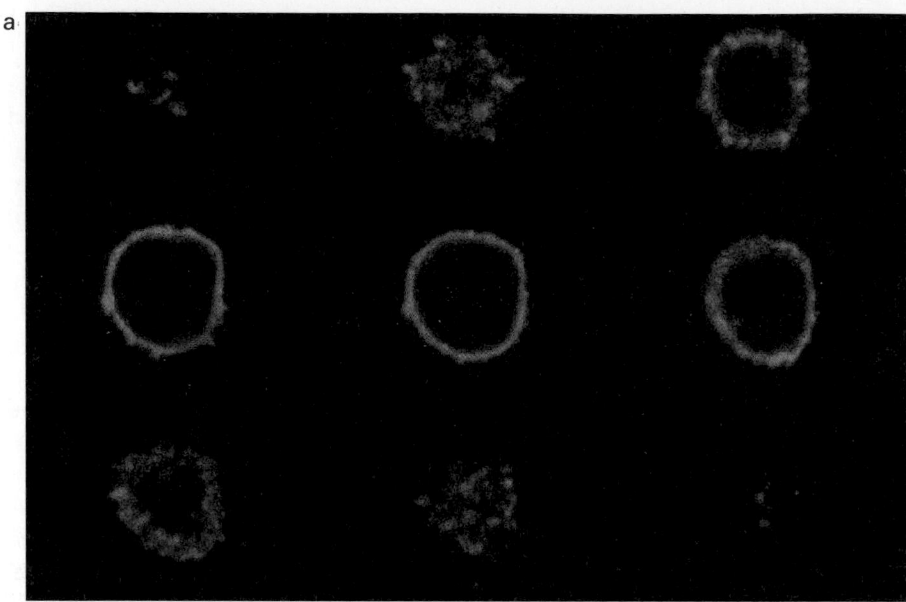

b

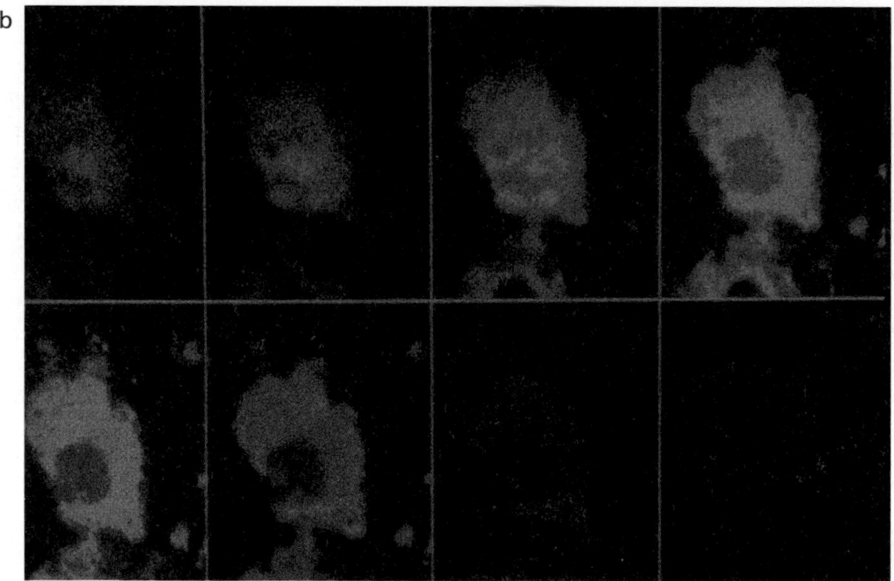

Figure 1. (a) Series of nine optical sections collected at 0.5 μm increments in the *z* axis of a single lymphocyte, showing the characteristic display of surface immunoglobulin. (b) *z*-series (eight images) collected as in (a), showing intracytoplasmic CD21 antigen in a follicular dendritic cell. Images were collected on a Bio-Rad 600 fitted with a krypton-argon laser at a microscope magnification of × 400.

revealing the presence of all features having a short vertical depth, e.g. centromeres in a chromosome analysis. When viewed with offset images various forms of 3D display are possible, including stereo-anaglyphs which give a three-dimensional picture when viewed with appropriate viewing equipment. Further processing can be employed to produce animated rotating images that may be useful in the study of cellular processes, for example in applications relating to neurons. Three-dimensional imaging is regarded as a major feature of confocal microscopy especially in certain fields outside immunology and the reader will find more detailed consideration of this topic in ref. 7.

(d) The attribute that is undoubtedly unique to CLSM is the ability to construct an *xy* view at any point in the *y* axis from the total information contained in the *z*-series. This is equivalent to viewing the preparation at the level of the front of the microscope stage, and enables features of the immunological staining to be analysed in the vertical plane, including information resulting from multiple staining. This has proved to be of great value, for example in studies of adhesion phenomena and when it is required to determine whether a particular structure is overlying another: in *Figure 2* the *xz* view establishes that the cell identified as a follicular dendritic cell by its reactivity with the FDC-specific mAb BU-10 does not have a cell overlying it.

3.4 Multichannel analysis

The ability to obtain separate images of the same microscope field in order to identify the sites of immunoreactivity detected with different fluorochromes and then merge the images to analyse the degree of co-localization is a major advantage of CLSM over conventional fluorescence microscopy. Detection of immunogold labelling may also be achieved in the confocal mode with a reflector filter system. A further option is the use of a transmitted light pathway that provides a non-confocal image useful for demonstrating structures, e.g. as observed by phase-contrast microscopy, which may then be merged with images produced by immunofluorescence. The analysis of merged (appropriately colour coded) images is clearly more efficient than separately viewing the field with alternate filter systems by normal microscopy, and various CLSM configurations are now available for the detection of separate signals. Since the seminal paper of Coons and Kaplan in 1950 (3) fluorescein in different forms (but especially as the isothiocyanate) has continued to be the preferred label: the possibility of overcoming its photosensitivity (which would have presented a serious problem with laser excitation) by the simple expedient of adding an anti-fading agent, e.g. 1,4-diazabicyclo-(2,2,2)-octane (Dabco) (2) to the mountant, and recognition of its pH-dependence (8.6 optimum) have contributed to its continued usefulness as the principle immunological marker in CLSM. Many new alternative dyes with different emission

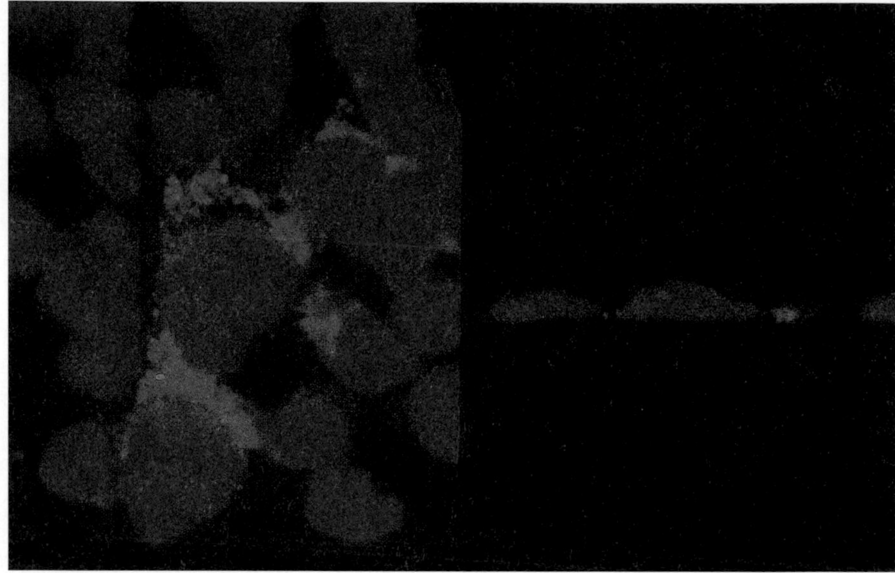

Figure 2. *Left*: standard *xy* view of tonsil cells showing a follicular dendritic cell identified with BU-10 mAb (green) and nuclei in red. *Right*: *xz* view confirming that there is no cell overlying the nucleus of the dendritic cell. Images were collected on a Bio-Rad 600 fitted with a krypton-argon laser at a microscope magnification of × 400.

characteristics are now available, their fluorescence extending over the entire range of the visible spectrum. It must be stressed that the development of technology to exploit these signals is directly attributable to the ability of the optical coating industry to produce precisely tailored filter systems—dichroic mirrors, primary and secondary filters—matching the spectral characteristics of the fluorochromes, and of the laser excitation lines now available.

The argon ion laser provides two excitation wavelengths—488 nm appropriate for fluorescein, and a second line at 514 nm which provides a suitable compromise for simultaneous (two channel) imaging of fluorescein and dyes emitting in the mid-red range, especially Texas Red™ and Cy3™. However it should be noted that excitation of rhodamine compounds (peak absorbance 555 nm) is poor at this wavelength. When the 514 nm line of the argon ion laser is employed for dual imaging of FITC and a red label the red secondary emission of the fluorescein image may be detected in the red channel together with the specific red signal. The strength of this 'cross-talk' due to the inevitable red component of the FITC fluorescence image is directly related to:

(a) The efficiency of excitation, and the intensity of the fluorescein signal.
(b) The photomultiplier gain employed to image the specific red fluorochrome.

It follows that cross-talk will be high when specific red fluorescence is low, necessitating a high gain setting. This situation also applies in dual FACS analysis where the inappropriate red signal from fluorescein is gated-out by establishing a threshold above which specific red fluorescence is identified. The problem of cross-talk is dealt with in CLSM analysis by use of the image-subtract facility as follows: having determined the optimal gain settings for both channels a control preparation stained only with fluorescein is imaged in both channels. The relative intensity of positive staining—high in the green, low in the red—is measured (see below) and the ratio determined. When it is desired to correct the red image from a double-stained preparation obtained *under the same gain settings as the control* the specific red image is produced by subtraction of the appropriate proportion of the green image. Having produced a suitable pair of images they may be combined—'merged'—to study their relative localization. When it is necessary to verify co-localization in discrete areas it may be useful to apply a re-alignment command in order to displace the overlying images by one or two pixels.

Co-localization may also be demonstrated by adding the third screen colour (blue) to the red-green image: this has the effect of identifying double-stained areas in white, provided the intensity of the red image is comparable to that of the green (*Figure 3*).

The krypton-argon laser provides three excitation wavelengths—488, 568, and 647 nm. This permits the separate excitation of fluorescein and a mid-red dye, thus avoiding the cross-talk problem described above. The third line at 647 nm is very close to the absorbance maximum (650 nm) of the far-red fluorochromes Allophycocyanin™ and Indocarbocyanine™ which offer the possibility of a third specific immunological signal: although their emission is near the limit of the retinal sensitivity these dyes produce a very potent signal, Indocarbocyanine™ being the more stable when exposed to the laser energy. When a merged image is produced by combining images from all three channels the third (far-red) signal is identified with the blue pseudo-colour option (*Figure 4*). It should be noted that the point-of-focus in the z axis is a function of the wavelength of the light employed for excitation, and it may therefore be necessary to adjust the focusing for each separate signal in order to obtain correct coincidence of serial images. The possibility of subtracting one image from a coincident image collected in a different channel is especially useful in studies involving translocation of immunological features within a tissue/cell: for example migration of a cellular constituent from the nucleus to the cytoplasm, where the antigen is identified with FITC and nuclei are counterstained with propidium iodide. The total antigen (detected in the green channel) contained in the area occupied by the cell is first quantified as described below. The red image representing the nucleus is then enhanced to an intensity $\sim$ 100% with a ramp threshold of $\sim$ 20% and 'fixed': the threshold adjustment is important in order to avoid enlargement of the nuclear area. Subtraction of the adjusted red image from the green

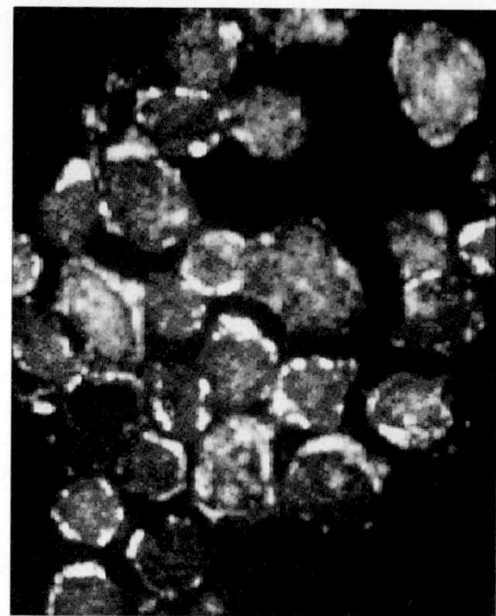

Figure 3. Tonsil cells dual-stained with antibody to bcl-2 (FITC) and mitochondria (T. Red™). Blue pseudo-colour was added to the merged red image so that coincident staining appears white: this demonstrates that the proto-oncogene is not restricted to mitochondria. Images were collected on a Bio-Rad 600 fitted with a krypton-argon laser at a microscope magnification of × 400.

image results in the nuclei being blacked-out so that when measurement of the remaining green image is performed the relative amounts of intra-/extra-nuclear antigen may be determined by comparing the two readings. Clearly, in this example the analysis is best performed on optical sections corresponding—in the *z* axis—to the central plane of the nuclei in the vertical axis. In *Figure 5* the subtraction process is demonstrated on autoantibody showing a perinuclear staining pattern.

3.5 Quantitative image analysis

Immunological features present in samples ranging from single cells to low power views of complex tissue sections may be comprehensively quantified by use of appropriate software programmes. The fluorescence intensity of defined areas ranging from full screen image to a single pixel (the smallest screen area on which data are recorded) may be measured on a scale based on the 0–255 computer range. The area may be selected by use of a default format of predetermined size, or it may be precisely outlined by a cursor drawn on the screen. Intensity of staining may be related to standard linear, area, depth, and volume measurements. The product of mean intensity and

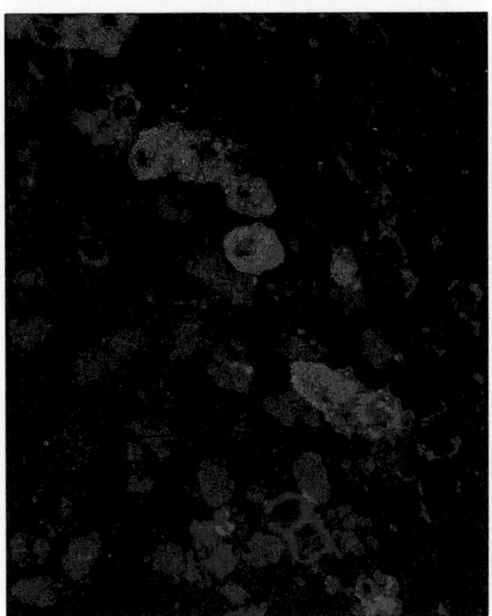

Figure 4. Triple-staining of a tonsil section showing plasma cells in green, nuclear proliferation antigen in red, and activated T cells in blue. Images were collected on a Bio-Rad 600 fitted with a krypton-argon laser at a microscope magnification of × 160.

area provides the 'integrated intensity' value which is a measure of the total amount of analyte in the selected area. The actual processing steps will obviously be determined by the software incorporated in the system which will also include programming for on-screen analysis of the data. Thus intensity may be measured along a defined linear pathway of predetermined width, e.g. across the full diameter of a single cell, and the data displayed as a graph (*Figure 6*); the distribution of pixel intensities in a defined area may similarly be displayed in graphic form.

Probably the most useful process for obtaining an immediate visual analysis of relative intensity of different features in an image is provided by colour-banding, either by the use of built-in 'look-up tables' (LUT) or user-programmed commands to identify specified levels of immunoreactivity (*Figure 7*). Special applications of this very versatile tool include the identification of peak levels in an image by a single colour linked to the top end of the intensity range on a sliding scale, and visualization of unstained structures at the bottom of the intensity scale by differential colour-banding of lowest levels. In *Figure 8* minimal cytoplasmic staining is positively identified—in comparison with the unstained background—in a cell stained with the nuclear counterstain ethidium bromide: lowest intensity levels are shown in

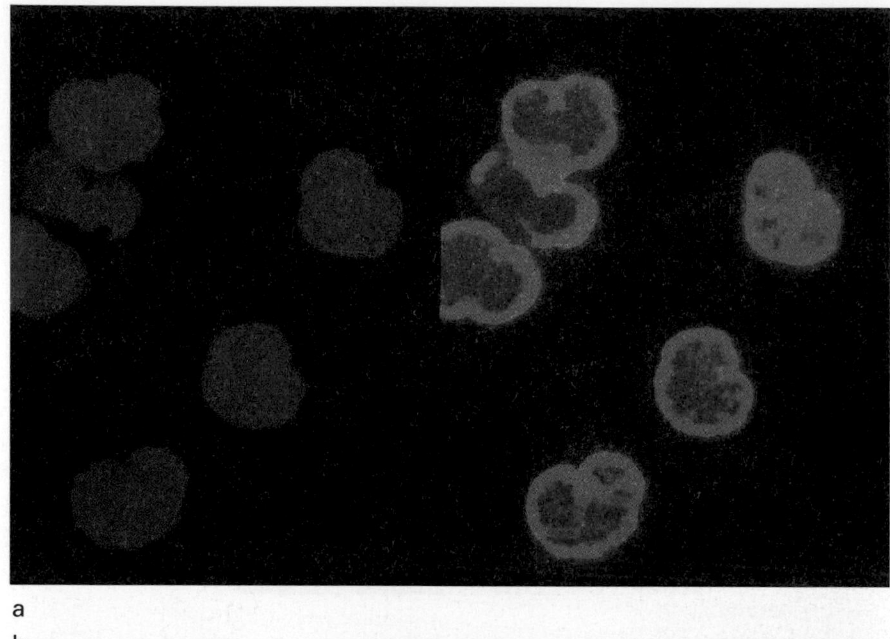
a

b
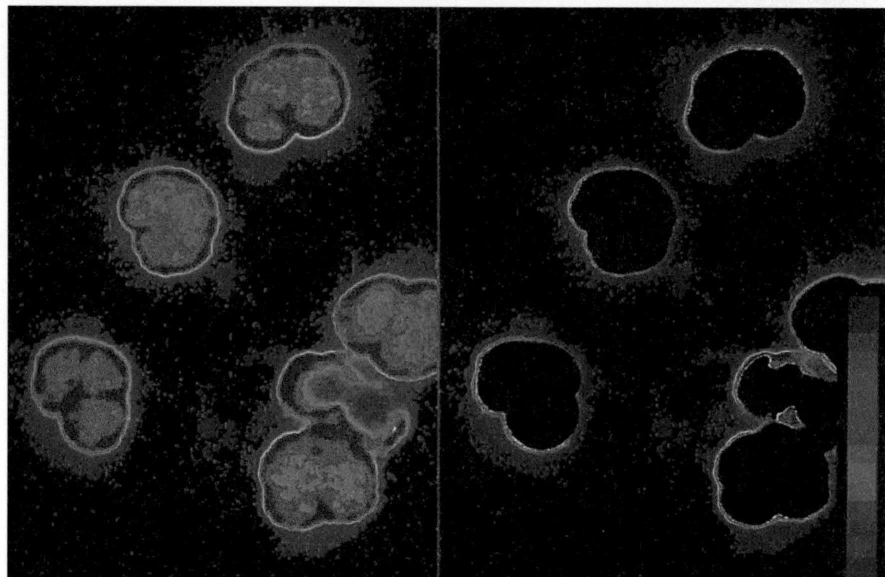

Figure 5. (a) Autoantibody staining of a neutrophil with FITC (*left panel*) counterstained with propidium iodide (*right panel*) to identify the nuclear area. (b) Intensity colour-banded image of the autoantibody staining before (*left*) and after subtraction of the nuclear PI image (*right*). This shows that there is very little extranuclear reactivity. Images were collected on a Bio-Rad 600 fitted with a krypton-argon laser at a microscope magnification of × 400.

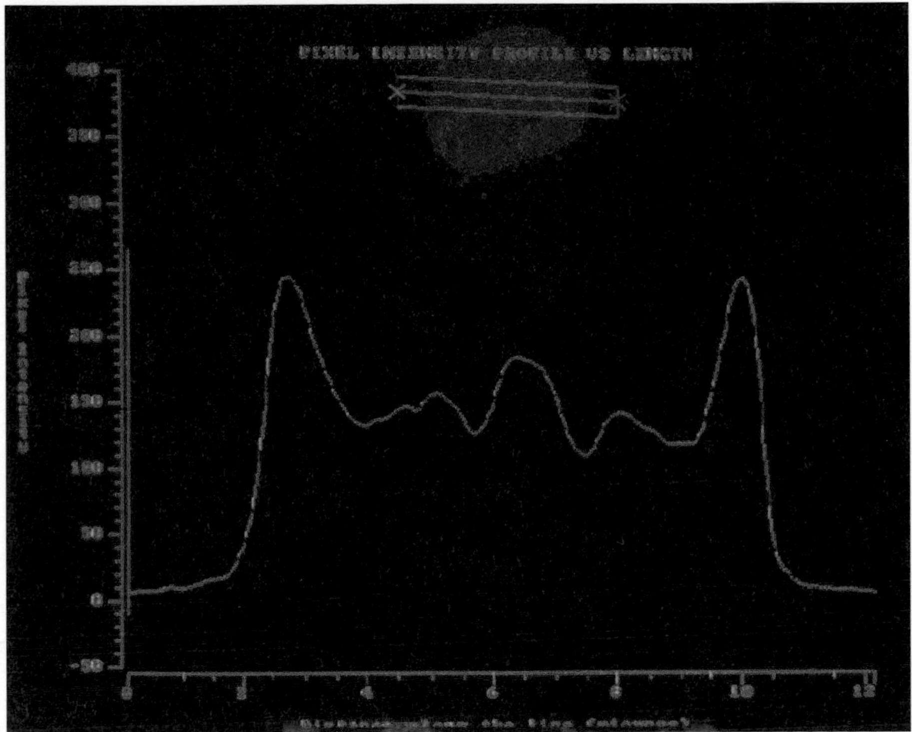

Figure 6. Plot of fluorescence intensity on a linear pathway, ten pixels wide, across a cell stained with the autoantibody shown in *Figure 5*. The total positively-stained area was colour-banded red. Enhanced intensity at the periphery of the nucleus is clearly seen. Images were collected on a Bio-Rad 600 fitted with a krypton-argon laser at a microscope magnification of × 400.

different shades of blue. Adjustment of the 'ramp parameters' produces a detailed visual analysis of the cytoplasmic area.

4. Summary

Image analysis is widely available for producing maximum information from two-dimensional images obtained by all forms of microscopy. When applied to the images produced by CLSM the possibility of exploiting the third dimension in the vertical (z) axis has great potential for studying immunological reactions—through its ability to produce optical sections of the area of interest which show enhanced resolution and lack of out-of-focus flare. This feature is available at all levels of microscope magnification normally employed—including additional zoom factors. It enables an objective view of immunological features to be obtained that is not possible by conventional fluorescence microscopy.

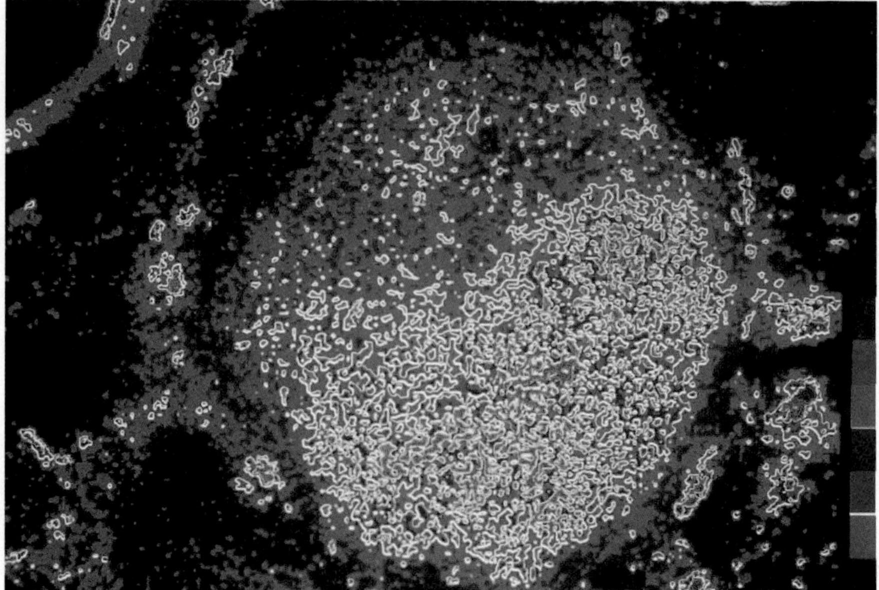

Figure 7. Analysis by intensity colour-banding of the distribution of CD77—Burkitt's lymphoma-associated antigen (BLA)—in a tonsil germinal centre. The antibody shows strongest reactivity with centroblasts in the dark zone, and with endothelial cells in vessels. Images were collected on a Bio-Rad 600 fitted with a krypton-argon laser at a microscope magnification of × 160.

4.1 Future prospects for CLSM in immunology

The continuing development of fluorescent dyes having distinctive spectral characteristics for use as protein labels—and for direct staining of isolated cell populations—calls for parallel development of the equipment employed for analysis, especially for specific discrimination between different signals which may not be present at comparable intensity levels. Video-enhanced light microscopy will clearly play an important role, and CLSM with its ability to generate optical sections of fixed or living tissues—and cell preparations—in which out-of-focus flare is virtually eliminated, enables the most precise analysis to be achieved. This clearly has enormous potential in immunological research for studying the three-dimensional organization of molecules involved in cell–cell interactions and especially the localization/co-localization of multiple macromolecules, e.g. adhesion molecules. The many options available for separately quantifying individual specific analytes in the context of a complex immunological event, combined with the possibility of enhancing the effective magnification of the optical microscope by a factor of 10 × will enable new information to be obtained which could not have been contemplated prior to the advent of CLSM. Areas of research involving antigen–

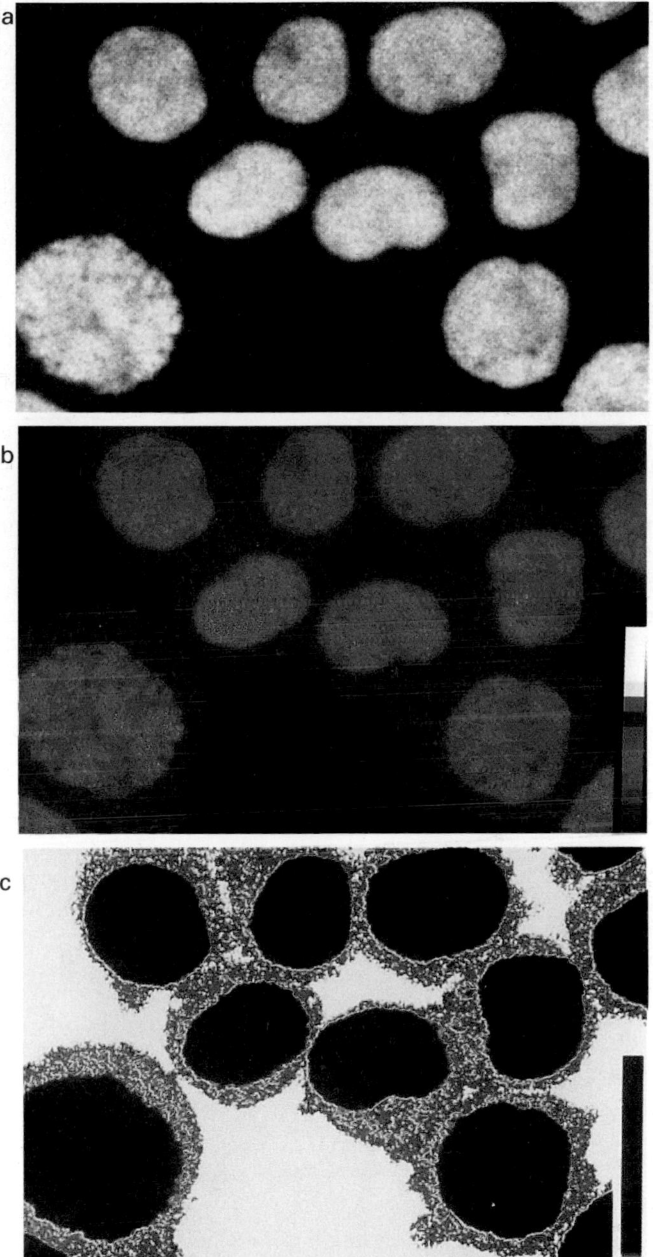

Figure 8. (a) Nuclear DNA stained by propidium iodide—standard grey-scale image. (b) The same image colour-banded to display differential intensity levels at the bottom of the range, revealing the unstained cytoplasm. (c) Adjustment of 'ramp parameters', to show the cytoplasmic structure in detail. Images were collected on a Bio-Rad 600 fitted with a krypton-argon laser at a microscope magnification of $\times$ 400.

antibody interaction(s) which will benefit from the new technology include: cytokine signalling, cell-cycle regulation and programmed cell death, interactions between cells and the extracellular matrix, the involvement of edothelial structures in cellular adhesion, cell signal transduction in relation to kinase pathways, and applications in cytogenetics involving chromosome analysis and fluorescent *in situ* hybridization.

References

1. Haugland, R. P. (1992). *Molecular probes: handbook of fluorescent probes and research chemicals*. Molecular Probes Inc., Eugene, USA.
2. Johnson, G. D., Davidson, R. S., McNamee, K. C., Russell, G., and Holborow, E. J. (1982). *J. Immunol. Methods*, **55**, 231.
3. Coons, A. H. and Kaplan, M. H. (1950). *J. Exp. Med.*, **91**, 1.
4. Shotton, D. M. (1989). *J. Cell Sci.*, **95**, 175.
5. Shotton, D. M. and White, N. (1989). *Trends Biol. Sci.*, **14**, 435.
6. Hardie, D. L., Johnson, G. D., Khan, M., and MacLennan, I. C. M. (1993). *Eur. J. Immunol.*, **23**, 997.
7. Lansing Taylor, D. and Wang, Y.-L. (ed.) (1989). *Methods in cell biology*,Vol. 30, Part B. Academic Press, California.

6

Flow cytofluorimetry

G. DAMGAARD, C. H. NIELSEN, and R. G. Q. LESLIE

1. Introduction

The employment of flow cytofluorimetry (FC) in both qualitative and quantitative investigations of cell phenotype and activity has increased explosively in recent years. The strength of the technique lies in the fact that detailed information is acquired on individual cells passing through the detector system: information which, upon acquisition of data from a predetermined number of cells, can be processed to provide a statistical profile for the cell population, or populations, of interest. Thus FC differs fundamentally from the traditional radiometric approach, which only provides information on the cell population as a whole. In addition, the technique has largely supplanted fluorescence microscopy in the study of single cell suspensions, because it is able to provide quantitative data on much greater numbers of cells very rapidly.

In practical terms, the primary advantages with FC lie in the modest requirement of cells for analysis (measurements can readily be performed with as few as 10^5 cells per sample), and in the fact that purification of particular cell subpopulations prior to analysis is unnecessary. Most of the flow cytometers in current use are capable of registering five parameters on a cell simultaneously; the cell's forward light scatter (FSC) and side light scatter (SSC) characteristics, reflecting the cell's size and granularity, respectively (see *Figure 1*) and the presence, on the cell, of up to three different fluorescent markers with emission peaks at different wavelengths. Thus, it is feasible to quantify a desired parameter (e.g. expression of a particular receptor) on a minor cell subpopulation in a mixed cell preparation, by identifying the cells on the basis of their morphological characteristics and the presence of up to two population-specific markers, and then carrying out the measurement, using an appropriate ligand labelled with a third type of fluorochrome.

The lower limit to the size of a minor cell subpopulation that is required to provide reliable information is dictated statistically. Given that an analysis is typically performed on 10^4 cells, a cell frequency of at least 5% (i.e. 500 cells) can be regarded as a minimum requirement for most purposes. In situations where this requirement is not satisfied, however, the problem can be circumvented if the flow cytometer is equipped with the option of selecting the cell

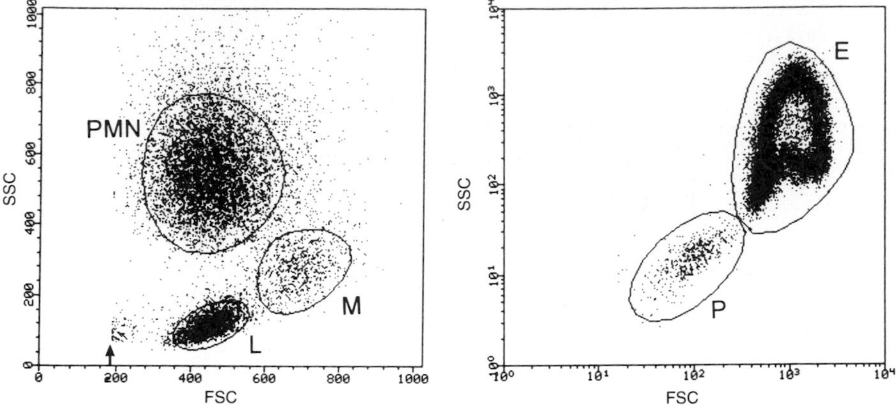

Figure 1. Forward scatter (FSC)/side scatter (SSC) dot plots reflecting size and granularity, respectively, of (*left*) polymorphonuclear leucocytes (PMN), lymphocytes (L), and monocytes (M) from a leucocyte preparation and acquired in linear mode, at a threshold set to exclude debris (vertical arrow), and (*right*) erythrocytes (E) and platelets (P) acquired in logarithmic mode.

subpopulation for analysis under data acquisition (so-called live gating, see *Protocol 1*). This being the case, the operator can then determine the size of the data group, independent of the frequency of the cell subpopulation in the sample under investigation. The live gating approach enables the measurement of cell subpopulations comprising less than 1% of the total sample; if the investigator has sufficient cells, and patience, for the task.

The lack of a need to purify the cells for investigation is advantageous, both in terms of saving labour and of reducing the risk of selecting, during the purification, an inadequately representative subgroup of the cells to be investigated. Furthermore, by virtue of its selective analytical capability, FC provides the possibility for performing studies that are virtually impossible by other means. Thus, it enables the investigator to measure, simultaneously, the expression of a given receptor on several different subpopulations in a complex cell mixture, or to study the individual responses of a variety of cell types to a signal they receive as a mixed cell population. Examples of the application of these approaches to the investigation of whole blood cells will be described later in the chapter.

2. Applications of flow cytofluorimetry

The earliest, and still most widespread, use of FC arises from its origin as a method developed to separate cells on the basis of surface markers (fluorescence activated cell sorting); namely, to provide cell population statistics based on surface phenotype. The massive production, particularly in the 80s, of innumerable monoclonal antibodies recognizing different CD markers on

Table 1. Clinical and research applications of flow cytofluorimetry

Primarily clinical

1. Determination of cell subpopulations on the basis of surface marker expression
2. Measurement of DNA content in malignant cells (ploidity determination)

Primarily research

3. Quantification of membrane receptors (or other glycoproteins) on cell subpopulations
4. Measurement of intracellular proteins and mRNA
5. Investigation of cellular activation
6. Investigation of cellular replication
7. Measurement of cellular uptake and ingestion of soluble and particulate materials
8. Investigation of phagocyte oxidative processes
9. Measurement of cell-mediated cytotoxicity and apoptosis

human leucocyte subpopulations has ensured the success of FC as the approach of choice in clinical investigations of blood cell population changes in a variety of disorders (e.g. malignancies, immunodeficiencies, autoimmune diseases)—see *Table 1*, point 1. A second approach, which has proved to be of considerable clinical importance, is the measurement of the nuclear DNA content in malignant cells, using the DNA-binding fluorochromes such as propidium iodide (PI), Hoechst 33342 or 4′,6-diamidino-2-phenylindole (DAPI) (*Table 1*, point 2). The application of FC in determining cell polyploidy for diagnostic purposes is now more or less universal. Since these areas of application have already been comprehensively described in numerous texts (see ref. 1, as source material), they will not be discussed further here.

The dramatic advance of FC as an investigative tool in the research laboratory is consequent upon developments of both a conceptual and a material nature. The primary conceptual development has been the realization that FC can provide just as precise data as the more traditional quantitative approaches, such as radioassays, with the additional advantages inherent in a method that provides information at a single cell level (see Section 1). This realization, in turn, has prompted the production of more advanced software for FC analysis. As a result, the use of FC in both quantitative and qualitative analysis of membrane-bound and intracellular proteins and, more recently, mRNA species, is now widespread (*Table 1*, points 3 and 4).

Credit for recent progress on the material front can largely be placed in the hands of the organic chemists, who have provided the investigator with an arsenal of fluorescent probes to measure an ever growing range of molecular species found within living cells. In addition to more suitable conjugatable fluorochromes for triple colour analysis at a single excitation wavelength, fluorochromes capable of registering cell membrane potential, intracellular pH, Na^{+} concentration, Ca^{2+} ion mobilization, lysosomal proton pump activity, protease activity, glutathione content, superoxide anion synthesis, and even cell division are now commercially available (*Table 1*, points 5, 6, and 8) (reviewed in ref. 2). Finally, it may be said that the investigator's fantasy has also played a vital role in devising evermore sophisticated and discriminatory procedures for investigating a variety of cell activities, such as phagocytosis, cell-mediated cytoxicity, and programmed cellular self-destruction (apoptosis) (*Table 1*, points 7 and 9).

The limitations of space do not permit a comprehensive description of all the above-mentioned applications of FC to research. It is the authors' intention, therefore, to focus on a few applications, with the purpose of illustrating the potential that lies in the FC approach.

3. Investigation of membrane glycoprotein expression and molecular interactions at the cell surface

The flow cytometer is an instrument fundamentally suited to quantitative analysis; in the sense that the size of the fluorescence signal it registers is directly related to the amount of light emitted by a cell upon passage through the excitatory laser beam. However, the application of FC to quantification of cell surface proteins has, until relatively recently, been hampered by a number of problems of both a physico-chemical and a technical nature, with the result that the potential of FC for this purpose remains comparatively unexplored.

3.1 Quenching and pH dependence

The major problems encountered at the chemical level are the pH dependence of the emission spectra for the fluorochromes employed and quenching. The latter complication arises when the fluorochrome comes into intimate (e.g. covalent) contact with another molecular species; for example, when it is coupled to a probing antibody. A proportion of the light emitted by the coupled fluorochrome is lost in the form of energy transfer to the associated protein, with the result that its specific fluorescent activity is diminished, compared to the free fluorochrome. For the most commonly employed fluorochrome, fluorescein isothiocyanate (FITC), quenching of 50% or more may be observed, depending on the nature of the conjugating protein and the fluorochrome : protein coupling ratio (3).

The problem of quenching can, however, be overcome relatively easily. The specific activity of the fluorescent protein conjugates, relative to the free fluorochrome, can be measured by spectrofluorimetry or, as an acceptable approximation, the specific activity can be estimated from the fluorochrome : protein (F/P) molar ratio, using a fluorescence quenching curve determined for a related protein (see *Protocol 1* and ref. 4).

The issue of pH dependence is discussed later in the chapter (see Section 7.3).

3.2 Calibration

Technically speaking, the primary obstacles to be faced are the lack of standardization between the various types of flow cytometers on the market, and the fact that the absolute magnitude of the signal registered is almost infinitely variable through adjustment of the photomultiplier tube (PMT) voltage.

These obstacles are overcome by calibrating the flow cytometer with fluorochrome-coupled particles, such as latex beads, capable of providing constant well-defined signals. Two types of calibration beads are available: beads bearing different known amounts of fluorochrome (defined in terms of soluble fluorochrome equivalents, SFE), and beads bearing a predetermined

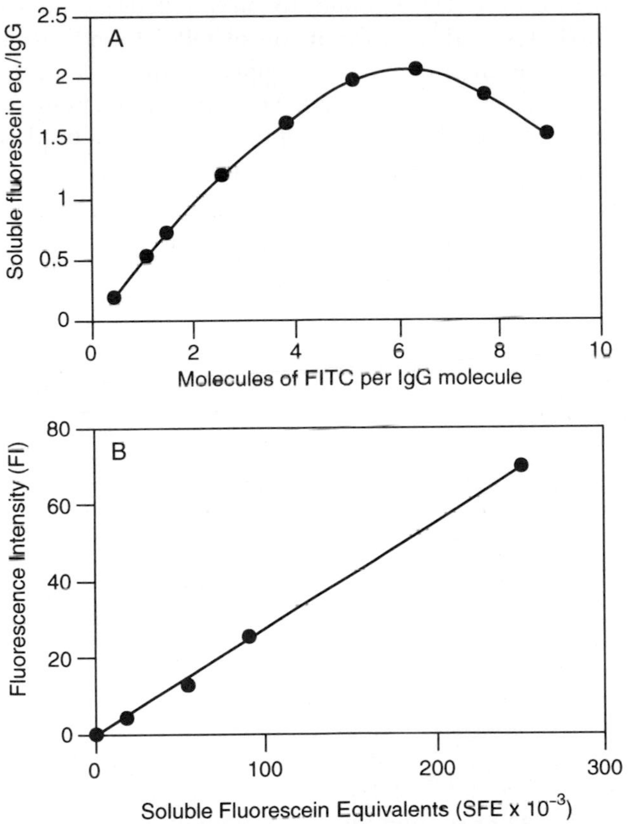

Figure 2. (A) Calibration curve for determining the specific fluorescence activity of FITC-conjugated IgG from the molar FITC : protein ratio of the conjugate (from ref. 4). (B) Calibration curve for converting the FCs arbitrary fluorescence intensity (FI) units to soluble fluorescein equivalents (SFE). These curves are used in *Protocol 1*, part A and D, respectively.

number of antibody molecules reactive with the fluorochrome-conjugated probe employed in the investigation. Both types of calibration beads are commercially available (from Flow Cytometry Standards). It is worth noting that the advantage with the fluorescent beads lies in the direct nature of the calibration and their applicability with an essentially unlimited range of correspondingly conjugated proteins, while the antibody-coated beads, though limited in use to conjugates containing the appropriate antigens, are unrestricted in terms of the type of fluorochrome employed.

3.3 Measurement of a membrane glycoprotein on blood leucocytes

In *Protocol 1*, the quantification of a membrane component, CD35, on B cells in a whole blood preparation is described. CD35, the receptor for complement fragment C3b (CR1), is found, to varying degrees, on all blood cells, including erythrocytes, and the proportion of CR1, found on the B cells in whole blood, is in the order of 0.1% (or approximately 2% of the leucocyte-borne CR1) (unpublished observations). The purpose of *Protocol 1* is to illustrate how live gating on the B cell population can be used to acquire a reliable estimate of CR1 expression on these cells.

Protocol 1. Determining the number of CR1 expressed on peripheral blood B cells

Equipment and reagents

- Fluorescein isothiocyanate (FITC) (Sigma), prepared as a 10 mg/ml solution (normally 100 μl) in conjugation buffer (see below)
- Murine monoclonal anti-CR1 antibody (HB8592, IgG1, ATCC) purified from the culture supernatant by affinity chromatography on protein G–Sepharose (Pharmacia)
- Murine IgG1 (Coulter Clone)
- Human IgG (Kabi)—to block Fc receptor-mediated binding
- Sheath fluid (Becton Dickinson)
- Phycoerythrin (R-PE)-conjugated murine anti-CD19 (Leu 12) (Becton Dickinson)
- Conjugation buffer: 0.225 M $NaHCO_3$, 0.025 M Na_2CO_3, 0.14 M NaCl pH 9.0
- Lysis buffer (10 × stock solution): 1.68 M NH_4Cl, 0.1 M $NaHCO_3$, 1 mM tetrasodium EDTA pH 7.3—the working dilution is prepared just before use
- Assay buffer (PBS/BSA): phosphate-buffered saline (PBS) pH 7.4, containing 0.5% (w/v) bovine serum albumin (BSA)
- Fluorescence calibration beads (Quantum 24, Flow Cytometry Standards)
- Flow cytometer (FACScan with Lysis 2 software, Becton Dickinson)

A. FITC labelling of HB8592 and murine IgG1, and determination of the specific fluorescence of the conjugates

1. Incubate HB8592 or murine IgG1 (1–5 mg/ml), equilibrated with conjugation buffer, with FITC (0.04 mg FITC per mg protein) for 4 h at room temperature in the dark with rotational mixing.
2. Dialyse the conjugates against two changes of PBS and then measure their absorbance at 276 nm and 493 nm.

3. Determine the protein concentrations and molar ratios of FITC : protein from these absorbance values using the following formulae:
   (a) $[IgG] = 0.714(A_{276} - 0.367 \times A_{493})/150\,000$ M.
   (b) $[FITC] = (6.5 \times 10^{-3} \times A_{493})/389$ M.
   (c) F/P ratio = [FITC]/[IgG].
4. The specific fluorescent activity (measured as soluble fluorescein equivalents, SFE, per antibody molecule) may be determined spectrofluorimetrically using FITC–lysine as standard and excitation and detection wavelengths of 493 nm and 520 nm, respectively, or by reference to the calibration curve shown in *Figure 2* (4).[a]

B. The assay[b]

1. Wash 1 ml of human blood taken in CPD anticoagulant three times with 10 ml PBS, centrifuging at 400 *g* for 10 min between washes.
2. Suspend the whole blood cells in PBS/BSA to the original blood volume and add 100 μl of the suspension to 100 μl of PBS/BSA containing the FITC-conjugated HB8592 or murine IgG1 (final concentrations = 2 μg/ml), human IgG (5 mg/ml), and the R-PE-conjugated B cell marker, Leu 12 (10 μl).
3. Incubate this mixture in the dark for 2 h at room temperature (or 4 h at 4°C).
4. Wash the cells once with 2 ml of ice-cold PBS/BSA and suspend the pellet (plus approximately 100 μl residual buffer) in 1.4 ml of cold lysis buffer.
5. Incubate on ice for 8 min and harvest the intact leucocytes by centrifugation for 10 min at 400 *g*. Wash the cells once with cold PBS (2 ml)[c] and suspend them in 1 ml sheath fluid.

C. Data acquisition

1. **Ungated.** Acquire data on the whole leucocyte preparation using an excitation wavelength of 488 nm with the FSC and SSC channels in linear mode and two fluorescence channels (FL1—green, 530 nm and FL2—orange, 585 nm) in log mode. Set a threshhold on the FSC channel to exclude small debris from analysis (see *Figure 1*) and acquire data on 10 000 cells.
2. **Live gating.** Set the axes on the dot plot, used to define acquisition conditions, to FL2 (abscissa) and SSC (ordinate). Under 'Setup' mode, acquire data from 2000 cells and draw an acquisition region around the B cells, which are characterized by low SSC and high FL2 (PE-anti CD19) fluorescence (R1 in *Figure 3A*). Acquire data under 'Live Gate' mode on 3000 cells lying within this region.

Protocol 1. *Continued*

D. Analysis

1. (a) **Ungated whole leucocyte population.** Call up an FL2 versus SSC dot plot and an FL1 histogram. The dot plot permits discrimination of four cell subpopulations: polymorphonuclear leucocytes (PMN), monocytes (M), non-B lymphocytes (L), and B cells (B) (see *Figure 3A*). The FL1 histogram displays a complex profile (*Figure 3B*), reflecting the variable expression of CR1 on the different leucocyte subpopulations. By setting a gate on the B cells in the dot plot, a histogram presenting the data on these cells alone can be called up (*Figure 3C*). Note that relatively few events are registered in this manner, reflecting the paucity of B cells in the leucocyte population.
   (b) **Live gated B cells.** Call up an ungated FL1 histogram presenting all the data acquired by live gating on B cells (*Figure 3D*).
2. Using the FCs statistics package, determine the arithmetic mean and the standard deviation for the fluorescence intensities (FI) of the B cells presented in the above-mentioned histograms. Determine the net (specific) FI for the investigated receptors (CR1) by subtracting signal obtained with the control IgG1[d] from that obtained with the specific antibody (HB8592).
3. Using the low level fluorescein calibration beads, bearing known numbers of SFE per bead, convert the mean FI signals for the cells to SFE/cell (*Figure 2B*). By dividing this value with SFE activity of the probing Ab (see part A, step 4), obtain the number of Ab bound per cell (see *Table 2*). This number is stoichiometrically related to the number of epitopes on the cell surface, most frequently in the ratio 1:1.

[a] It is important that the quantifying antibody and isotype control have similar specific activities, and that they are aggregate-free. FITC–IgG preparations should be either gel filtered or ultracentrifuged (100 000 *g* for 1 h) before use, and the protein concentration should be checked after aggregate removal.

[b] It should be noted that the surface expression of certain receptors (e.g. CR1 on monocytes and granulocytes) may be modulated as a consequence of the handling procedures (i.e. changes in temperature, washing, and even centrifugation) (5, and personal observations). It is, therefore most important, when comparing receptor expression on different cell samples, to ensure that the handling conditions are maintained as uniform as possible for all samples.

[c] Since erythrocytes outnumber leucocytes in whole blood by about 500 to 1, they have to be removed from the sample before FC analysis. Removal of erythrocytes, usually by lysis, may be performed either before or after incubation of the blood cells with the detector antibody (or antibodies). The advantage of performing the lytic step at the end of the incubation is that the preparative handling of the cells prior to reaction with the antibodies is reduced to a minimum. However, this has to be weighed against the fact that a certain degree of dissociation of the antibodies may occur during the subsequent lytic and washing steps.

[d] In our experience, the non-specific signal seen with control IgG is often indistinguishable from the autofluorescence of the leucocytes (i.e. the fluorescence signal obtained in the absence of any FITC-conjugated ligand), in which case the use of a fluorescence-matched isotype control may be omitted. However, it is most important to check, with each new antibody probe employed, whether this condition applies.

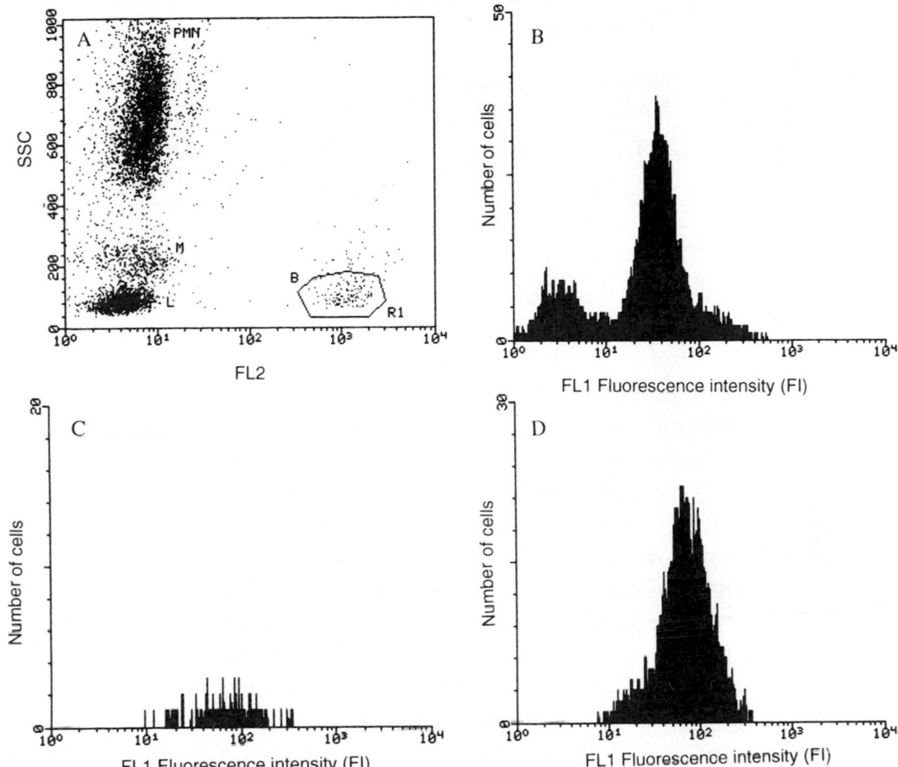

Figure 3. (A) Dot plot showing the side scatter (SSC) and orange fluorescence (FL2) characteristics of the whole leucocyte preparation investigated in *Protocol 1*. Polymorphonuclear leucocytes (PMN), monocytes (M), non-B lymphocytes (L), and B cells (B) appear as distinct populations. The region set for both B cell analysis on the whole leucocyte population and live gating is denoted R1. (B)–(D) FL1 histograms, showing the FITC–anti-CR1 staining of (B) the whole leucocyte population, (C) the B cells obtained from data acquisition on the the whole leucocyte preparation (10 000 cells), and (D) the B cells obtained by live gating during data acquisition (3000 cells).

3.3.1 General comments regarding membrane glycoprotein quantification

The importance of ensuring that the concentration of the probing conjugate is sufficient to achieve **saturation** of the investigated glycoprotein cannot be over-emphasized! Preliminary experiments designed to establish the incubation time required to reach equilibrium binding and the minimum conjugate concentration needed to reach the plateau for specific binding must be performed on each new probe employed.

If binding measurements are performed over a range of subsaturating concentrations, the data can be employed to determine the **binding affinity** of the probe using a modified version of the Scatchard plot (4).

Table 2. Expression of CR1 on B cells

Acquisition mode	Number of B cells	Mean FI (SD)	SFE/B cell[a] (SD)	Anti-CR1 Ab/B cell[b] (SD)
Ungated (MNC)	123	83.1 (64.3)	23 300 (18 000)	14 500 (11 300)
Live gated (B cells)	3000	79.3 (50)	22 200 (14 400)	13 900 (9000)

[a] 1 FI unit = 280 SFE, as determined from *Figure 2B*.
[b] F/P ratio = 3.9 : 1, equivalent to 1.6 SFE/Ab molecule, as determined from *Figure 2A*.

An initially disconcerting observation, with regard to the data provided by FC analysis of membrane proteins, is the **magnitude of the standard deviation (SD)** seen with almost any cell surface component examined (a coefficient of variance of 50% is by no means exceptional!). The high degree of variance is not simply an artefact of the FC approach since homogeneous target particles, such as the calibration beads or cell nuclei examined for DNA content, are registered as highly resolved peaks with low SD values. The most plausible explanation for the large SD is that it reflects heterogeneity in expression of the membrane glycoprotein within the cell population under study.

The choice of probes to quantify membrane components is not necessarily restricted to antibodies specific for the component in question. If the component is a **receptor** and its **ligand** is available as a pure product in sufficient amounts for conjugation, then FC analysis with the fluorochrome-labelled ligand can provide detailed information about the ligand–receptor interaction.

Quantification in absolute terms requires that the specific fluorescent activity of the probe as well as its combinatorial ratio with the investigated membrane component is known. This condition is normally met in studies of ligand–receptor interactions, or when monoclonal antibodies are used as probes. In situations where neither of these conditions is met (e.g. when the only available reagent is an IgG preparation from a polyclonal antiserum) a semi-quantitative estimate is obtainable in terms of the SFE of antibody bound per cell, for a given detection system.

The greatest **precision** in quantitative investigations is achieved using a direct labelling approach—i.e. where the probe itself is coupled to the fluorochrome. In situations where this is impracticable, the problem can be overcome by employing indirect staining (i.e. using a fluorescent secondary antibody) and calibrating the system using standard beads coated with antibodies against the primary probe. In this case, the beads are incubated successively with the primary probe and secondary antibody conjugate in precisely the same way as the cells under investigation.

The **sensitivity** of the system can, in theory, be varied almost infinitely by adjusting the PMT voltage on the fluorochrome detector. However a practical limit is imposed by the signal-to-noise ratio, where the noise level is largely determined by the autofluorescence of the cells under investigation. For cells with a low autofluorescence, such as erythrocytes, receptor numbers as low as a few hundred per cell can be reliably measured.

3.3.2 Applications

Quantitative studies of membrane glycoproteins, using monclonal antibodies as probes, include the C3 fragment-binding complement receptor and regulator proteins (CR1, CR2, DAF, and MCP) (6), MHC class II glycoproteins, the low affinity IgE receptor (CD23), CD3, CD4, CD5, CD8, CD20, CD28, CD38, CD45RA, CD45RO, and CD57 (7), while natural ligand binding studies have been performed on receptors for IgG (4), and IgE (8), as well as receptors for the complement fragment, C5a (9), and the bacterially-related peptide, fMLP (10).

3.4 Investigation of molecular interactions at the cell surface

Although fluorescence quenching is generally regarded as a complicating factor in FC analysis, the phenomenon can be exploited to reveal associations between different membrane glycoproteins. A pair of fluorochromes, chosen so that the emission wavelength of the one (the donor, e.g. FITC) corresponds to the excitation wavelength of the other (the acceptor, e.g. tetramethylrhodamine isothiocyanate, TRITC), may be coupled individually to the probes for two molecules of interest. If the two molecules are found in close steric proximity, energy transfer will occur between the fluorochromes, resulting in quenching of the signal from the donor and an increase in fluorescence of the acceptor. It should be noted, however, that quantitative investigations of this energy transfer require an FC equipped for dual wavelength excitation (i.e. for both the donor and acceptor excitation wavelengths).

3.4.1 Applications

The principle has been applied to study the association of surface molecules such as CD4 with the TCR (11), the low affinity IL-2 receptor with MHC class I molecules (12), and ICAM-1 with the IL-2 receptor and class I and II MHC molecules (13), as well as in the investigation of micronuclei (14) and endosomal fusion events (15).

4. Measurement of intracellular proteins and mRNA

In principle, the approach employed to quantify the expression of cell surface components can equally well be applied to measurement of intracellular components, provided that the cell membranes have been permeabilized to permit entry of the macromolecular fluorescent probes (e.g. antibodies) into the cytoplasm and intracellular organelles. However, to ensure that the cells' integrity is maintained during permeabilization and subsequent handling, fixation of the cells is also necessary.

4.1 Detection of intracellular proteins

The primary technical problems encountered in measuring intracellular proteins using specific antibodies as probes are:

(a) The significantly greater non-specific uptake of the antibodies by the permeabilized cells, as compared to intact cells.

(b) The risk of epitope loss by masking or conformational change during fixation and permeabilization of the cells under study.

4.1.1 Non-specific uptake of the probing antibody

The non-specific uptake can be minimized in two ways. For the first, the binding of the antibody probe to sites other than the cognate antigen can reduced by including serum proteins from the same animal species at high concentration in the incubation mixture. Thus, dilution of the antibody in 50% heat inactivated, delipidated, and 0.2 μm filtered serum in PBS should be suitable for most purposes, although some adjustment of the serum concentration may be required to achieve optimal blocking (16). Secondly, it is important to ensure that the concentration of the probe employed is just sufficient for the purpose of the study, rather than in a 'comfortable' excess. Thus, the lowest concentration required to achieve saturation, or even a concentration that gives an experimentally determined level of subsaturation (e.g. 80% or 90%) is preferable to the employment of supersaturing concentrations. Finally, it is essential in this type of study to include a concentration- and isotype-matched control to determine the non-specific binding contribution which has to be deducted from the signal obtained with the probing antibody.

4.1.2 Epitope loss during fixation

An inevitable consequence of cell fixation is that epitopes containing amino acid residues reactive with the fixing agent are likely to be masked by the procedure. This problem may be somewhat reduced by employing a fixative which forms a mixture of both irreversible and reversible covalent linkages with the cellular proteins (16). Hydrolysis of the latter during the subsequent steps of the staining procedure may thus lead to re-exposure of epitopes on the intracellular target protein. For this reason, formaldehyde, which is reported to form reversible methylene bridge linkages with proteins (17), is frequently employed as a fixative.

4.1.3 Permeabilization and denaturation

Permeabilization may be achieved either with detergents or the lower alcohols (methanol, ethanol). While both types of reagents cause some denaturation of cellular proteins, the degree of denaturation is most pronounced with alcohols, although the damage may be minimized by performing the permeabilization at very low temperatures (−20 to −70 °C). On the other hand, the alcohols, by virtue of their denaturing properties, can lead to dissociation of intracellular complexes, leading to the exposure of hidden epitopes. Thus, while detergent permeabilization may be the method of choice when probing for epitopes known to be dependent on the protein's conformational integrity, alcohol permeabilization may be advantageous in the investigation of non-conformational determinants. The most commonly employed permeabilization procedures involve pre-fixation with formaldehyde followed by treatment with Triton X-100, saponin, lysolecithin, digitonin, or *n*-octyl-β-D-glucopyranoside (18–21) or by treatment with methanol, ethanol, or acetone, either with or without formaldehyde pre-fixation (22–24).

4.1.4 Applications

While the primary focus for intracellular FC studies has been the proteins associated with cell proliferation (e.g. PCNA, Ki67, myc, c-fos, p53, p34cdc2kinase—reviewed in ref. 16), the approach is applicable generally to all intracellular proteins for which specific antibodies are available. The most extensively investigated proteins of immunological interest have been the cytokines, including IFN-γ, IL-2, IL-4, and IL-10 (25–27), although investigations of other proteins, such as complement components (28) and virally-encoded proteins (29), have also been undertaken.

4.2 Measurement of intracellular enzymatic activity

An alternative approach in the study of intracellular proteins is the measurement of enzymatic activity using fluorogenic substrates. For this purpose, the ideal substrate is one which is non-fluorescent, lipophilic, and non-toxic but yields a fluorescent highly polar product upon cleavage by the appropriate enzyme. Thus the substrate should be able to permeate freely into the intact cell while the fluorescent product, by virtue of its polarity, remains efficiently trapped within the cell. Derivatives on both fluorescein and rhodamine 110 have proven to be highly suitable in this regard, while substrates based on the fluorophores naphthol, naphthylamine, quinolines, methylumbelliferone, and monochlorobimane have also been employed.

4.2.1 Applications

Among the enzymes investigated by this approach are the serine- and cysteine-proteases, esterases, lipases, sulfatases, phosphatases, glucoronidases, transferases, peroxidases, glycosidases, and glutathione *S*-transferases. For further information about some of these applications, the reader is referred to the reviews by Klingel *et al.*, Turek and Robinson, and Watson and Dive (30–32).

4.3 Measurement of mRNA

The increasing focus on gene transcription and mRNA metabolism, as indicators of cellular differentiation and activation, has also been reflected in recent developments within the field of FC.

4.3.1 Total mRNA

The selective measurement of total mRNA (as distinct from ribosomal or transfer RNA) has proven to be a relatively straightforward task, involving cell fixation and permeabilization, in a manner similar to that for intracellular protein studies, followed either by direct probing with FITC-conjugated oligo(dT) (oligodeoxythymidine), which hybridizes with the polyadenylate tail of mRNA (fluorescent *in situ* hybridization, FISH) (see *Figure 4,1A*), or by constructing a fluorescent complementary polynucleotide sequence on the poly(A) using an oligo(dT) primer, reverse transcriptase, and FITC–dUTP to generate the complementary strand (primed *in situ* labelling, PRINS) (*Figure 4,2*) (33).

4.3.2 Specific mRNA

The measurement of individual mRNA species, on the other hand, presents greater problems in that the number of mRNA copies per cell is generally low (< 1000/cell), compared to its protein product, and that each mRNA molecule will only bind a single molecule of the specific oligonucleotide probe, in contrast to the binding of multiples of FITC–oligo(dT) to the poly(A) tails of total mRNA. Thus the sensitivity demands of this approach are extreme. One solution to the problem has been to employ fluorescence activated cell sorting to purify the desired cell population and then perform quantitative PCR on the mRNA extracts from these cells (reviewed in ref. 34). However, the challenge of using FC directly for specific messenger measurements has also been met with some success by performing FISH with mixtures of oligonucleotide probes recognizing different sequences in the mRNA (thereby 'painting' the whole molecule) (*Figure 4,1B*), or even by reverse transcribing the target mRNA and then amplifying the gene by PCR within the cell itself before detecting by FISH (*Figure 4,3*) (34).

4.4 General remarks regarding the investigation of intracellular components

It should perhaps be stressed that, with the possible exception of the abovementioned assays for enzymatic activity (see Section 4.2), intracellular measurements by FC can, at best, only be regarded as semi-quantitative; because the fixation and permeabilization procedures invariably lead, in the case of protein targets, to partial loss of antigenic activity as a result of chemical modification and alterations in tertiary structure, and because target molecules

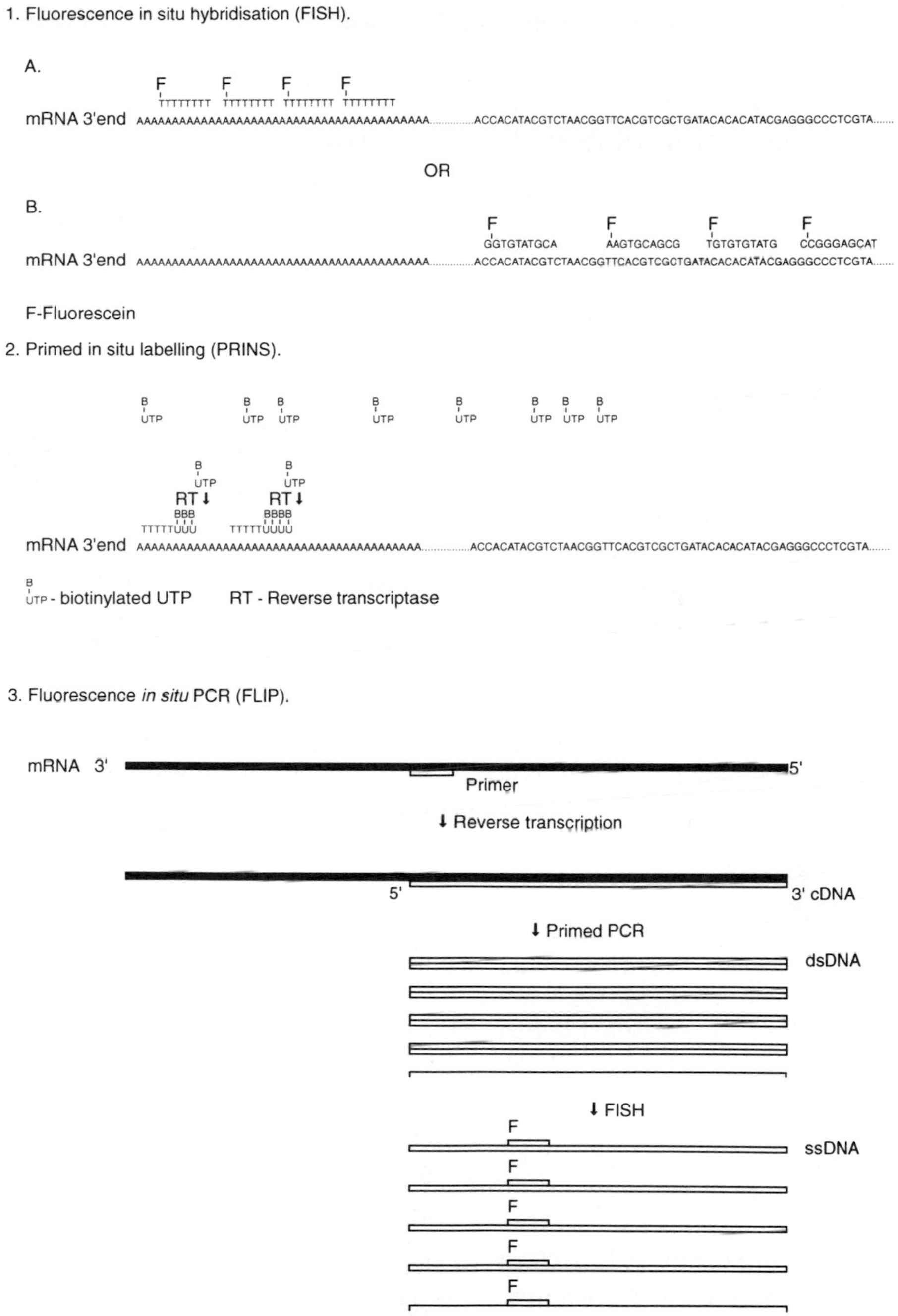

1. Fluorescence in situ hybridisation (FISH).

A.

F F F F

TTTTTTTT TTTTTTTT TTTTTTTT TTTTTTTT

mRNA 3'end AAAAAAAAAAAAAAAAAAAAAAAAAAAAAAAAAAAAAAAAAA...............ACCACATACGTCTAACGGTTCACGTCGCTGATACACACATACGAGGGCCCTCGTA.......

OR

B.

F F F F

GGTGTATGCA AAGTGCAGCG TGTGTGTATG CCGGGAGCAT

mRNA 3'end AAAAAAAAAAAAAAAAAAAAAAAAAAAAAAAAAAAAAAAAAA...............ACCACATACGTCTAACGGTTCACGTCGCTGATACACACATACGAGGGCCCTCGTA.......

F-Fluorescein

2. Primed in situ labelling (PRINS).

B UTP B UTP B UTP B UTP B UTP B UTP B UTP B UTP

B UTP RT ↓ B UTP RT ↓

BBB BBBB

TTTTTUUU TTTTTUUUU

mRNA 3'end AAAAAAAAAAAAAAAAAAAAAAAAAAAAAAAAAAAAAAAAA...............ACCACATACGTCTAACGGTTCACGTCGCTGATACACACATACGAGGGCCCTCGTA.......

B UTP - biotinylated UTP RT - Reverse transcriptase

3. Fluorescence *in situ* PCR (FLIP).

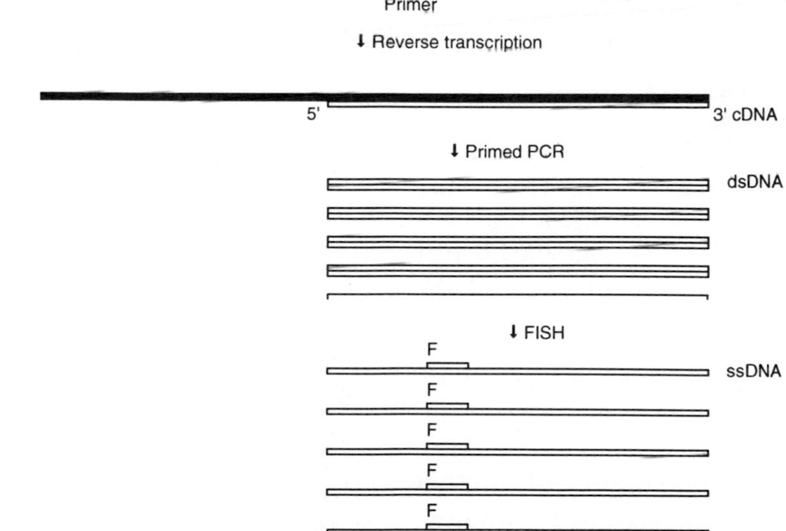

Figure 4. Strategies for detecting mRNA by FC. It should be noted that the probes (ss or dsDNA, RNA, or oligonucleotides) actually employed in the hybridizations normally range from 60 bp to 300 bp in length.

may diffuse out of the permeabilized cells during handling procedures (e.g. during *in situ* amplification of cDNA by PCR).

5. Investigation of cellular activation

Among the innumerable changes that occur in a cell's constitution upon activation, there are two which are eminently suited to FC analysis; mobilization of intracellular calcium and alterations in surface phenotype.

5.1 Measurement of intracellular calcium ions

Calcium-sensitive fluorochromes are convenient tools for measurement of intracellular ionized calcium concentration $[Ca^{2+}]_i$, and thereby early cell activation events. If one has access to a UV laser or a mercury arc-based flow cytometer, indo-1 is a useful fluorochrome, with a Ca^{2+}-dependent excitation maximum of approximately 350 nm and a shift in emission spectrum upon binding of Ca^{2+}. The fluorescence signals of calcium-bound and calcium-free indo-1 are usually detected at 405 nm and 485 nm, respectively. The ratio between the fluorescence signals at these wavelengths is proportional to the intracellular Ca^{2+} concentration. The loading and calibration procedures for indo-1, data treatment, and potential pitfalls are thoroughly described by June and Rabinowitch (35).

If only a standard argon laser is available, the fluorescein derivative fluo-3 (36), having an excitation maximum of 488 nm, is suitable. Due to emission characteristics similar to FITC, it can be used in combination with almost all other fluorochromes normally employed in multicolour analyses. A major disadvantage of fluo-3, however, is the lack of shift in emission wavelength upon binding of Ca^{2+}, which renders it less readily quantifiable. This problem may be overcome by simultaneous loading with dyes with markedly different emission wavelengths which are taken up, distributed, and converted in a equivalent manner to fluo-3, but do not exhibit increases in fluorescence intensity upon cell activation. Two such dyes are the seminaphthorhodafluor (SNARF-1) (37), with a pH-dependent emission spectrum between 550 and 650 nm, and Fura-Red (35,38), which has an emission maximum at 660 nm and displays decreased fluorescence intensity upon binding of Ca^{2+}. Thus, the fluo-3/SNARF-1 ratio or the fluo-3/Fura-Red ratio may be used to measure $[Ca^{2+}]_i$, the latter combination giving a greater response than indo-1 and allowing simultaneous detection of PE-labelled probes (38).

5.2 Measurement of surface activation markers

Another approach to FC assessment of cellular activation is measurement of appropriate cell surface activation markers. Antibodies reactive with a number of such markers are commercially available for direct or indirect staining techniques. The most commonly employed markers of lymphocyte activation are CD69 (an early activation marker) (39), CD25 (the low affinity IL-2 receptor), and HLA-DR. Moreover, CD45RO may be employed as a memory cell marker, while CD23 is often used as a marker for B cell activation. Expression of CD71, the receptor for transferrin, is measured as a marker of proliferation (40). Finally, platelet activation can be readily measured by FC with antibodies against CD62 or CD63 (41).

6. Investigation of cellular replication

FC offers a unique opportunity to investigate cell division within a cell subset in a heterogeneous cell population, by combining registration of the replicative event with detection of a surface marker specifically expressed by the cells of interest. The replication can be measured using three different approaches:

(a) By detecting cells in S phase on the basis of the non-covalent association of proliferating cellular nuclear antigen (PCNA) with the replicating DNA.
(b) By measurement of DNA synthesis, based on the incorporation of 5′-bromo-2-deoxyuridine (BrdU).
(c) By following cell division registered as the twofold dilution of macromolecular intracellular markers (e.g. fluorescently-labelled intracellular proteins) that occurs on completion of each cell cycle.

The first two approaches are usually supplemented by concurrent measurement of the DNA content of cells, using intercalating dyes such as propidium iodide (PI), to provide additional information regarding the cell cycle kinetics.

The three approaches provide quite different types of information about cellular proliferation, and this should be taken into account before adopting a particular procedure. Thus PCNA measurement combined with PI staining gives an instantaneous picture of the distribution of cells between G_0/G_1, S, and G_2/M phases. BrdU incorporation, on the other hand, records all cells that have been in S phase within a particular time window, including those that enter or leave S phase during the labelling period. Pulse chase experiments with BrdU incorporation in combination with PI are used to provide detailed information about cell cycle kinetics (42). Finally, the macromolecular marker dilution approach gives a full historical record of all the cells undergoing division from the moment of fluorescein labelling. On the other hand, this approach is uninformative about events within a single cell cycle.

Since numerous descriptions of the first two approaches already exist in the literature (reviewed in ref. 43), they will only be discussed briefly in this section, while the third approach will be handled in greater detail.

6.1 PCNA and BrdU approaches

Superficially, the two methods bear striking similarities: they both involve antibody probing for antigens present in the nucleus and at the cell surface (for subset identification), combined with DNA staining. Thus, it is necessary to use detergent or alcohol treatment to permeabilize the plasma and nuclear membranes and, since one wishes to preserve cellular integrity as much as possible, some form of fixation (see also Section 4.1). However, the widely different natures of the nuclear antigens require that quite distinct procedures be used for their detection.

In the case of PCNA detection, one has to allow for the fact that only a small proportion of the total PCNA in the cells is actually bound in the replication sites; the rest forming a loosely-associated pool from which it is recruited by the replicating DNA. This unbound pool must be selectively removed to avoid the staining of quiescent cells (44). The combination of 100% cold methanol as fixative and NP-40 as detergent has proven to be effective in selectively extracting the unbound PCNA (45). In addition, it should be borne in mind that if PI staining is included in the procedure, treatment of the cells with RNase is also necessary, since RNA also takes up intercalating dyes.

Detection of BrdU incorporation into DNA requires that the double-stranded (ds) DNA be denatured to permit access of the anti-BrdU antibody. This denaturation can be accomplished using different approaches, the most commonly employed being heating or acid treatment. The denaturation can, however, interfere with the detection of a surface marker protein, as acid treatment may denature the membrane markers and destroys the fluorochromes commonly employed in conjugates for second and third colour fluorescence, such as the haem-containing R-phycoerythrin (R-PE). The problem can be circumvented by labelling the cells with biotinylated antibody prior to fixation of the cells and then incubating with a streptavidin–fluorochrome conjugate just before FC analysis. Finally, it should be noted that the denaturation of the DNA for detecting BrdU incorporation has to be only partial, as the DNA dyes used to measure quantitative DNA content intercalates with double-stranded DNA.

6.2 The macromolecular dilution approach

The macromolecular dilution approach for investigation of cell division relies on stable fluorescence labelling of long-lived intracellular molecular species. This requires a fluorochrome precursor which:

(a) Is non-polar, to enable it to readily permeate the cell.

(b) Is rapidly hydrolysed to a polar product that remains trapped within the cell.

(c) Possesses a moderately reactive side chain capable of forming stable linkages with intracellular proteins.

In the case of 5-(and-6)-carboxy-2′,7′-dichlorofluorescein diacetate succinimidyl ester (CFSE), the charged fluorescein is masked as a diacetate derivative that allows the compound to penetrate the membrane and, once in the cell, the CFSE is cleaved to the polar fluorescent form. Due to the succinimidyl ester group, CFSE binds covalently to intracellular macromolecules and this covalent binding ensures that the dye persists for a long period inside the cells.

CFSE labelling was originally used to follow lymphocyte migration *in vivo* (46) but has also great potential as a means of recording cell proliferation over several generations (47). In addition, the CFSE technique is simple and rapid compared to the two previously described approaches. As the cells are already charged with CFSE at the beginning of the study, the only additional step upon harvesting is to identify the cells of interest with a fluorescent antibody towards a surface marker. *Protocol 2* describes application of this approach to the investigation of B cell proliferation in a mononuclear cell preparation from whole blood upon stimulation with pokeweed mitogen (PWM).

Protocol 2. Measurement of B and T cell division in a mononuclear cell preparation stimulated with PWM

Equipment and reagents

- Complete medium: RPMI 1640 supplemented with 10% FCS, 2 mM L-glutamine, 1 mM sodium pyruvate, and penicillin/streptomycin (10 IU/ml)
- 5 mM CFSE (Molecular Probes) in DMSO—diluted to 20 μM in PBS just before use
- Lymphoprep (Nycomed), density: 1.077 g/ml
- PWM (100 ng/ml, Sigma) in complete medium
- R-PE anti-CD19 (DAKO)
- Human IgG (165 mg/ml) (Kabi)
- Flow cytometer (FACScan, Becton Dickinson)

A. *Cell labelling*

1. Dilute 3 ml human blood with CPD as anticoagulant with 3 ml PBS in a 10 ml centrifuge tube.
2. Carefully layer 3–4 ml of Lymphoprep under the blood with a syringe and centrifuge the cells at 700 *g* for 20 min at room temperature.
3. Transfer the interface with the mononuclear cells (MNC) to a 50 ml polyethylene centrifuge tube containing PBS and wash the cells twice in PBS, centrifuging at 400 *g* for 10 min. Resuspend the final cell pellet in 10 ml PBS.
4. Add 1 ml of diluted CFSE to the cells (to give a final CFSE concentration of 2 μM) and incubate for 10 min at 37 °C. Centrifuge the cells at 400 *g* for 10 min and discard the supernatant.
5. Wash the cells twice at room temperature; once in RPMI 1640 alone

Protocol 2. *Continued*

and once in complete medium. Count the cells and adjust to 1×10^6 cells/ml in complete medium.

6. Add an equal volume of PWM (100 ng/ml) in complete medium to the cell suspension resulting in a final concentration of 50 ng/ml PWM in the culture flasks.
7. Culture the cells for three or five days in an incubator with 5% CO_2, humidified air at 37 °C.
8. Transfer 1 ml aliquots of the cells to the sample tubes for FC analysis, spin down at 400 *g* for 10 min at room temperature, and wash twice in PBS.
9. Resuspend the cells in 100 µl PBS, add 10 µl R-PE anti-CD19, and 10 µl human IgG, and incubate the mixture for 30 min at room temperature.
10. Spin the cells down, wash twice in PBS, and resuspend in 1 ml sheath fluid.

B. *Data acquisition and analysis*

1. Acquire data on 10 000 cells, either ungated or with live gating on the B cells (see *Protocol 1* for details).
2. Call up a dot plot of FL1 versus FL2. This shows the cells divided into two tiers, the lower tier representing non-B cells (T cells, NK cells, and monocytes) and the upper tier representing B cells (*Figure 5*).
3. Create FL1 histogram on the upper tier, or on the live gated B cells. Markers can be set which define B cells displaying $\frac{1}{2}$, $\frac{1}{4}$, $\frac{1}{8}$, etc. of the maximal fluorescence, representing first, second, third, and subsequent generations of dividing B cells. The FC statistics package can be used to determine the per cent of cells represented in each generation (see *Table 3*).

7. Measurement of cellular uptake and ingestion of soluble and particulate materials

FC is unique in its ability to provide a multiparameter analysis of the kinetics of interaction between a complex ligand and mixed cell populations. This situation is exemplified in immunological terms by the binding of opsonized immune complexes or opsonized micro-organisms to whole blood cells and their ingestion by phagocytes. FC analysis of certain aspects of these processes are described below.

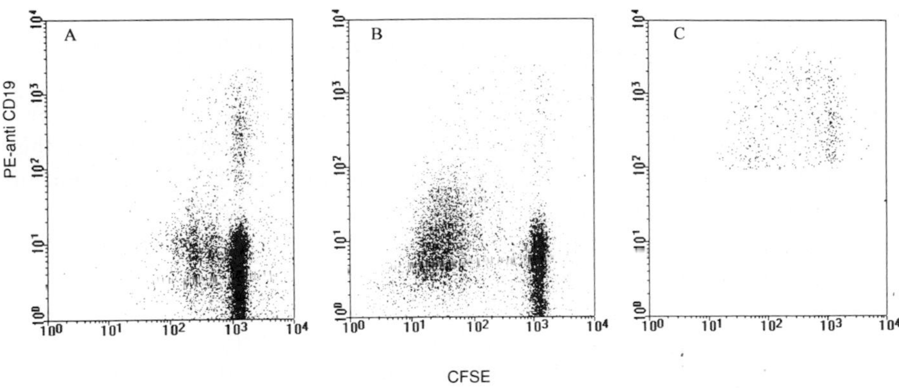

Figure 5. MNC charged with CFSE and stimulated to proliferate with PWM. B cells are detected with PE-conjugated anti-CD19 antibody. (A) MNC cultured for three days. (B) MNC cultured for five days. (C) Live gated B cells from the five day MNC culture. As seen in (A), a substantial proportion of the non-B cells have begun to proliferate and up to three rounds of division can be discerned. In (B) the non-B cells show proliferation for up to seven rounds of division. (C) B cell proliferation can best be observed after live gating.

Table 3. Percentage of B cells undergoing cell division after stimulation with PWM

No. of divisions	0	1	2	3	4	5	6	7
B cells								
Day 3	85	10	5	–	–	–	–	–
Day 5	38	13	10	10	14	12	3	–
Non-B cells								
Day 5	50	3	3	4	8	11	14	7

7.1 Binding of opsonized immune complexes to whole blood cells

Immune complexes (IC) are potent activators of the classical pathway of the complement cascade and covalently bind fragments of complement components 3 (C3) and 4 (C4), for which a variety of receptors exist on blood cells. Erythrocytes express complement receptor type 1 (CR1) in low numbers (< 500/cell), whereas leucocytes express CR1 in higher numbers (5000–20 000/cell). In addition, leucocytes bear other complement receptors (CR3 and CR4 on myeloid cells, CR2 on B lymphocytes) and Fc receptors for the constituent antibodies in the IC. As fragments of C3 and C4 are enzymatically degraded they shift binding specificity from CR1 to the other complement receptors.

7.1.1 Quantification of opsonized IC binding to whole blood cells

Quantification of IC binding to whole blood cells can be performed using FITC-labelled antibody or antigens, in much the same way as described for receptor quantitation using monoclonal antibodies. In practical terms, this requires that data acquisition is performed in two stages. First, a portion of the sample is diluted 1000-fold and analysis is performed on the erythrocytes, and then the rest of the sample is subjected to erythrolysis (see *Protocol 1*), and data is collected on the leucocytes. Given that erythrocytes and the leucocytes bind, on a per cell basis, widely divergent amounts of IC, it is necessary to acquire the data using different PMT voltages in the two stages of analysis. However calibration of the system with standard beads enables the data to be harmonized in terms of the mean numbers of antigen (or antibody) taken up per cell, for each of the examined cell subpopulations. Upon multiplication of the obtained mean values with the relative numbers of the respective cell populations, determined using an automated cell counter, a complete picture of the total IC binding to blood cells at the sampling time point can be derived (*Figure 6*). Thus, it can be seen that E, due to their numerical preponderance, account for the vast majority of cell-bound IC after 1 min, but that, at later time points, the major proportion of IC is associated with leucocytes, mainly PMN (73).

7.1.2 Assessment of heterogeneity in binding of opsonized IC to whole blood cells

Whereas radioassays only give information about the mean binding per cell, FC analysis is informative about the distribution of IC on individual cells.

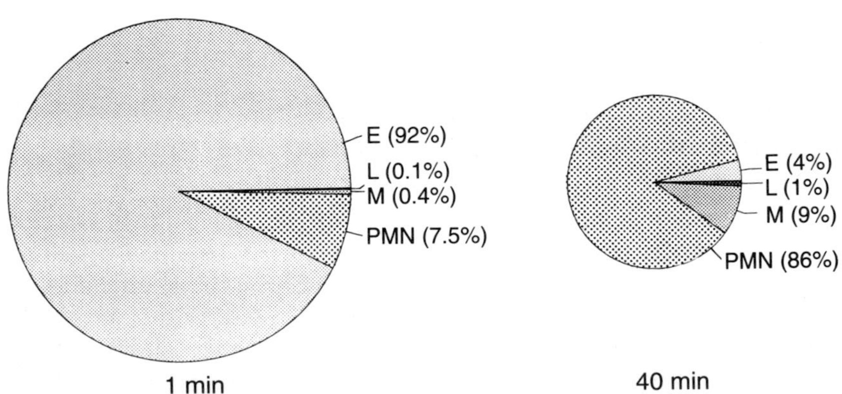

Figure 6. Pie diagram showing the proportional binding of pre-formed FITC–tetanus toxoid/anti-tetanus toxoid complexes to the individual cell populations in whole blood upon incubation for different times with autologous serum. The total amount of cell-associated IC is reflected by the size of the pies.

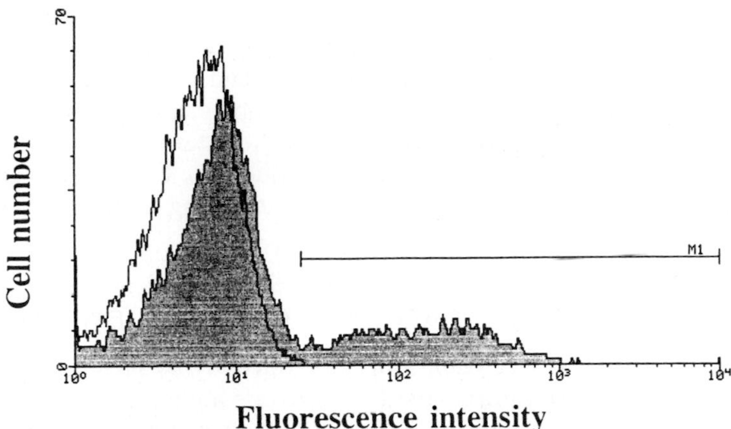

Figure 7. Fluorescence histogram showing the binding of pre-opsonized FITC–bovine serum albumin/anti-bovine serum albumin complexes to erythrocytes in a whole blood cell preparation, resuspended in autologous serum (shaded). The background fluorescence peak (unshaded) was obtained by incubating IC with serum containing 10 mM EDTA in order to abrogate complement activation. The marker, M1, indicates the IC-positive cells.

Thus FC measurement of IC uptake by blood cells reveals that PMN bind IC relatively homogeneously while monocytes and particularly lymphocytes exhibit heterogeneous binding characteristics, related in the latter case to the differential binding capacities of B cells, T cells, and NK cells (48).

The most pronounced heterogeneity, with respect to IC binding, is observed with erythrocytes. Thus, in the example shown in *Figure 7*, the IC binding per erythrocyte varies from zero to approximately 50 000 bound antigens per erythrocyte, with only 22% of the cells accounting for almost the entire binding (48).

7.2 Measurement of binding and ingestion by phagocytes

Binding of opsonized bacteria, viruses, or fungi (or IC) to phagocytes at 37 °C is followed by rapid ingestion of the bound material in a surface membrane envelope (phagosome). Fusion of the phagosomes with acidic lysosomes results in a decrease in pH in the phagolysosome and, consequently, partial quenching of the fluorescent label that may be attached to the ingested target (49). Thus, total uptake of a fluorescent target at physiological temperatures will be underestimated unless the quenching effect is countered. This can be achieved in two ways: either by inclusion of cytochalasin b in the assay, which disrupts microfilaments and hinders internalization (50), or by the addition of monensin, which is a proton ionophore that leads to neutralization of the acidic phagolysosomes (51). Monensin is cytotoxic and should, therefore, be added at the end of the assay, just before data acquisition.

In assays of phagocytic function, it is often desirable to distinguish between the degree of target binding and the degree of ingestion. This can be achieved by measuring, sequentially, the total and residual uptake, respectively, before and after the release of surface-bound target with detergent (52), or by selectively quenching the signal of the externally attached particles with a non-permeating dye, such as Trypan Blue (53). Using either approach, one should ideally correct for pH-mediated quenching of the signal from the ingested material.

8. Measurement of phagocytic oxidative processes

A variety of stimuli induce respiratory burst activity by phagocytes. The initial product of the respiratory burst is superoxide anion, $\cdot O_2^-$, which is generated through mono-electronic reduction of O_2 by a membrane-bound enzyme complex, NADPH oxidase. $\cdot O_2^-$ dismutates either spontaneously or through the action of superoxide dismutase to hydrogen peroxide, H_2O_2. In neutrophils, the generated H_2O_2 may be converted in the phagolysosomes by myeloperoxidase, derived from azurophilic granula, to the highly microbicidal hypochlorous acid and chloramines, or it may, in all phagocytes, be reconverted to O_2 and water by catalase. Alternatively, $\cdot O_2^-$ and H_2O_2 may be released to the extracellular environment.

Flow cytometry offers the possibility of measurement, at the single cell level, of $\cdot O_2^-$ and H_2O_2 production by means of probes that become fluorescent upon oxidation by these species. Dihydrorhodamine 123 (DHR 123) (54) and 2',7'-dichlorofluorescein-diacetate (DCFH-DA) (55), of which the former is the more sensitive (56,57), are two such probes, which diffuse readily into phagocytes and are oxidized during the respiratory burst to the green fluorescent rhodamine 123 (emission wavelength: 500–540 nm) and 2′,7′-dichlorofluorescein, respectively. These derivatives are charged and therefore trapped within the cell. Thus, the fluorescence intensity of a given cell is proportional to its respiratory burst activity from cell stimulus to measurement or arrest, e.g. by cooling on ice. DHR 123 and DCHF-DA are oxidized mainly by H_2O_2-dependent mechanisms (56,57). It should be noted that azide is a haem inhibitor that inhibits myeloperoxidase and catalase activities and therefore enhances the fluorescence of DHR 123 and DCFH-DA considerably, even at relatively low concentrations (57). Azide, or cyanide, may also be utilized in blocking mitochondrial oxidation, which is the main source of spontaneous oxidation.

Another probe, hydroethidine is oxidized by $\cdot O_2^-$ to the red fluorescent ethidium bromide (emission maximum $>$ 600 nm), which is then trapped in the nucleus upon intercalation with DNA (58).

For induction of respiratory burst in phagocytic cells, 12-myristate 13-acetate (PMA) (56) or zymosan may be used as stimulating agents. Natural stimuli include opsonized bacteria, complement fragment C5a, soluble immune complexes, or *N*-formyl-Met- Leu-Phe. Combined measurements of oxidative burst activity and phagocytosis may be performed using hydroethidine and fluorescein-labelled opsonized bacteria (59).

9. Measurement of cell-mediated cytotoxicity and apoptosis

Techniques for measuring cell death are of fundamental importance in studying two quite distinct aspects of the immune response; cell-mediated cytotoxicity and apoptosis. The former relates to the clearance of virally-infected and malignant cells from the host, and involves intimate physical contact between the target cell and the cytotoxic effector cell (primarily cytotoxic T cells and NK cells, with or without the assistance of antibodies). The latter is the process whereby non-functional or autoreactive lymphocytes are removed from the immune system and may be described as a form of programmed self-destruction into which the cells enter when they fail to receive the appropriate signals for survival from accessory cells.

In addition to differences in initiation, the two processes may be distinguished by the manner in which death occurs. In the case of cell-mediated cytotoxicity, loss of integrity of the cell membrane is an early event which results in rapid release of the cytoplasmic contents of the cell, followed by more gradual destruction of intracellular organelles and the nucleus. Apoptosis, on the other hand, is characterized by rapid DNA fragmentation and programmed destruction of intracellular organelles with gradual loss of cytoplasmic contents. The surface membrane remains intact until relatively late in the process, though loss of membrane polarity may occur (60). As might be expected from the marked differences in the mode of cell death, the processes of cytotoxicity and apoptosis can readily be distinguished experimentally (see below).

9.1 Cell-mediated cytotoxicity

The basic requirements in an FC assay for cell-mediated cytotoxicity are a means of distinguishing between the target cell and the effector cell (or cells) and a means of detecting dead cells. Registering of dead cells is usually performed using a non-permeable dye such as PI, whilst a number of different approaches have been employed to discriminate between target and effector cells. Thus tumour cell targets have been distinguished on the basis of morphology (high FSC and SSC values) and high autofluorescence (61), whilst cell combinations not displaying such marked differences in natural characteristics may be distinguished by labelling the target cells or effector cells, or both, with fluorescent lipophilic dyes (such as PKH26, red and PKH2, green) (62), FITC (63), permeable fluorogenic substrates which become converted to non-permeable products intracellularly (e.g. conversion of calcein-AM to the highly fluorescent calcein by the target cell esterase) (64), or by using specific fluorescently-labelled antibodies directed against epitopes on the target or effector cells.

9.1.1 Measurement of NK cell cytotoxic activity

As an elegant example of the last-named approach, a cytotoxicity assay involving discrimination of the effector cells by their expression of MHC class I antigens is presented in *Protocol 3*. In this procedure, target cells (the human erythroleukemic cell line, K562) are mixed with effector cells (human peripheral blood mononuclear cells) at appropriate effector-to-target (E/T) ratios for various periods of time. The cells are then labelled with murine anti-MHC class I antibody, to label all nucleated effector cells (K562 is negative for MHC class I antigens), and PI, to label dead cells.

Protocol 3. Measurement of NK cell cytotoxicity against the tumour cell line, K562

Equipment and reagents

- K562 cells cultured in complete RPMI 1640 medium (see *Protocol 2*)
- Peripheral blood mononuclear cells (PBMC) (see *Protocol 2*)
- Polystyrene 96-well microtitre plates (Nunc)
- FITC-conjugated murine anti-human MHC class I (Seralab)
- Propidium iodide (PI) (Sigma)
- Carriers for plate centrifugation
- Flow cytometer (Coulter Elite)

A. *The assay*

1. Preparation of target cells. Wash the K562 cells once in complete RPMI 1640 medium, centrifuge (5 min, 200 *g*, room temperature), and resuspend in medium at 10^4 cells/ml.
2. Preparation of PBMC. Wash the cells three times and resuspend in RPMI 1640 at cell densities of 10^5, 5×10^5, and 10^6 cells/ml.
3. Add 100 μl of target cells to triplicate wells containing one of the following:
   - 100 μl RPMI 1640 (spontaneous kill)
   - 100 μl effector cells (10^5/ml)
   - 100 μl effector cells (5×10^5/ml)
   - 100 μl effector cells (10^6/ml)

   resulting in E:T ratios of 10 : 1, 50 : 1, and 100 : 1, respectively.
4. Centrifuge the plates for approx. 30 sec at 200 *g*, to promote contact between effector and target cells, and then incubate at 37 °C for the desired time periods (between 1–6 h).[a]
5. Centrifuge the plates at 200 *g* for 5 min.

6. Remove 100 μl of supernatant from each well and replace with 10 μl of FITC-conjugated murine anti-human MHC class I antibody (diluted 1/40).
7. Resuspend the cells and incubate for 30 min at room temperature in the dark.
8. Wash the plates twice by adding 100 μl RPMI 1640, centrifuging for 5 min at 200 *g*, and then removing 100 μl supernatant.
9. Add PI (final concentration = 1 μg/ml) to each well just before processing for FC analysis.

B. *Data processing*

1. Call up a FL1 versus FL2 dot plot (see *Figure 8A*). Four populations of events can be discerned: those without fluorescence (lower left) representing live target cells (A), those showing high FL2 fluorescence only (upper left) representing dead target cells (B), those showing high FL1 fluorescence only (lower right) representing live effector cells (C), and a few showing high FL1 and FL2 fluorescence (D) representing dead effector cells.
2. Determine per cent cytotoxicity as: events in B/(events in A + B) × 100. The data from a representative experiment employing this approach is shown in *Figure 8B*.[b]

[a] Effector cells will bind to the targets cells at room temperature but target cell lysis will not begin before the temperature is increased to 37 °C.
[b] This protocol and the accompanying data was kindly provided by Dr Marianne Hokland, Department of Medical Microbiology, Bartholin Institute, Århus University, Århus, Denmark.

9.1.2 General comments regarding FC measurement of cell-mediated cytotoxicity

A potential weakness of the FC approach is that when the dead cells become completely disrupted they may fail to register at all in the detection system. Thus the FC measurements may be an underestimate, especially in assays involving long incubation periods. One approach that has been devised to minimize this error is to add to each sample a fixed number of distinctively labelled standard cells and use these to compute, on a ratio basis, the absolute numbers of target cells, living or dead, remaining in the sample (62).

The strength of the FC approach lies in the fact that it can be used to register contact between individual effector and target cells. Thus if each of the two cell populations is labelled with a distinctive marker, effector/target conjugates will be registered as events displaying both markers. By using subpopulation-specific markers, it is thus possible to determine the phenotype of the effector cell involved in a particular cytotoxicity assay (see ref. 64 for a fuller description of this approach).

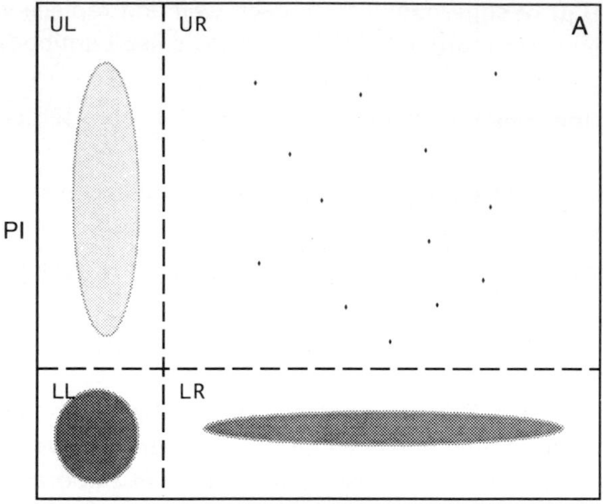

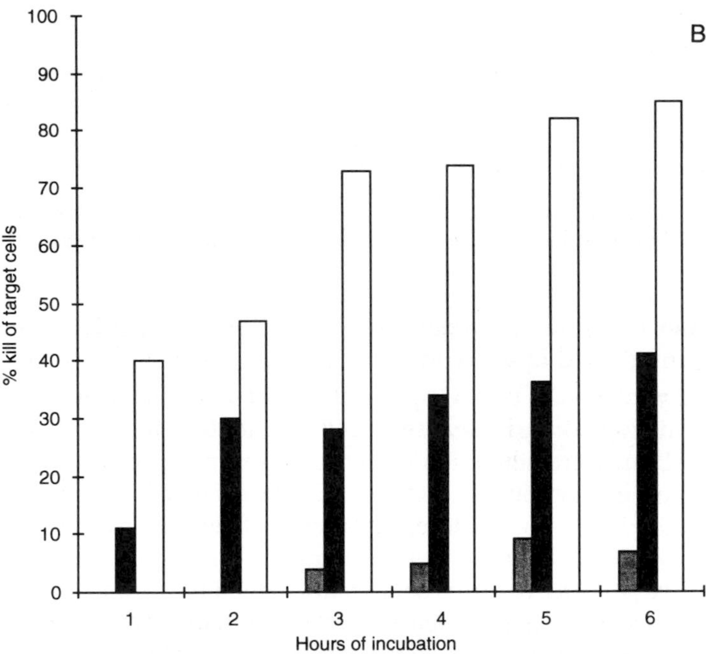

Figure 8. (A) Schematic contour plot showing the FL1 (FITC–anti-MHC class I) and FL2 (PI DNA-staining) characteristics of live K562 target cells (LL), dead targets (UL), live effector cells (LR), and dead effector cells (UR). (B) An example of the data derived from the cytotoxic assay described in *Protocol 3*. The grey, black, and white columns represent cytotoxicity at E:T ratios of 10 : 1, 50 : 1, and 100 : 1 respectively (courtesy of M. Hokland, Århus University, Denmark).

9.2 Measurement of apoptosis

The primary characteristic of apoptosis is the rapid fragmentation of nuclear DNA to segments of approximately 180 base pairs in length, and it is this feature that has most commonly been exploited in FC analysis.

9.2.1 DNA staining on ethanol-fixed cells

One of the first approaches to be employed was ethanol fixing of the cells under investigation combined with PI staining (reviewed in ref. 65), with the result that apoptotic cells registered as being hypodiploid. Fixation with reagents that caused cross-linking of intracellular components failed to give the same result, indicating that the success of the approach lay in the fact that ethanol fixation permitted controlled leakage of DNA fragments from the apoptotic cells.

9.2.2 DNA staining on unfixed cells

An alternative approach involving bulk DNA staining has been to use permeable fluorescent stains on unfixed cells. In this case, apoptosis is registered as an increase in staining intensity, related partially to the greater accessibility of the DNA following fragmentation and the concomitant loss of chromatin structure (66), and in part to a slight increase in membrane permeability permitting more rapid entry of the dye (67). One great advantage of this approach has been that, by using a combination of permeable and non-permeable DNA dyes, it has proven possible to discriminate between apoptotic cells which take up elevated amounts of the permeable dye alone and necrotic cells which take up both dyes.

9.2.3 Nick translation and 3′ end-labelling

In an effort to improve the sensitivity of detection of early fragmentation, two approaches, based on incorporating fluorescent markers in the DNA breaks, have been developed. In one approach, fluorescein-conjugated nucleotides have been incorporated by nick translation with DNA polymerase on the fixed cells (68,69), whilst the other approach involves incorporation of biotinylated thymidine using terminal deoxythymidine transferase (tdTt) followed by probing with streptavidin–FITC (70–72).

9.2.4 Membrane lipid translocation

Finally, a promising new development in the detection of apoptosis has arisen with the demonstration that translocation of phosphatidylserine (PS) from the inner to the outer lammella of the plasma membrane occurs very early in the apoptotic process. Using FITC-labelled annexin, which binds specifically to PS, in combination with a non-permeable DNA dye, it has thus been possible to discriminate between apoptotic cells and necrotic cells, which also display PS translocation at a very early stage (60).

References

1. Darzynkiewicz, Z., Robinson, J. P., and Crissman, H. A. (ed.) (1944). *Flow cytometry, parts A and B*, 2nd edn. In *Methods in cell biology*, Vol. 41 and 42. Academic Press, New York.
2. Haugland, R. P. (1994). In *Methods in cell biology*, Vol. 42, p. 662. Academic Press, New York.
3. Tengerdy, R. P. (1965). *Anal. Biochem.*, **11**, 272.
4. Christensen, J. and Leslie, R. G. Q. (1990). *J. Immunol. Methods*, **132**, 211.
5. Fearon, D. T. and Collins, L. A. (1983). *J. Immunol.*, **130**, 370.
6. Marquart, H. V., Svehag, S.-E., and Leslie, R. G. Q. (1994). *J. Immunol.*, **153**, 307.
7. Lenkel, R. and Andersson, B. (1995). *J. Immunol. Methods*, **183**, 267.
8. Chen, X.-J., Juluisson, S., Aldedborg, F., and Enerbäck, L. (1994). *J. Immunol. Methods*, **177**, 139.
9. Van Epps, D. E. and Chenowith, D. E. (1984). *J. Immunol.*, **132**, 2862.
10. Allen, C. A., Broom, M. F., and Chadwick, V. S. (1992). *J. Immunol. Methods*, **149**, 159.
11. Chuck, R. S., Cantor, C. R., and Tse, D. B. (1990). *Proc. Natl. Acad. Sci. USA*, **87**, 5021.
12. Harel-Bellan, A., Krief, P., Rimsky, L., Farrar, W. L., and Mishal, Z. (1990). *Biochem. J.*, **268**, 35.
13. Bene, L., Balazs, M., Matko, J., Dierich, M. P., Szollosi, J., and Damjanovich, S. (1994). *Eur. J. Immunol.*, **24**, 2115.
14. Schreiber, G. A., Beisker, W., Bauchinger, M., and Nusse, M. (1992). *Cytometry*, **13**, 90.
15. Hammond, T. G., Majewski, R. R., Muse, K. E., Oberly, T. D., and Morrissey, L. W. (1994). *Am. J. Physiol.*, **267**, F1021.
16. Bauer, K. D. and Jacobberger, J. W. (1994). In *Methods in cell biology*, Vol. 41, p. 352. Academic Press, New York.
17. Pearse, A. G. E. (1980). In *Histochemistry: theoretical and applied* (ed. A. G. E. Pearse), Vol. 1, p. 97. Churchill Livingstone Press, New York.
18. Rabin, H., Trimpe, K. L., and Hamer, P. J. (1989). *Cancer Cells*, **7**, 157.
19. Dent, G. A., Leglise, M. C., Pryzwansky, K. B., and Ross, D. W. (1989). *Cytometry*, **10**, 192.
20. Anderson, P., Blue, M., O'Brien, C., and Schlossman, S. F. (1989). *J. Immunol.*, **143**, 1899.
21. Hallden, G., Andersson, U., Hed, J., and Johansson, S. G. O. (1989). *J. Immunol. Methods*, **124**, 103.
22. Jacobberger, J. W., Fogleman, D., and Lehman, J. M. (1986). *Cytometry*, **7**, 356.
23. Gerdes, J., Leuke, H., Baisch, H., Wacker, H. H., Schwab, U., and Steen, H. (1984). *J. Immunol.*, **133**, 1710.
24. Landberg, G., Tan, E. M., and Roos, G. (1990). *Exp. Cell. Res.*, **187**, 111.
25. Sander, B., Andersson, J., and Andersson, U. (1991). *Immunol. Rev.*, **119**, 65.
26. Jung, T., Schauer, U., Heusser, C., Neumann, C., and Rieger, R. U. (1993). *J. Immunol. Methods*, **159**, 197.
27. Kreft, B., Singer, G. C., Diaz-Gallo, C., and Kelly, R. U. (1994). *J. Immunol. Methods*, **156**, 125.

28. Heltand, G., Garred, P., Mollnes, T. E., and Størvold, G. (1991). *J. Immunol. Methods*, **140**, 167.
29. Heyman, C. A. and Holzer, T. J. (1992). *J. Immunol. Methods*, **152**, 25.
30. Klingel, S., Rothe, G., Kellermann, W., and Valet, G. (1994). In *Methods in cell biology*, Vol. 41, p. 449. Academic Press, New York.
31. Turek, J. J. and Robinson, J. P. (1994). In *Methods in cell biology*, Vol. 41, p. 461. Academic Press, New York.
32. Watson, J. V. and Dive, C. (1994). In *Methods in cell biology*, Vol. 41, p. 469. Academic Press, New York.
33. Belloc, F. and Durrieu, F. (1994). In *Methods in cell biology*, Vol. 42, p. 59. Academic Press, New York.
34. Li, B. D., Timm, E. A. Jr, Riedy, M. C., Harlow, S. P., and Stewart, C. C. (1994). In *Methods in cell biology*, Vol. 42, p. 96. Academic Press, New York.
35. June, C. H. and Rabinowitch, P. S. (1994). In *Methods in cell biology*, Vol. 41, p. 149. Academic Press, New York.
36. Minta, A., Kao, J. P. Y., and Tsien, R. Y. (1989). *J. Biol. Chem.*, **264**, 8171.
37. Rijkers, G. T., Justement, L. B., Griffioen, A. W., and Cambier, J. C. (1990). *Cytometry*, **11**, 923.
38. Novak, E. J. and Rabinowitch, P. S. (1994). *Cytometry*, **17**, 135.
39. Testi, R., D'Ambrosio, D., De Maria, R., and Santoni, A. (1994). *Immunol. Today*, **15**, 479.
40. Brekelmans, P., van Soest, P., Leenen, P. J., and van Ewijk, W. (1994). *Eur. J. Immunol.*, **24**, 2896.
41. Tschoepe, D., Spangsberg, P., Esser, J., Schwippert, B., Kehrel, B., Roesen, P., *et al.* (1990). *Cytometry*, **11**, 652.
42. Dolbeare, F., Gratzner, H., Pallavicini, M. G., and Gray, J. W. (1983). *Proc. Natl. Acad. Sci. USA*, **80**, 5573.
43. Ormerod, M. G. (1994). In *Flow cytometry: a practical approach*, 2nd edn, p. 69. IRL Press, Oxford.
44. Bravo, R. and Macdonald-Bravo, H. (1987). *J. Cell. Biol.*, **105**, 1549.
45. Landberg, G. and Roos, G. (1991). *Cancer Res.*, **51**, 4570.
46. Weston, S. A. and Parish, C. R. (1990). *J. Immunol. Methods*, **133**, 87.
47. Lyons, A. B. and Parish, C. R. (1994). *J. Immunol. Methods*, **171**, 131.
48. Nielsen, C. H., Svehag, S.-E., Marquart, H. V., and Leslie, R. G. Q. (1994). *Scand. J. Immunol.*, **40**, 228.
49. Geisow, M. J. (1984). *Exp. Cell. Res.*, **150**, 29.
50. Leslie, R. G. Q. (1980). *Eur. J. Immunol.*, **10**, 799.
51. Midoux, P., Roche, A. C., and Monsigny, M. (1987). *Cytometry*, **8**, 327.
52. Wilson, R. M., Galvin, A. M., Robins, R. A., and Reeves, W. G. (1985). *J. Immunol. Methods*, **76**, 247.
53. Hed, J., Hallden, G., Johansson, S. G. Q., and Larsson, P. (1987). *J. Immunol. Methods*, **101**, 119.
54. Emmendörffer, A., Hecht, M., Lohmann-Matthes, M.-L., and Roesler, J. (1990). *J. Immunol. Methods*, **131**, 269.
55. Bass, D. A., Parce, J. W., DeChatelet, L. R., Szejda, P., Seeds, M. C., and Thomas, M. (1983). *J. Immunol.*, **130**, 1910.
56. Rothe, G., Emmendörffer, A., Oser, A., Roesler, J., and Valet, G. (1991). *J. Immunol. Methods*, **138**, 133.

57. Smith, J. A. and Weidemann, M. J. (1993). *J. Immunol. Methods*, **162**, 261.
58. Rothe, G. and Valet, G. (1990). *J. Leukoc. Biol.*, **47**, 440.
59. Perticarari, S., Presani, G., Mangiarotti, M. A., and Banfi, E. (1991). *Cytometry*, **12**, 687.
60. Vermes, I., Haanen, C., Steffens-Nakken, H., and Reutelingsperger, C. (1995). *J. Immunol. Methods*, **184**, 39.
61. Papa, S. and Valentin, M. (1994). In *Methods in cell biology*, Vol. 42, p. 193. Academic Press, New York.
62. Fleger, D., Gruber, R., Schlimok, G., Reiter, C., Pantel, K., and Reithmüller, G. (1995). *J. Immunol. Methods*, **180**, 1.
63. Karawejew, L., Jung, G., Wolf, H., Michael, B., and Ganzel, K. (1994). *J. Immunol. Methods*, **177**, 119.
64. Papadopoulos, N. G., Dedoussis, G. V. Z., Spanakos, G., Gritzapis, A. D., Baxevanis, C. N., and Papamichail, M. (1994). *J. Immunol. Methods*, **177**, 101.
65. Telford, W. G., King, L. E., and Fraker, P. J. (1994). *J. Immunol. Methods*, **172**, 1.
66. Miller, T., Beausang, L. A., Meneghini, M., and Lidgard, G. (1993). *Bio-Techniques*, **15**, 1042.
67. Ormerod, M. G., Sun, X.-M., Snowden, R. T., Davies, R., Fernhead, H., and Cohen, G. M. (1993). *Cytometry*, **14**, 595.
68. Jonker, R. R., Baumann, J. G. J., and Visser, J. M. W. (1992). In *New developments in flow cytromtery*, p. 30. NATO Advanced Study Institutes Programme Lectures, Opt. C, CNRS, Villejuif.
69. Zhang, L., Wang, C., Radvanyi, L. G., and Miller, R. G. (1995). *J. Immunol. Methods*, **181**, 17.
70. Gorzyca, W., Bruno, S., Darzynkiewicz, R. J., Gong, J., and Darzynkiewicz, Z. (1992). *Int. J. Oncol.*, **1**, 639.
71. Gorzyca, W., Traganos, F., Jesianowska, H., and Darzynkiewicz, Z. (1993). *Exp. Cell. Res.*, **207**, 202.
72. Dolzhansky, A. and Basch, R. S. (1995). *J. Immunol. Methods*, **180**, 131.
73. Nielsen, C. H., Matthiesen, S. H., Lyng, I., and Leslie, R. G. Q. (1997). *Immunology*, **90**, 129.

7

Analysis of soluble adhesion molecules

M. G. BOUMA, M. P. LAAN, M. A. DENTENER, and W. A. BUURMAN

1. Introduction

Adhesion of leucocytes to endothelial cells, and their subsequent trans-endothelial migration into target tissues are crucial events in the development of an inflammatory reponse. This leucocyte–endothelial interaction is mediated by specific adhesion molecules, expressed on the endothelial cell surface, that recognize and bind to their specific ligands on leucocytes. During the last decade, a number of endothelial adhesion molecules have been identified, including E-selectin, intercellular adhesion molecule-1 (ICAM-1), and vascular cell adhesion molecule-1 (VCAM-1), which mediate the successive steps of the adhesion process (1). Expression of these adhesion molecules can be induced by a wide range of inflammatory mediators, thereby tightly controlling leucocyte recruitment during inflammatory responses. Also, adhesion molecules are believed to play an important role in the invasive and metastatic cellular processes in the development of cancer (2).

While E-selectin, ICAM-1, and VCAM-1 were identified originally as transmembrane glycoproteins, during recent years soluble isoforms of these adhesion molecules have been demonstrated in various human body fluids. The presence of soluble adhesion molecules in the circulation of patients with a variety of both acute and chronic inflammatory disease states as well as several cancers (3), has raised the possibility that serum levels may reflect disease activity. Also, serum levels of soluble E-selectin (sE-selectin), soluble ICAM-1 (sICAM-1), and soluble VCAM-1 (sVCAM-1) have been correlated with clinical outcome in a number of studies. As a consequence, accurate determination of the concentration of soluble adhesion molecules in serum, as well as in other human samples such as broncho-alveolar lavage fluid, cerebrospinal fluid, urine, various effusions, and ascites, has become an important tool for monitoring disease activity and predicting clinical outcome. Nevertheless, a full understanding of the physiological and pathophysiological role of circulating adhesion molecules is still lacking.

In this chapter, the potential physiological roles of shedding of the adhesion molecules E-selectin, ICAM-1, and VCAM-1, and the possible significance of circulating adhesion molecules in various diseases are briefly discussed. Furthermore, as an example to illustrate the specific problems that might occur with ELISAs for soluble adhesion molecules, a detailed description is given of a sensitive ELISA to quantitate levels of sICAM-1 in culture supernatants and various human biological fluids. Finally, we will conclude with some general remarks on important issues to keep in mind when determining soluble adhesion molecules in human samples by ELISA.

2. E-selectin

E-selectin (CD62E), formerly known as ELAM-1, is an adhesion molecule exclusively expressed on activated vascular endothelial cells. Surface expression of E-selectin *in vitro* is maximal 4–6 h after stimulation with inflammatory cytokines such as tumour necrosis factor-α (TNF-α), interleukin-1β (IL-1β), or with lipopolysaccharide (LPS), and then declines to basal levels within 24 h. To date, two mechanisms of down-regulation of E-selectin have been reported. First, Von Asmuth *et al.* (4) have presented evidence that TNF-α-induced cell surface E-selectin is rapidly internalized by human umbilical vein endothelial cells *in vitro*, at a rate of approximately 1.7% of membrane E-selectin per minute. This then results in 90% of cell surface E-selectin being internalized within one hour. They have proposed that binding and subsequent endocytosis of soluble ligands for E-selectin could be a major function of E-selectin internalization, suggesting that endocytosis would be a mechanism by which E-selectin might clear circulating adhesion inhibiting factors in situations of severe immunological challenge. Secondly, it has been reported by several authors that E-selectin is released into the supernatants of cytokine-activated cultured endothelial cells (5–7). Immunoprecipitation studies have revealed that the molecular weight of soluble E-selectin is lower than that of its membrane-bound form (6,7). While there is no evidence that an alternative spliced form of E-selectin, lacking the transmembrane domain, exists, it is generally considered that E-selectin is shed from the cell membrane by cleavage of the extracellular part of the molecule. Since E-selectin is only present on activated endothelium, in contrast to other adhesion molecules, the presence of sE-selectin in blood would be strongly indicative of endothelial activation in a variety of inflammatory diseases. However, even in the absence of any overt inflammatory processes, sE-selectin is released into the circulation, since detectable levels are present in normal individuals (2,7,8). In an experimental human study by Kuhns *et al.* (9), strongly elevated serum levels of sE-selectin were detected after intravenous administration of endotoxin in healthy volunteers, the elevation of sE-selectin being linear to the endotoxin dose administered. In line with this, increased sE-selectin concentrations were found in the serum of critically ill patients with sepsis, and could be correlated to disease severity and mortality (7,10,11). Also, in patients with inflammatory disorders such as scleroderma (12), Kawasaki's disease (13), polyarteritis nodosum, and giant cell arteritis (8), elevated serum levels of sE-selectin have been found, but without a direct correlation to disease activity. Furthermore, elevated levels of sE-selectin in patients with diabetes mellitus (14) and essential hypertension (15), have been interpreted as markers of endothelial injury or activation.

3. ICAM-1

ICAM-1 (CD54), a member of the immunoglobulin superfamily, is present on the surface of cells such as lymphocytes, macrophages, epithelial, and endothelial cells (16). During immune and inflammatory responses ICAM-1 promotes leucocyte adhesion by binding to its ligands the leucocyte function-associated antigen-1, MAC-1, and CD43 (17–19). The quantitative expression of ICAM-1 on various cell types *in vitro* can either be induced, or extensively enhanced after stimulation with inflammatory mediators, like TNF-α, interferon-γ, or IL-1 (16,20,21).

ICAM-1 is not only present in a membrane-bound form, but also in soluble form, which contains all five extracellular domains of membrane-bound ICAM-1 (22–24). *In vitro* stimulation of human umbilical vein endothelial cells with cytokines not only increases the cell membrane expression of ICAM-1, but also results in release of sICAM-1, which increases in parallel with ICAM-1 cell surface expression (5,6). In contrast to E-selectin, ICAM-1 is only mimimally internalized by endothelial cells (4). The release of sICAM-1 is not restricted to endothelial cells of different vascular beds, but has also been reported to occur *in vitro* in human peripheral blood mononuclear cells (22) and various types of human non-haematopoietic cells, such as keratinocytes (25,26), synovial cells (27), hepatocytes (28), and several carcinoma cells (29,30), as well as melanoma cells (31,32).

Of the three soluble adhesion molecules discussed in this chapter, sICAM-1 was the first circulating adhesion molecule to be described and has consequently been studied most extensively. While sICAM-1 can be detected in the circulation of normal human individuals (22), there is now quite a large number of studies to demonstrate that levels of sICAM-1 in various human body fluids are elevated in a wide variety of inflammatory and infectious diseases, as well as in cancers. In a prospective cohort study, Cowley and co-workers demonstrated increased plasma levels of sICAM-1, as well as sE-selectin and sVCAM-1, in patients with the systemic inflammatory response syndrome, and even higher levels when organ dysfunction was present (10). In line with this, Law *et al.* reported elevated levels of sICAM-1 correlating with the development of multiple organ failure in severely injured trauma patients (33), while sICAM-1 levels also appear to correlate with mortality in such critically ill patients (11,34). In a wide range of organ-specific inflammatory diseases, such as idiopathic pulmonary fibrosis (35), chronic hepatitis C (36), inflammatory bowel disease (37), psoriasis (38), scleroderma (12), and chronic B lymphocytic leukaemia (39), serum levels of ICAM-1 have been reported to be elevated and to correlate with disease activity. Furthermore, circulating levels of ICAM-1 are indicative of disease progression of various malignant tumours (40–43). In human samples other than blood, sICAM-1 has also proven to be useful in monitoring inflammatory activity. Determination of sICAM-1 in urine of renal allograft recipients may serve as a diagnostic tool for assessment of allograft rejection (44), whereas sICAM-1 in cerebrospinal fluid of patients with AIDS-defining diseases could serve as a marker for immune activation (45).

4. VCAM-1

VCAM-1, another member of the immunoglobulin superfamily and previously designated as INCAM-110, is variably present on resting endothelial cells, and is up-regulated on endothelial cells after stimulation with inflammatory cytokines, such as TNF-α, IL-1β, and IL-4 (46,47). As a result of alternative splicing of the mRNA, two forms of VCAM-1 are expressed on activated endothelial cells, either with six or seven Ig-like domains (48,49). While found primarily on vascular endothelial cells, VCAM-1 is also expressed by non-endothelial cells including lymphoid dendritic cells, tissue macrophages, and renal tubular endothelial cells (50,51). VCAM-1 serves as a counter-receptor for the VLA-4 (α4β1) integrin (CD49d/CD29), which is primarily expressed on monocytes, lymphocytes, and eosinophilic neutrophils (46,51). Therefore, it is thought that the most important function of VCAM-1 is to mediate leucocyte–endothelial interactions, although it may also serve as a receptor for melanoma cells (52) and other VLA-4-bearing tumour cells of myeloid lineage, thereby playing a role in tumour progression and metastasis.

As reported by Pigott *et al.* (6) and Cartwright *et al.* (53), sVCAM-1 is released, in truncated form, by cytokine-activated human endothelial cells in culture.

Similar to sE-selectin and sICAM-1, sVCAM-1 levels are significantly elevated in septic and critically ill patients, and are positively correlated with organ dysfunction (10) and fatal outcome (11). In both serum and urine of renal allograft recipients, sVCAM-1 may reflect its histological distribution in corresponding graft biopsies, thus providing valuable information with regard to the severity of allograft rejection (3,44,54). Similarly, in patients with scleroderma (12), systemic lupus erythematosus (55), and Wegener's granulomatosis (56), sVCAM-1 levels in serum correlate well with clinical disease activity. Soluble VCAM-1 in cerebrospinal fluid of patients with multiple sclerosis correlates with elevated serum VCAM-1 during exacerbation of the disease (57).

5. Potential roles of soluble adhesion molecules in health and disease

With regard to the possible physiological roles of circulating adhesion molecules, two major concepts have emerged, which are not mutually exclusive. First, if the shed molecules retain their ability to bind their specific ligands on leucocytes, the release of these adhesion molecules may induce a decrease in the potential adhesiveness of leucocytes by competing with the membrane-bound receptors for their ligands. Indeed, recombinant sE-selectin has been shown to inhibit leucocyte adhesion both *in vitro* (58) as well as *in vivo* (59). Similarly, it has been suggested that sICAM-1 (27,60) and sVCAM-1 (53) may play a role in down-regulating adhesive interactions between leucocytes and membrane-bound forms of these adhesion molecules. Interestingly, sICAM-1 is also able to inhibit rhinovirus infection of cells by inhibiting the interaction between cell surface ICAM-1 and rhinoviruses (61).

Secondly, soluble adhesion molecules can act as co-stimulatory factors, triggering a response in a ligand-bearing cell. Recombinant sE-selectin has been shown to be a neutrophil chemoattractant and to play a role in activating the CD11b/CD18 integrin on circulating neutrophils by binding to the ligand of E-selectin on these cells (62,63). Likewise, sICAM-1 has been demonstrated to deliver chemokinetic signals to lymphocytes (25). Furthermore, sICAM-1 enhances cytokine production and T cell proliferative responses stimulated by alloantigen in mixed lymphocyte cultures (64). On the other hand, while circulating adhesion molecules can serve as co-stimulatory signals for their ligand-bearing cells, it is also conceivable that shedding of adhesion molecules in locally high concentrations may act to interrupt proper co-stimulation, leading to a diminished response of immunocompetent cells (65). The presence of sE-selectin, sICAM-1, and sVCAM-1 in the circulation of normal healthy individuals, would define the events described above as part of the normal, physiological host defense. However, the regulatory mechanisms that determine the release of soluble adhesion molecules, both in health and in inflammatory diseases, still remain to be elucidated. From a clinical perspective, the issue whether elevated plasma levels of soluble adhesion molecules in pathological inflammatory conditions are either of benefit for, or detrimental to patients, is still open and needs to be addressed in further experimental human studies.

6. ELISA for sICAM-1

With the steadily increasing interest in the role of soluble adhesion molecules both in health and disease, a growing number of commercial ELISA kits for the detection of soluble adhesion molecules in various human body fluids has become available, while many research groups themselves have developed specific ELISAs for experimental and clinical use. The general design of these assays is that of a two-site sandwich ELISA, using two different specific antibodies, each recognizing topographically distinct epitopes on the molecule to be assayed. The first antibody is attached to plastic to capture the antigen, whereas the second antibody, conjugated to an enzyme, is used for quantification of the captured antigen. We describe here (*Protocol 1*), as an example, a sensitive and reproducible ELISA, which allows for quantification of sICAM-1 in biological fluids. Furthermore, some technical issues are addressed, which are of importance when determining levels of soluble adhesion molecules in biological fluids by ELISA.

Protocol 1. ELISA for sICAM-1

Equipment and reagents

- 96-well immunomaxisorp microplates (Nunc)
- PBS
- BSA (Sigma)
- Anti-sICAM-1 mAbs HM.2 and biotin-labelled HM.1[a]
- sICAM-1 standard[b]
- Streptavidin–peroxidase conjugate (Dakopatts)
- 3,3′,5,5′-tetramethylbenzidine (TMB; Kirkegaard & Perry Lab., Gaithersburg, MD)
- 1 M H_2SO_4

Method

1. Coat a 96-well immunosorp plate overnight at 4°C with anti-sICAM-1 mAb HM.2 (3 μg/ml) in PBS (100 μl/well).
2. Prevent non-specific binding by blocking the plates for 1 h at room temperature (RT) with 125 μl/well PBS/1% (w/v) BSA.
3. Wash the plate five times using PBS/0.1% BSA as wash buffer, and shake the plate dry.
4. Add sICAM-1 standard (0.1–12.5 ng/ml) in duplicate, add samples and controls to four to eight wells per plate (100 μl/well), using PBS/0.1% BSA as dilution buffer. Incubate for 1 h at RT.[c]
5. Wash the plate five times with PBS/0.1% BSA, and shake it dry.
6. Add 100 μl/well biotinylated anti-sICAM-1 mAb HM.1, and incubate for 1 h at RT.
7. Wash the plate five times with PBS/0.1% BSA, and shake it dry.
8. Add 100 μl/well streptavidin–peroxidase conjugate, and incubate for 1 h at RT.
9. Wash the plate five times with PBS/0.1% BSA, and shake it dry.
10. Add 100 μl/well TMB as substrate and allow it to react for 10–15 min. Stop the reaction with 100 μl 1 M H_2SO_4.

11. Measure absorbance at 450 nm, using a micro-ELISA autoreader (*Figure 1*).[d]

[a]Both anti-sICAM-1 mAb HM.1 and HM.2 are of IgG1 isotype, and are produced by hybridomas, obtained after immunization of BALB/c mice with an ICAM-1–Fc construct, consisting of five Ig-like domains of ICAM-1 fused to a human IgG1–Fc portion. HM.1 recognizes Ig-like domain 4, whereas HM.2 recognizes Ig-like domain 2 of the sICAM-1 molecule.
[b]Human sICAM-1, produced by NSO sICAM-1/2 cells (kindly provided by Dr M. Robinson, Celltech, Slough, UK), is used as standard in this ELISA. It contains all five extracellular domains of ICAM-1.
[c]The influence of the length of the incubation period of sICAM-1 standard on the sensitivity of the ELISA was investigated. These experiments were performed with a constant incubation period of 1 h for the biotin-labelled detector mAb HM.1 as well as for streptavidin–peroxidase conjugate. Increasing the incubation time of sICAM-1 standard from 1 h to 2–3 h did not enhance sensitivity (data not shown). Therefore, an incubation time of 1 h is recommended.
[d]The sensitivity of the ELISA is arbitrarily defined as the lowest detectable sICAM-1 concentration giving rise to an absorbance higher than the mean background absorbance + 3 × standard deviation (SD) of background. The sensitivity of this ELISA, defined as such, is 400 pg/ml.

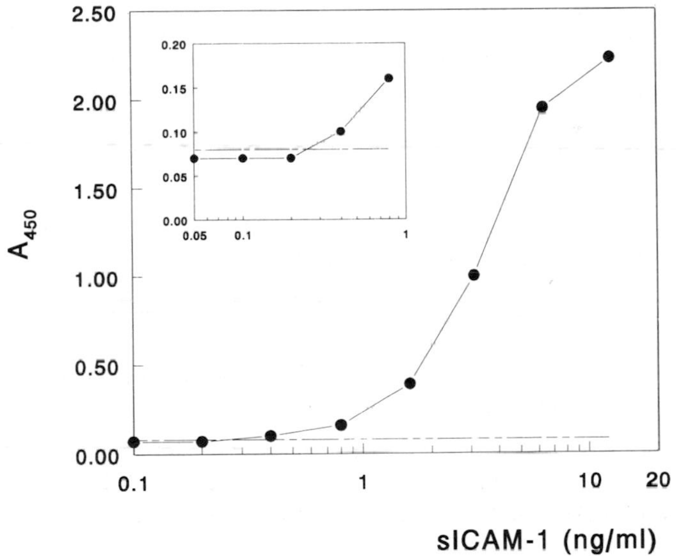

Figure 1. Representative standard curve of sICAM-1. Values were determined in duplicate. One representative experiment from a series of seven experiments is shown. Mean background A_{450} + 3 × SD is indicated by a dashed line.

For validation of the sICAM-1 ELISA, the intra- and interassay variance (*Protocol 2*), as well as the recovery of spiked sICAM-1 (*Protocol 3*) must be determined.

For determination of the intra- and interassay variance, the reproducibility of standard sICAM-1 values within individual experiments and between experiments have to be compared.

Protocol 2. Determination of intra- and interassay variance of sICAM-1 assay

Equipment and reagents

- ELISA for sICAM-1 (see *Protocol 1*)

Method

1. Prepare a standard stock solution of sICAM-1 of 5 μg/ml in PBS/0.1% BSA, aliquot it into polypropylene tubes, and store at −20°C.
2. Thaw an aliquot of sICAM-1 standard, and make a series of seven dilutions in the concentration range of 0.1–12.5 ng/ml. Apply this serial dilution in sextuplicate to a 96-well microtitre plate.
3. Repeat the procedure described in step 2 five times. Thaw a new aliquot of sICAM-1 standard for each procedure.
4. Determine the mean A_{450} of the first two standard curves of each plate (*Protocol 1*), and use it as a reference curve to calculate the sICAM-1 concentrations of the next four standard curves in the same microtitre plate.
5. Calculate, for each sICAM-1 concentration in each microtitre plate, the mean of the corresponding four calculated sICAM-1 concentrations in the same microtitre plate.
6. Determine the intra-assay variance[a] by calculating the coefficients of variance (SD/mean) for each microtitre plate (*Table 1*).
7. Determine the interassay variance[b] by calculating the coefficients of variance of the mean sICAM-1 levels measured in the five separate microtitre plates (*Table 1*).

[a] The mean intra-assay variance of this sICAM-1 ELISA is 6.2%.
[b] The mean interassay variance of this sICAM-1 ELISA is 10.5%. The intra- and interassay coefficients of variance achieved with this ELISA are comparable with those reported for other immunoassays (66,67).

Protocol 3. Estimation of recovery of exogenous sICAM-1

Equipment and reagents

- Evacuated blood collection tubes (Sherwood Medical, St. Louis, MO), containing either 0.1 ml 15% (w/w) EDTA, or 0.1 ml 500 IU/ml Leo Heparin (Leo Pharmaceutical Products BV, Weesp, The Netherlands)
- Evacuated integrated serum separator tubes (Sherwood Medical)
- ELISA for sICAM-1 (see *Protocol 1*)

Method

1. To obtain fresh human EDTA plasma and heparinized plasma, draw blood from a healthy volunteer into evacuated blood collection tubes, containing 0.1 ml 15% (w/w) EDTA or 0.1 ml 500 IU/ml Leo Heparin, respectively. Immediately after collection, separate the plasma from blood cells by centrifugation of the tubes at 1500 *g* for 10 min.
2. To obtain fresh human serum, draw blood from a healthy volunteer into an integrated serum separator tube, and allow the blood to coagulate for 1 h at RT. Then separate the serum from blood cells by centrifugation of the tubes at 1500 *g* for 10 min.
3. Add 50 μl/well of the plasma and serum samples to a microtitre plate. Add 50 μl of sICAM-1 standard in PBS/0.1% BSA to a final concentration of 100 ng/ml and 200 ng/ml, resulting in a 1/2 dilution of the plasma and serum samples. For determination of the endogenous sICAM-1 content, dilute the plasma and serum samples 1/2 in PBS/0.1% BSA, without adding sICAM-1 standard. Incubate the samples for 45 min at RT.
4. Dilute the samples 1/60 and determine the sICAM-1 content (*Protocol 1*).
5. Calculate the percentage recovery of spiked sICAM-1 (100 or 200 ng/ml), after correction for endogenous sICAM-1 content (*Table 2*).

Table 1. Intra- and interassay variance of sICAM-1 ELISA

sICAM-1 (ng/ml)	**Intra-assay[a] Mean (ng/ml)**	**SD**	**CV[c] (%)**	**Interassay[b] Mean (ng/ml)**	**SD**	**CV[c] (%)**
6.3	6.0	0.2	2.8	5.8	0.2	3.2
3.1	3.0	0.1	3.9	2.8	0.1	4.0
1.6	1.5	0.1	3.4	1.5	< 0.1	1.3
0.8	0.6	0.1	8.7	0.7	0.1	11.0
0.4	0.2	< 0.1	12.2	0.3	0.1	33.2

[a] Results of one representative experiment from a series of five experiments is shown. Mean and SD of sICAM-1 concentrations measured in quadruplicate, in one 96-well microtitre plate, are presented.
[b] Mean and SD of sICAM-1 concentrations measured in five separate experiments are shown.
[c] CV= SD/mean × 100%.

When determining soluble adhesion molecules in biological fluids by ELISA, the presence of inhibitory factors interfering with the assay, or disturbing matrix effects have to be considered. Also, the influence of sample storage conditions on the detection of soluble adhesion molecules must be determined.

To investigate whether the determination of sICAM-1 in blood is in-

Table 2. Recovery of exogenous sICAM-1 in plasma and serum

Sample	Endogenous *n*	sICAM-1[a]	Recovery (%)[b] sICAM-1 spike 100 ng/ml	200 ng/ml
EDTA plasma	10	90 ± 24[c]	108 ± 18[d]	96 ± 19
Heparinized plasma	10	92 ± 24	106 ± 23	116 ± 12
Serum	10	76 ± 6	101 ± 16	119 ± 13

[a] Endogenous sICAM-1 levels in non-treated fresh plasma and serum samples.
[b] Percentage recovery of spiked sICAM-1 was calculated after correction for endogenous sICAM-1 levels.
[c] Data are presented as mean ± SD (ng/ml).
[d] Data are presented as mean ± SD (%).

fluenced by the collection system, generating different matrices, compare sICAM-1 levels in EDTA plasma, heparinized plasma, and serum of healthy individuals. For obtaining and handling of plasma and serum samples, see *Protocol 3*. Dilute all samples 1/20 in PBS/0.1% BSA before analysis in ELISA (*Protocol 1*). As an example, *Table 3* shows that the highest level of sICAM-1 was measured in EDTA plasma, with a mean level of 103 ng/ml. In heparinized plasma and serum, 83% (86 ng/ml) and 61% (63 ng/ml), respectively, of the sICAM-1 level as determined in EDTA plasma were detected. Similar ratios of sICAM-1 levels in EDTA plasma, heparinized plasma, and serum were observed for each individual (*Figure 2*). In conclusion, a difference was observed between the sICAM-1 levels as detected in serum and in EDTA plasma. The fact that samples to be measured had to be diluted at least 20 times, indicates that matrix effects should be minimal. The differences observed between EDTA plasma and serum may therefore be caused by trapping of sICAM-1 in the clot formed during coagulation. The observation that recovery of exogenous sICAM-1 was not different in plasma and in serum samples (*Table 2*), supports this hypothesis.

To determine the influence of sample storage conditions on detection of sICAM-1, aliquot and store fresh plasma and serum samples of healthy individuals (for obtaining and handling of plasma and serum samples, see *Protocol 3*) at 4°C, −20°C, or −70°C for two weeks. Subject the samples stored at −20°C to several freeze–thaw cycles. After two weeks, determine the

Table 3. Soluble ICAM-1 levels in plasma and serum of healthy individuals[a]

Sample		Mean	SD
EDTA plasma	(n = 32)	103 ng/ml[b]	38
Heparinized plasma	(n = 32)	86 ng/ml	35
Serum	(n = 32)	63 ng/ml	34

[a] sICAM-1 levels were determined in freshly prepared plasma and serum samples.
[b] Samples were assayed in duplicate.

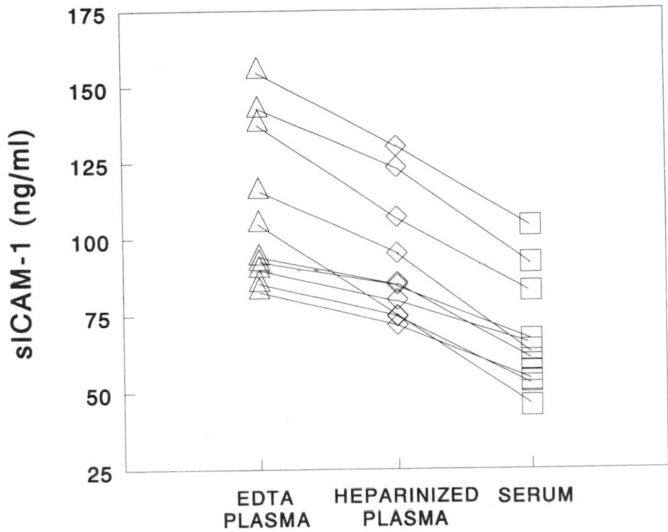

Figure 2. sICAM-1 levels of ten healthy volunteers (from a group of 32 volunteers, described in *Table 3*) in EDTA plasma, heparinized plasma, and serum. The sICAM-1 values of each individual are linked. Data are presented as mean of duplicate determinations.

sICAM-1 levels by ELISA (*Protocol 1*). As an example, *Table 4* shows that in samples stored at −70°C the highest sICAM-1 levels were measured, whereas after storage at −20°C reduced sICAM-1 levels were detected. Repeated freezing and thawing of the samples did not reduce recovery of sICAM-1. The effects of storage conditions on recovery of sICAM-1 were constant for each individual (data not shown). These data indicate that standard storage conditions for samples are necessary. When samples were stored at −70°C, sICAM-1 levels corresponded well with sICAM-1 levels measured in fresh samples.

To illustrate that the ELISA described in this chapter is useful for detection of sICAM-1 content in biological fluids of patients, sICAM-1 was determined

Table 4. Influence of sample storage conditions on sICAM-1 detection in serum and plasma[a]

Sample		**Storage temperature** 4°C	–20°C	–20°C f/t[b]	–70°C
EDTA plasma	(n = 12)	87[c]	87	87	102
Heparinized plasma	(n = 12)	81	73	79	87
Serum	(n = 12)	82	70	76	74

[a]Samples were stored for two weeks before analysis in ELISA.
[b]–20°C f/t: samples stored at –20°C, were subjected to five freeze–thaw cycles.
[c]sICAM-1 in ng/ml. All samples were assayed in duplicate.

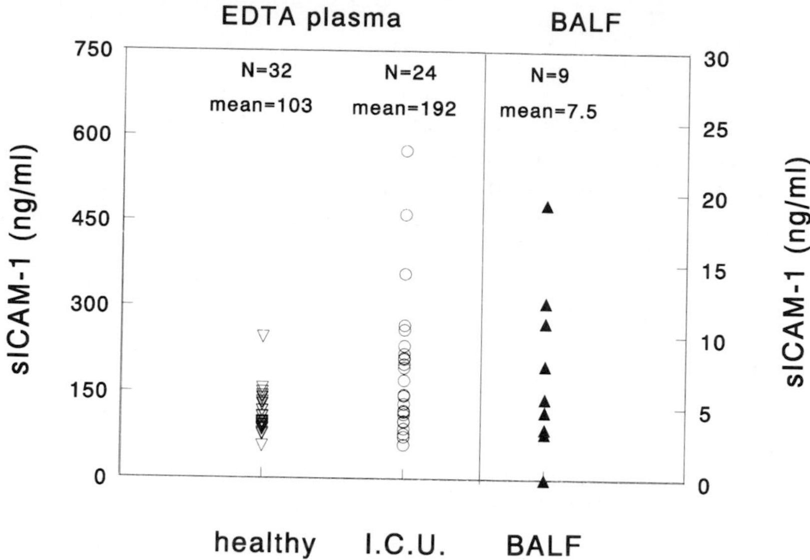

Figure 3. sICAM-1 levels in EDTA plasma of healthy individuals and critically ill patients at I.C.U., and sICAM-1 levels in BALF. Each value represents the mean of duplicate determinations.

in EDTA plasma of 24 critically ill patients at the I.C.U., and in broncho alveolar lavage fluid (BALF) obtained from nine patients undergoing a diagnostic fibre-optic bronchoscopy (*Figure 3*). These human studies were approved by the Ethical Committee of the University Hospital Maastricht.

EDTA plasma of 24 critically ill patients at the intensive care unit (I.C.U.) was collected, as described in *Protocol 3*, on the first day of admission, regardless of diagnosis, and stored at −20°C until analysed. For comparison, EDTA plasma was obtained from healthy volunteers between 20 and 40 years of age. As shown in *Figure 3*, the sICAM-1 levels measured in EDTA plasma of the I.C.U. patients were significantly higher than sICAM-1 levels measured in healthy volunteers (192 ng/ml ± 120 versus 103 ng/ml ± 38).

Furthermore, sICAM-1 levels were determined in BALF obtained during diagnostic fibre-optic bronchoscopy from nine patients with a suspected peripheral lung tumour (*Figure 3*). Further clinical diagnostic evaluation revealed that these patients did not have a malignancy. Lavage was performed in the following way: 200 ml of physiological fluid was instilled into the segment suspected to contain the tumour, in four aliquots. Each aliquot was aspirated immediately after inspiration. The aliquots 2, 3, and 4 were pooled and the BALF was centrifuged to remove cells and debris, and stored at −20°C until analysed. In the BALF of these patients, sICAM-1 was detectable, with a mean value of 8 ± 6 ng/ml.

7. Potential pitfalls

When determining levels of soluble adhesion molecules in culture supernatants or human body fluids, there are some important caveats with regard to the interpretation of such data (3). First, the absolute concentrations measured should be interpreted with caution, since they may vary considerably, depending on the particular ELISA kit used. Due to differences both in antigen specificity of the antibodies, as well as in the standards used in the various ELISAs available, cross-laboratory comparison of results may be hampered. Secondly, although circulating adhesion molecules may serve as good markers for inflammatory activity, the pathophysiological significance of such levels is still unclear for several reasons. An issue of major importance in this respect is whether or not the soluble adhesion molecules detected are biologically active. It is conceivable that a significant fraction of the molecules shed will bind to ligand-bearing cells, and as a result, will either escape detection in ELISA or become biologically inactive. Furthermore, there may be a difference in the systemic and local biological activity of shed adhesion molecules. The concentrations at local sites of production may very well be much higher than those determined in the circulation by ELISA. Consequently, local biological activity may not be reflected by average systemic levels. Finally, little is known about the clearance of circulating adhesion molecules. Impaired clearance due to liver or kidney failure could result in higher detectable serum levels, however, without a direct relation to biological activity.

Acknowledgements

The authors are grateful to Dr A. Craig (Institute of Molecular Medicine, University of Oxford, UK) for providing us with the ICAM-1–Fc construct and for determining the domains of sICAM-1 to which the anti-sICAM-1 mAbs HM.1 and HM.2 were reactive. For providing biological fluids of patient groups, we thank Drs A. Froon and J. Staal-Van den Brekel (Department of Surgery and Department of Pulmonology, University Hospital Maastricht, Maastricht, The Netherlands).

References

1. Stad, R. K. and Buurman, W. A. (1994). *Cell Adhes. Commun.*, **2**, 261.
2. Rougon, G., Durbec, P., and Figarella-Branger, D. (1992). *Cancer J.*, **5**, 137.
3. Gearing, A. J. H. and Newman, W. (1993). *Immunol. Today*, **14**, 506.
4. Von Asmuth, E. J. U., Smeets, E. F., Ginsel, L. A., Onderwater, J. J. M., Leeuwenberg, J. F. M., and Buurman, W. A. (1992). *Eur. J. Immunol.*, **22**, 2519.
5. Leeuwenberg, J. F. M., Smeets, E. F., Neefjes, J. J., Shaffer, M. A., Cinek, T., Jeunhomme, T. M. A. A., *et al.* (1992). *Immunology*, **77**, 543.

6. Pigott, R., Dillon, L. P., Hemingway, I. H., and Gearing, A. J. H. (1992). *Biochem. Biophys. Res. Commun.*, **187**, 584.
7. Newman, W., Beall, L. D., Carson, C. W., Hunder, G. G., Graben, N., Randhawa, Z. I., *et al.* (1993). *J. Immunol.*, **150**, 644.
8. Carson, C. W., Beall, L. D., Hunder, G. G., Johnson, C. M., and Newman, W. (1993). *J. Rheumatol.*, **20**, 809.
9. Kuhns, D. B., Alvord, W. G., and Gallin, J. I. (1995). *J. Infect. Dis.*, **171**, 145.
10. Cowley, H. C., Heney, D., Gearing, A. J. H., Hemingway, I., and Webster, N. R. (1994). *Crit. Care Med.*, **22**, 651.
11. Boldt, J., Wollbruck, M., Kuhn, D., Linke, C., and Hempelmann, G. (1995). *Chest*, **107**, 787.
12. Gruschwitz, M. S., Hornstein, O. P., and Vondendriesch, P. (1995). *Arthritis Rheum.*, **38**, 184.
13. Kim, D. S. and Lee, K. Y. (1994). *Scand. J. Rheumatol.*, **23**, 283.
14. Steiner, M., Reinhardt, K. M., Krammer, B., Ernst, B., and Blann, A. D. (1994). *Thromb. Haemostasis*, **72**, 979.
15. Blann, A. D., Tse, W., Maxwell, S. J. R., and Waite, M. A. (1994). *J. Hypertension*, **12**, 925.
16. Dustin, M. L., Rothlein, R., Bhan, A. K., Dinarello, C. A., and Springer, T. A. (1986). *J. Immunol.*, **137**, 245.
17. Marlin, S. D. and Springer, T. A. (1987). *Cell*, **51**, 813.
18. Diamond, M. S., Staunton, D. E., De Fougerolles, A. R., Stacker, S. A., Garcia-Aguilar, J., Hibbs, M. L., *et al.* (1990). *J. Cell. Biol.*, **111**, 3129.
19. Rosenstein, Y., Park, J. K., Hahn, W. C., Rosen, F. S., Bierer, B. E., and Burakoff, S. J. (1991). *Nature*, **354**, 233.
20. Pober, J. S., Gimbrone, M. A. Jr, Lapierre, L. A., Mendrick, D. L., Fiers, W., Rothlein, R., *et al.* (1986). *J. Immunol.*, **137**, 1893.
21. Myers, C. L., Desai, S. N., Schembri-King, J., Letts, G. L., and Wallace, R. W. (1992). *Am. J. Physiol.*, **262**, C365.
22. Rothlein, R., Mainolfi, E. A., Czajkowski, M., and Marlin, S. D. (1991). *J. Immunol.*, **147**, 3788.
23. Seth, R., Raymond, F. D., and Makgoba, M. W. (1991). *Lancet*, **338**, 83.
24. Kirchhausen, T., Staunton, D. E., and Springer, T. A. (1993). *J. Leukocyte Biol.*, **53**, 342.
25. Nakayama, F., Wakita, H., Tokura, Y., Satoh, T., Maeda, M., and Takigawa, M. (1994). *Eur. J. Dermatol.*, **4**, 641.
26. Budnik, A., Trefzer, U., Parlow, F., Grewe, M., Kapp, A., Schopf, E., *et al.* (1992). *Exp. Dermatol.*, **1**, 27.
27. Shingu, M., Hashimoto, M., Ezaki, I., and Nobunaga, M. (1994). *Clin. Exp. Immunol.*, **98**, 46.
28. Thomson, A. W., Satoh, S., Nussler, A. K., Tamura, K., Woo, J., Gavaler, J., *et al.* (1994). *Clin. Exp. Immunol.*, **95**, 83.
29. Giavazzi, R., Nicoletti, M. I., Chirivi, R. G. S., Hemingway, I., Bernasconi, S., Allavena, P., *et al.* (1994). *Eur. J. Cancer*, **30A**, 1865.
30. Hansen, A. B., Lillevang, S. T., and Andersen, C. B. (1994). *Urol. Res.*, **22**, 85.
31. Giavazzi, R., Chirivi, R. G. S., Garofalo, A., Rambaldi, A., Hemingway, I., Pigott, R., *et al.* (1992). *Cancer Res.*, **52**, 2628.

32. Becker, J. C., Dummer, R., Hartmann, A. A., Burg, G., and Schmidt, R. E. (1991). *J. Immunol.*, **147**, 4398.
33. Law, M. M., Cryer, H. G., and Abraham, E. (1994). *J. Trauma*, **37**, 100.
34. Froon, A. H. M., Greve, J.-W. M., Van der Linden, C. J., and Buurman, W. A. (1996). *Eur. J. Surg.*, **162**, 287.
35. Shijubo, N., Imai, K., Aoki, S., Hirasawa, M., Sugawara, H., Koba, H., *et al.* (1992). *Clin. Exp. Immunol.*, **89**, 58.
36. Nouriaria, K. T., Koskinas, J., Tibbs, C. J., Portmann, B. C., and Williams, R. (1995). *Gut*, **36**, 599.
37. Nielsen, O. H., Langholz, E., Hendel, J., and Brynskov, J. (1994). *Digest. Dis. Sci.*, **39**, 1918.
38. Ameglio, F., Bonifati, C., Carducci, M., Alemanno, L., Sacerdoti, G., and Fazio, M. (1994). *Acta Derm. Venereol. Suppl. Stockh.*, **186**, 19.
39. Christiansen, I., Gidlof, C., Wallgren, A., Simonsson, B., and Totterman, T. H. (1994). *Blood*, **84**, 3010.
40. Tsujisaki, M., Imai, K., Hirata, H., Hanzawa, Y., Masuya, J., Nakano, T., *et al.* (1991). *Clin. Exp. Immunol.*, **85**, 3.
41. Harning, R., Mainolfi, E., Bystryn, J.-C., Henn, M., Merluzzi, V. J., and Rothlein, R. (1991). *Cancer Res.*, **51**, 5003.
42. Altomonte, M., Colizzi, F., Esposito, G., and Maio, M. (1992). *N. Eng. J. Med.*, **327**, 959.
43. Gruss, H.-J., Dölken, G., Brach, M. A., Mertelsmann, R., and Herrmann, F. (1993). *Leukemia*, **7**, 1245.
44. Bechtel, U., Scheuer, R., Landgraf, R., Konig, A., and Feucht, H. E. (1994). *Transplantation*, **58**, 905.
45. Heidenreich, F., Arendt, G., Jander, S., Jablonowski, H., and Stoll, G. (1994). *J. Neuroimmunol.*, **52**, 117.
46. Osborn, L., Hession, C., Tizard, R., Vassallo, C., Luhowskyj, S., Chi-Rosso, G., *et al.* (1989). *Cell*, **59**, 1203.
47. Masinovsky, B., Urdal, D., and Gallatin, W. M. (1990). *J. Immunol.*, **145**, 2886.
48. Cybulsky, M. I., Fries, J. W., Williams, A. J., Sultan, P., Davis, V. M., Gimbrone, M. A. Jr, *et al.* (1991). *Am. J. Pathol.*, **138**, 815.
49. Hession, C., Tizard, R., Vassallo, C., Schiffer, S. G., Goff, D., Moy, P., *et al.* (1991). *J. Biol. Chem.*, **266**, 6682.
50. Freedman, A. S., Munro, J. M., Rice, G. E., Bevilacqua, M. P., Morimoto, C., McIntyrem, B. W., *et al.* (1990). *Science*, **249**, 1030.
51. Rice, G. E., Munro, J. M., Corless, C., and Bevilacqua, M. P. (1991). *Am. J. Pathol.*, **138**, 385.
52. Rice, G. E. and Bevilacqua, M. P. (1989). *Science*, **246**, 1303.
53. Cartwright, J. E., Whitley, G. S., and Johnstone, A. P. (1995). *Exp. Cell Res.*, **217**, 329.
54. Wellicome, S. M., Kapahi, P., Mason, J. C., Lebranchu, Y., Yarwood, H., and Haskard, D. O. (1993). *Clin. Exp. Immunol.*, **92**, 412.
55. Spronk, P. E., Bootsma, H., Huitema, M. G., Limburg, P., and Kallenberg, C. G. M. (1994). *Clin. Exp. Immunol.*, **97**, 439.
56. Stegeman, C. A., Tervaert, J. W. C., Huitema, M. G., De Jong, P. E., and Kallenberg, C. G. M. (1994). *Arthritis Rheum.*, **37**, 1228.
57. Doreduffy, P., Newman, W., Balabanov, R., Lisak, R. P., Mainolfi, E., Rothlein, R., *et al.* (1995). *Ann. Neurol.*, **37**, 55.

58. Lobb, R. R., Chi-Rosso, G., Leone, D. R., Rosa, M. D., Bixler, S., Newman, B. M., *et al.* (1991). *J. Immunol.*, **147**, 124.
59. Ulich, T. R., Howard, S. C., Remick, D. G., Yi, E. H. S., Collins, T., Guo, K. Z., *et al.* (1994). *Inflammation*, **18**, 389.
60. Welder, C. A., Lee, D. H., and Takei, F. (1993). *J. Immunol.*, **150**, 2203.
61. Marlin, S. D., Staunton, D. E., Springer, T. A., Stratowa, C., Sommergruber, W., and Merluzzi, V. J. (1990). *Nature*, **344**, 70.
62. Lo, S. K., Lee, S., Ramos, R. A., Lobb, R., Rosa, R., Chi-Rosso, G., *et al.* (1991). *J. Exp. Med.*, **173**, 1493.
63. Kuijpers, T. W., Hakkert, B. C., Hoogerwerf, M., Leeuwenberg, J. F. M., and Roos, D. (1991). *J. Immunol.*, **147**, 1369.
64. McCabe, S. M., Riddle, L., Nakamura, G. R., Prashad, H., Mehta, A., Berman, P. W., *et al.* (1993). *Cell. Immunol.*, **150**, 364.
65. Secor, W. E., Dosreis, M. G., Ramos, E. A. G., Matos, E. P., Reis, E. A. G., Docarm, T. M. A., *et al.* (1994). *Infect. Immunol.*, **62**, 2695.
66. Engelberts, I., Möller, A., Schoen, G. J. M., Van der Linden, C. J., and Buurman, W. A. (1991). *Lymphokine Cytokine Res.*, **10**, 69.
67. Secchi, C., Berrini, A., and Borromeo, V. (1991). *J. Immunol. Methods*, **136**, 17.

8

Immunochemical assays for complement components

R. WÜRZNER, T. E. MOLLNES, and B. P. MORGAN

1. Introduction

1.1 The complement system

The complement system consists of more than 25 different plasma proteins. Most components are circulating in the blood in an inactive form. Classical or alternative pathway activation of the complement system results in the generation of multiple complement proteolytic cleavage products, recruited from these inactive precursor molecules in a sequentially proceeding cascade (1). This leads to an alteration of their antigenic pattern and thus to the consumption of the native molecule. Concomitantly, complement activation initiates formation of multimolecular complexes which function as convertases within the cascade or express other functions such as the membranolytic effects of the membrane attack complex, the terminal complement complex (TCC) generated on biological membranes. Such activation-dependent changes can be revealed by the appearance of neoepitopes, and by the disappearance of native-restricted epitopes (2), and are usually assessed by means of monoclonal antibodies in enzyme immunoassays (abbreviated as EIAs or ELISAs). The present chapter focuses on sensitive and specific quantitation of complement proteins, fragments, and complexes to reliably assess complement activation *in vivo*. *Figure 1* gives an overview of the complement system and indicates the proteins on which neoepitopes have been found upon activation.

1.2 Clinical importance of the complement system

The physiological importance of complement is graphically illustrated by the syndromes which result from deficiencies of complement components. The wider availability and improved performance of complement assays has resulted in a greatly increased recognition of complement deficiencies. Deficiencies of each component and of virtually all regulatory proteins of the complement

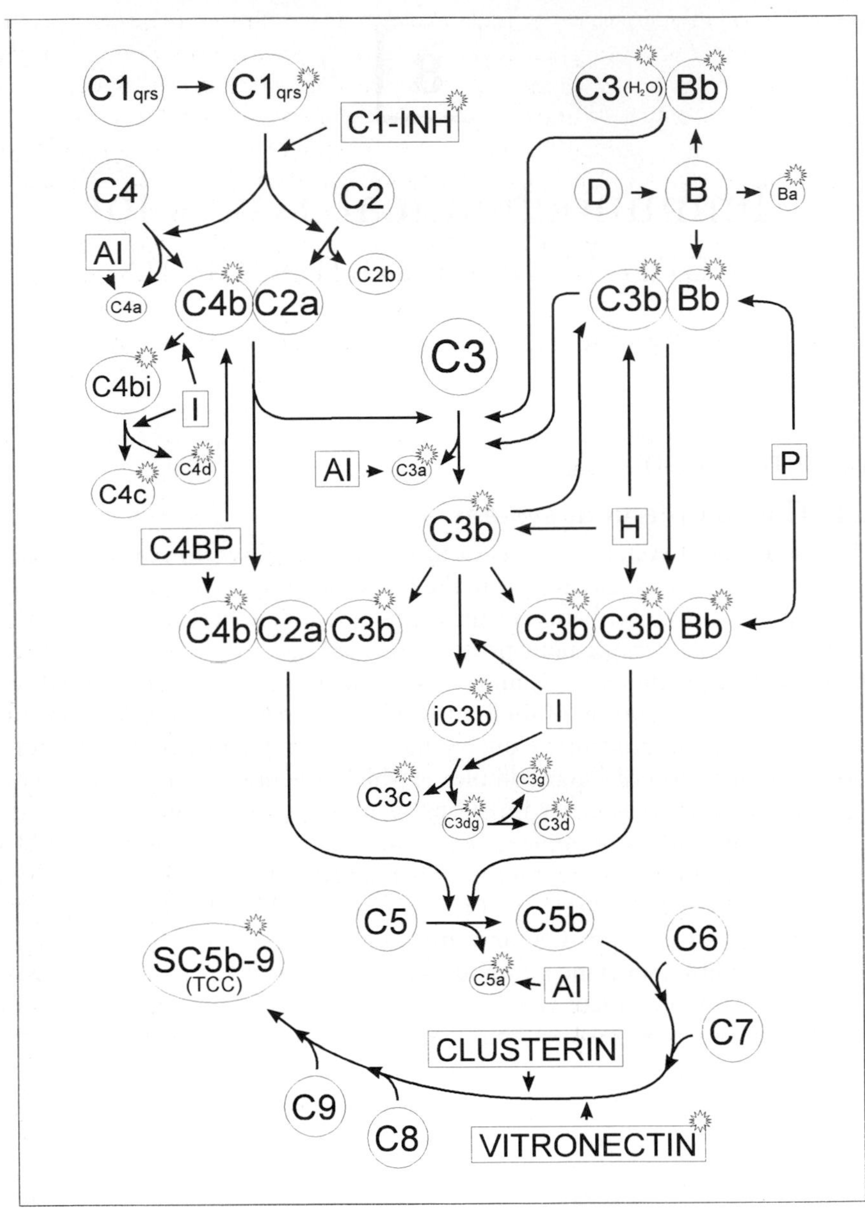

Figure 1. Appearance of neoepitopes (shown by asterisks) within the complement cascade upon activation. (From ref. 2 with permission.)

system have now been described. Depending on the component involved, these deficiencies predispose to immune complex diseases and/or bacterial infections. Several excellent reviews on complement deficiencies have appeared in recent years and the interested reader is referred to these (3–7).

The development of improved assays of complement activation in biological fluids and reagents to detect complement activation products in tissues has also caused an enormous increase in the number of clinical conditions in which complement is implicated. Evidence has included the detection of complement activation products in biological fluids or tissues and information from animal models of disease where complement can be efficiently inhibited. *Table 1* presents an incomplete summary of these many conditions. In almost all of these conditions complement is not the cause but is one of

Table 1. Complement in disease[a]

System	Disease	Evidence		
		Assay[b]	Histology[c]	Model[d]
Renal	Lupus nephritis	Yes	Yes	Yes
	Membranoproliferative GN	Yes	Yes	Yes
	Membranous nephritis	Yes	Yes	Yes
Rheumatological	Rheumatoid arthritis	Yes	Yes	Yes
	SLE	Yes	Yes	Yes
	Behcet's syndrome	Yes	Yes	No
	Juvenile rheumatoid arthritis	Yes	No	No
	Sjogren's syndrome	Yes	No	No
Neurological	Myasthenia gravis	Yes	Yes	Yes
	Multiple sclerosis	Yes	Yes	Yes
	Cerebral lupus	Yes	No	No
	Guillain–Barré syndrome	Yes	Yes	Yes
	Alzheimer's disease	No	Yes	No
Dermatological	Pemphigus/pemphigoid	No	Yes	No
	Phototoxic reactions	Yes	Yes	Yes
	Vasculitis	Yes	Yes	No
Biocompatibility/shock	Post-bypass syndrome	Yes	Yes	Yes
	Catheter reactions	Yes	Yes	No
	ARDS	Yes	Yes	Yes
	Anaphylaxis	Yes	No	No
	Transplant rejection	Yes	Yes	Yes
	Pre-eclampsia	Yes	Yes	No
Others	Atheroma	Yes	Yes	No
	Bowel inflammation	Yes	Yes	No
	Thyroiditis	Yes	Yes	Yes
	Infertility	Yes	Yes	No

[a] Modified from ref. 8.
[b] Evidence from measurement of complement activation products in biological fluids.
[c] Evidence from detection of complement products in diseased tissue.
[d] Evidence from animal models of disease.

several factors involved in pathogenesis; nevertheless, the contribution of complement may be important and perhaps amenable to therapy. A discussion of the roles of complement in diverse disease is beyond the scope of this chapter but has been the subject of several recent reviews (1,8,9).

1.3 Assays for the assessment of complement activation

The methods in use may be divided into immunochemical assays, assessing the presence and integrity of a protein and functional tests determining its activity and functional form. The former comprise radial immunodiffusion (Mancini), electroimmunodiffusion (rocket electrophoresis, Laurell), and enzyme immunoassays (EIAs), whereas the latter include methods that measure, by assessing the haemolytic capacity of the system, the functional integrity of classical, alternative, or terminal pathway or the concentrations of single active components. Detailed protocols for these methods which are widely used are compiled elsewhere (10,11).

Different rates of synthesis, degradation, and renal or hepatic clearance of the individual components, as well as multiple interactions of these complement factors with other serum proteins or cellular receptors may warrant a specific assessment of the concentration of each single component (native protein, cleavage product, or multimolecular complex) (12). Multiple studies have shown that the decrease in concentration of the uncleaved component is less sensitive for assessing complement activation than the increase in cleavage products of the complement activation or the complexes containing that particular component. This is easily understood: a rise of a particular concentration from 1% to 5% is much easier to detect (fivefold increase!) than a decrease from 99% to 95% (which is within the error of the assay). Nevertheless, an accurate assessment of complement activation *in vivo* requires the simultaneous determination of both native and activated complement proteins: low amounts of native proteins in the first place cannot generate as much activation product as high concentrations. Most quantitations, however, are hampered by the fact that the majority of antibodies recognize both native and activated forms. Furthermore, the removal of either form by immunochemical or functional means such as immunoprecipitation methods is error-prone as it can never be complete. Hence a sensitive assay for the assessment of activated complement molecules may additionally measure 5–10% of contaminating native molecules if these have not been depleted in the preceding step. This is the reason why mAbs specific for activation-dependent epitopes are preferred in order to distinguish reliably between activated and native states of complement proteins (2).

During activation, complement split products or complexes are not only released into the fluid phase where they can be readily measured but are also generated or deposited on biological membranes. Immunofluorescence with specific antibodies is the preferred method to detect complement *in situ*. To discriminate local complement activation from passive trapping of complement components neoepitope-specific mAbs have to be used.

1.3.1 Application of specific complement assays to human body fluids

Complement assays are *in vitro* tests that yield a good index of complement activation *in vivo*. They are used to follow the course of a disease, to reveal exacerbations, and to evaluate the success of a treatment. In particular, these assays have been used to assess the biocompatibility of extracorporeal membranes. In addition, these assays may be used to ascertain an arrest at a particular stage since complement activation does not necessarily involve the whole cascade. Concentrations of the individual components usually exhibit wide normal ranges which obscure minor deviations. The acute phase behaviour of most of the complement components will further cloud any changes. Complement deficiencies, however, can be easily assessed using the quantitative methods available but discrimination between subtotal and complete deficiency usually requires sensitive EIAs. However, it is wrong to assume that approximately half normal concentrations indicate heterozygous deficiency—even obligate heterozygous subjects, e.g. parents or children of complement deficient subjects, sometimes present with almost normal concentrations of the component in question.

Some of the mAbs discussed below and some of the assays can also be used to determine complement activation in animal models as detailed elsewhere (12). This, however, is only possible when the mAbs are directed against an epitope which is conserved in the animal counterpart protein.

2. Collection and preservation of samples

Complement undergoes a continuous low-grade activation under physiological conditions. Thus, complement activation products are normally present in low amounts in plasma and can be detected by the EIAs described. In order to obtain reliable results which reflects the *in vivo* situation as closely as possible it is crucially important to avoid *in vitro* activation of complement. Sample collection and preservation should be performed only by specially trained personnel who are aware of the consequences of incorrect handling. There are three basic criteria for correct sample collection:

(a) Preferably EDTA (ethylenediaminetetraacetic acid), inhibiting both the classical and the alternative pathway by binding calcium and magnesium, should be used and must be added to the tube before venepuncture.

(b) The sample temperature must be kept low throughout the whole procedure.

(c) The time from collection to final preparation should be as short as possible.

The effects of these three factors on *in vitro* activation have been investigated systematically (13). Based on these results the following guidelines for sampling should be followed (see *Protocol 1*).

Protocol 1. Guidelines for collection and preservation of samples to be analysed for complement activation products

Equipment and reagents

- Vacutainer or other tubes containing EDTA giving a final concentration of 10 mM after sampling
- Cryotubes or other tubes suitable for storage of plasma at –70 °C

Method

1. Draw blood directly into a tube containing EDTA (final concentration 10 mM) and turn tube gently three or four times to ensure sufficient mixing. Be careful to avoid air bubbles.
2. Place tube immediately on ice or in refrigerator (within 30 min!).
3. Centrifuge for 15 min at 1500 *g*, preferably at 4 °C.
4. Remove plasma carefully (avoid cellular elements), use cryotubes, and store immediately at –70° C. If several activation products are to be measured at different time points, split the plasma sample into small aliquots before freezing—avoid freeze–thaw cycles.

It is most important to keep the samples cold from collection until they are safely stored in the freezer. If the sample has to be stored for a short period during the handling procedure, be sure to keep it cool and never leave it on the bench. The samples can be centrifuged at room temperature if a cooled centrifuge is not available, but in that case be sure to cool the samples immediately after centrifugation. Samples can be stored at –70 °C for several years provided that they are stored at a place where the temperature does not fluctuate due to opening of the freezer (thus, for long-term storage, keep the samples deep in a freezer which is not frequently used). Storage at –20 °C will lead to antigenic changes and exposure of neoepitopes, at least for C3, after a few weeks and must be avoided.

The susceptibility to *in vitro* activation differs between the various components. The C3 and C4 molecules are rather labile *in vitro* and will give false positive results unless the strict guidelines for sampling and storage are followed. In contrast, TCC is rather stable *in vitro* and false positive results due to inappropriate storage are much less common than for products of the early components. The strict guidelines should, however, be followed in any case to avoid *in vitro* activation after sampling; if they are not, results may be highly unreliable.

These guidelines are restricted to complement activation assays. Haemolytic assays can be performed in normal serum frozen at –70 °C within 24 h after sampling. Antigenic quantitation of single components using polyclonal antisera in nephelometry or gel precipitation techniques can be done in serum without special precautions since these techniques do not usually distinguish between native and activated components but measure the total amount of antigen in the sample.

3. EIAs for the assessment of complement activation

A general introduction to enzyme immunoassays (EIA) is given in a preceding chapter. The focus of this paragraph is the methodology of EIAs used to quantitate complement proteins. The optimal design uses the most specific, usually native-restricted or neoepitope-specific mAb as coating antibody. The sample to be assayed is added in an appropriate dilution and measured by means of a second antibody. This antibody is either directly labelled with the enzyme (as detailed in *Figure 2*) or detected via an enzyme-labelled anti-species antibody, or in the case of a biotinylated second antibody, by an enzyme-labelled streptavidin conjugate.

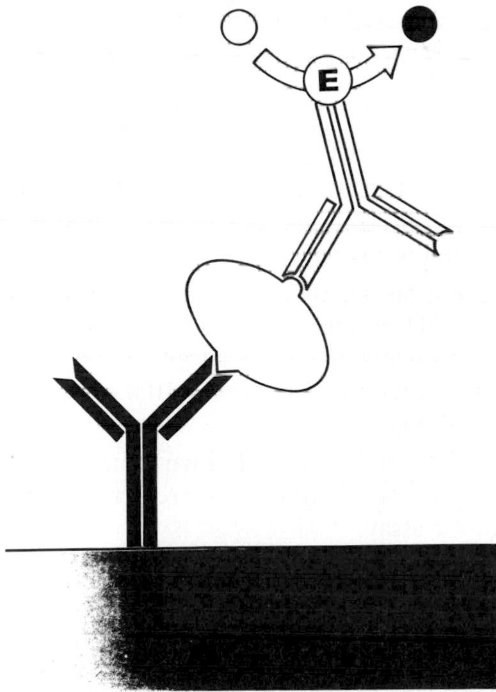

Figure 2. Optimal design for a sensitive and specific EIA: the most specific, preferably activation-dependent mAb is used as coating antibody (black). The sample containing the antigen to be assayed is added in an appropriate dilution and measured by means of an enzyme (E)-labelled second antibody (white) which facilitates substrate turnover (white circle, black circle). (Figure kindly provided by Dr R. Gieseler, University of Göttingen, Germany.)

This design has many advantages over others:

(a) Coating—coat the most specific mAb to the solid phase:

i. It ensures that the epitope in question is bound to the solid phase via the coating mAb and is thus in a less denatured form.

ii. It avoids saturation of the solid phase with irrelevant fragments or the native molecule.

iii. It avoids potentially denaturing procedures for separating native components from activation products.

iv. Antibody-coated plates can generally be stored longer (at least one week at 4 °C) than antigen-coated plates.

Do not coat the antigen directly:

i. It may lead to false results due to a possible denaturation of the protein by adsorption to the solid phase.

ii. It increases the background since other serum proteins are coated as well unless 100% pure preparations are used and this markedly reduces sensitivity.

(b) Blocking—block the solid phase with gelatin, skimmed milk, or bovine serum albumin but only after a very careful titration (incubation of a 0.5% solution of these substances for about 30 min is usually sufficient). In fact, most EIAs work well without any blocking step whereas others may even work better without. The rationale behind blocking is to reduce non-specific adsorption of all reagents applied in later steps to the solid phase but this may not necessarily occur.

(c) Sample application—apply each sample in different dilutions in a buffer containing a mild detergent, such as Tween 20, 0.05%–0.2%, but never undiluted (if virtually undiluted samples have to be used because of low antigen concentration add 10% of a 10 x concentrated stock solution of the dilution buffer):

i. It allows quantitation of unknown concentrations, as at least one of the dilutions are likely to yield results which are within the linear range of the assay.

ii. The detergent will help to reduce non-specific adsorption to the solid phase possibly making the preceding blocking step redundant.

Apply each sample in duplicate or triplicate in order to increase the reliability (intra-assay variation).

(d) Detection—use a labelled, preferably biotinylated, detection antibody:

i. It increases the sensitivity due to the provision of multiple binding sites for the (streptavidin)-conjugate in the following step.

ii. It reduces cross-reactions by avoiding anti-species antibodies in the next step which may react with the solid phase mAb.

Use either a monoclonal or a polyclonal antibody:

i. A mAb of the same species as the coating mAb will yield no cross-reaction, but has to recognize its epitope when the antigen is presented by the coating mAb.

ii. A polyclonal antibody may cross-react with the coating antibody. This can be reduced by incubating it with IgG from the same species as that of the coating mAb prior to its use in the EIA, but this should be considered only as a last resort. If a polyclonal antibody cross-reacts it is preferable that it be replaced by another.

Protocol 2 describes the general equipment and procedure used for EIAs to ascertain complement activation. The details of EIAs for complement components are listed in *Protocols 3–5*.

Protocol 2. Sandwich EIA for the quantitation of complement components

Equipment and reagents

- Spectrophotometer capable of reading absorbance in 96-well microtitre plates at 405 or 410 nm and 490 nm (reference filter)
- Optional: automatic washer for 96-well microtitre plates
- Multichannel pipette
- 96-well flat-bottom microtitre plates
- Phosphate-buffered saline (PBS)
- Optional: coating buffer consisting of 0.2 M sodium carbonate pH 10.6
- Optional, and only after careful titration: blocking buffer consisting of coating buffer or PBS, supplemented with 0.5–1% of gelatin or bovine serum albumin
- Normal human plasma or serum, preferably supplemented with EDTA, as control
- Incubation and washing buffer consisting of PBS supplemented with 0.05–0.2% Tween 20 (Sigma) (the addition of 10 mM EDTA is recommended when incubating the sample to be tested)
- Peroxidase system (other systems, i.e. the one using 1,2-phenylenediamine (Dako), also work well): use 0.5–2 mM ABTS (2,2 azino-di(3-ethyl)-benzthiazoline sulfonate) (e.g. (Boehringer Mannheim, 102946) in 0.1 M acetate buffer (alternatively: supplemented with 0.05 M sodium phosphate), pH 4.0–4.2, to which H_2O_2 (2.5 mM, 30 μl of 3% H_2O_2 per 10 ml acetate buffer) is added immediately before use
- Optional: 10% H_2SO_4 as stop solution

Method

For details see *Protocols 3–5*.

1. Coat the wells of a standard microplate by overnight incubation at 4–8 °C (superior to shorter incubation times or higher incubation temperatures) with 100 μl of coating mAb diluted in coating buffer or PBS. Do not coat the outer wells of the plate as they usually yield less reliable results even if the plate is always placed in a moisture box as recommended for all steps. Seal the plate with Parafilm (American National Can) to reduce evaporation effects. Use the plates within one or two weeks.
2. If no blocking step is required move to step 3. If blocking is considered advantageous, remove the coating buffer by deflecting the

Protocol 2. *Continued*

plate but do not wash with incubation/washing buffer containing a detergent (Tween) as it may affect the following blocking step. Use 150 µl blocking buffer in order to avoid non-specific adsorption to those parts of the wells which become exposed when the plate is not held or placed exactly horizontally (e.g. when you carry the plate). Block for about 30 min at room temperature.

3. Wash plate with washing buffer at room temperature, at least three times between all incubation steps, using 200–300 µl per well. Wash by hand using a multichannel pipette or a plastic bottle, or use an automatic washer. An experienced worker will be faster and as reliable as an automatic washer which is advantageous only when many plates are being used.
4. Apply samples appropriately diluted in incubation buffer (preferably supplemented with 10 mM EDTA, in duplicate). If you have to use virtually undiluted samples (e.g. when testing deficient subjects), add more Tween in a smaller volume of incubation buffer. Titrate the standard serum and apply in duplicate in the same buffer. Keep buffer and samples cool (on crushed ice). Incubate for at least one hour, preferably at 4°C, as this temperature will yield the least *in vitro* complement activation.
5. Wash the plate three times but be careful at the first wash, as some wells may contain very high concentrations of the antigen and others very low. Under these circumstances, even a very short exposure of the latter well with higher amounts of antigen from a neighbouring well may yield falsely positive results.
6. Apply detection antibody diluted in incubation buffer.
7. Wash plate.
8. Apply conjugate diluted in incubation buffer.
9. Wash plate.
10. Add substrate (ABTS, 100 µl per well) rapidly and incubate at room temperature until the upper standard reaches an absorbance of approx. 1.0. Add 100 µl of stop solution if measurement is not possible within the desired time. Read in a spectrophotometer for 96-well microtitre plates at 405/410 nm using 490 nm as reference filter.

There is general agreement that all EIA results obtained using native-restricted mAbs should be expressed in SI units rather than in arbitrary units whenever possible. The situation is rather more complex for EIAs using neoepitope-specific mAbs, because the same epitope can be present in several heterogeneous activation fragments or complexes of that particular component. This is particularly the case for C4 and C3, where some mAbs are reacting with several fragments. However, SI units based on molar concentrations are advantageous as they give an estimate of the actual amounts present and allow comparison between data from different laboratories. Indeed, three anti-TCC assays based on different C9 neoepitope-specific mAbs yielded comparable normal ranges. In the long-term the same standardized reference samples (not yet available) should be used by all laboratories.

4. Native-restricted and neoepitope-specific mAbs

Polyclonal antibodies directed to complement proteins or to their fragments are difficult to standardize and require the storage of a large pool obtained from several animals. Once this stock is used up the new batch has to be assessed again. Most importantly, even if these antibodies were generated by immunizing with either native or activated proteins, they will mostly react with both forms, as an adsorption of the entire unwanted activity is virtually impossible. Thus, mAbs should be used which are specific for native monomeric uncleaved proteins, termed native-restricted mAbs, or which recognize complement components only in their activated configuration, called neoepitope-specific mAbs (14). Both have been described for several complement components.

If it is intended to produce suitable mAbs for EIAs, two steps should be followed. The first involves a selective screening system for hybridoma culture supernatants whereby the solid phase is coated with activated or native serum in adjacent wells. By comparing the reactivities of the culture supernatants in both sets of wells, the few clones showing different patterns can be separated from the others and thus singled out at the very first step (15). The chosen hybridoma culture supernatants can then be further examined for their specificity and suitability in EIA procedures, which is also possible at this early stage (16).

4.1 The classical pathway (*Table* 2)

4.1.1 C1

Binding of C1q to an exposed binding site within an immunoglobulin or another C1q binding molecule induces both loss of antigenic activity and expression of neoepitopes, particularly in the collagenous portion of C1q. Of several anti-C1q mAbs developed by Golan *et al.* (17) mAbs 239E12 and 239G7 were directed against neoepitopes exposed in bound C1q whereas mAbs 241F11 and 242G3 bound to native-restricted epitopes of C1q. Changes in C1q after binding leads to activation of C1r which in turn activates C1s. The latter activation induces conformational changes of the protein without cleavage and a C1s neoepitope is exposed closely related to the esterolytic activity since the neoepitope-specific mAb M241 inhibited the activity markedly (18).

Table 2. Monoclonal antibodies to activation-dependent epitopes in the components of the classical pathway

Antibody	Specificity	Reference
239E12	C1q, collagenous portion; NE[a]	17
239G7	C1q, collagenous portion; NE	17
241F11	C1q, collagenous portion; NRE[b]	17
242G3	C1q, collagenous portion; NRE	17
M241	C1s; NE related to the esterolytic activity	18
242	C4b; NE	19
α-C4d	C4d; NE	20
CLB anti-C4–1	iC4, C4b, iC4b, C4c; NE	21
A1 121/6	C4 and C4d, but not C4b	22
C2-S3	C2; NRE	23
C2-S9	C2; NRE	23

[a] NE, neoepitope.
[b] NRE, native-restricted epitope.

4.1.2 C4

C4 is cleaved during activation into C4b and C4a. C4b is further degraded to iC4b, C4c, and C4d. Neoepitopes are expressed in C4b (mAb 242) (19) and in C4d (a-C4d) (20), whereas C4a is one of the few complement activation products for which there are, as yet, no monoclonal antibodies reacting with neoepitopes. Recently, an interesting anti-C4 mAb (CLB anti-C4–1) has been described reacting with a neoepitope in the C4c part of the molecule after disruption of the thioester bond. This antibody reacts with hydrolysed C4 (iC4), C4b, iC4b, and C4c, but not with native C4, and can successfully be used for the detection of C4 activation products (21). Upon treatment of C4 with activated C1s or methylamine an epitope identified by mAb A1 121/6 is exposed in native C4 and in C4d, but not in C4b or methylamine-treated C4 (22). Thus, this is a linear epitope which is hidden during activation of C4 but reappears in the final C4d fragment.

4.1.3 C2

mAbs to neoepitopes in C2 activation fragments have not been described, but a few native-restricted C2 specific antibodies (C2-S3, C2-S9) have been developed (23).

Assays for complexes of components from the classical pathway have also been described using antibodies specific for C1rs/C1 inhibitor complexes (24). Recently, complexes between C4 and C3 were detected (25) using the neoepitope-specific mAb 13/15 (identifies C3b, iC3b, and C3dg) (26) and a conventional mAb to C4 (M4d2). A review on mAbs to activation-dependent epitopes in components of the classical pathway is recommended for further reading (27).

4.2 C3 and the alternative pathway (*Table 3*)

Table 3. Monoclonal antibodies to neoepitopes in the components of the alternative pathway

Antibody	Specificity	Reference
H13	C3a, C3a-desArg	28
H453, H454	C3a, C3a-desArg	29
H466	C3a-desArg	30
Anti-C3a	C3a, C3a-desArg	31
2900	C3a	32
Anti-C3–5	iC3, C3a	33
Anti-C3–9	iC3, C3b, iC3b, C3c	33
Anti-C3–11	iC3, C3b, iC3b, C3d	33
bH6	C3b, iC3b, C3c	34
I3/15	C3b, iC3b, C3dg	26
7D84.1, 7D264.6	Surface bound iC3b	35
7D323.1	iC3b	35
nn/A209	iC3b	Quidel
130	iC3b, C3dg, C3d	36
105	C3b, iC3b, C3c	37
C-5G	C3b, C3c	38
G-3E	iC3b, C3dg, C3d	38
Clone 9	iC3b, C3dg, C3g	39
D22/3	Ba	40
014–11, 014III-221	Ba	41
032B-22, 032B-39, 032B-49, 032B-71	Bb	41

4.2.1 C3

The central and most abundant component C3 can be activated and split into C3a and C3b either by the classical (C4bC2a) or the alternative (C3bBb) pathway convertase. C3b is further degraded by factors I and H to iC3b, C3c, and C3dg. Continuous hydrolysis of the internal thioester bond of C3 generates a particular form of the molecule called C3(H_2O) or iC3. During hydrolysis the molecule undergoes conformational changes rendering it 'C3b-like' although C3a is not split off. This molecule can bind factor B and thus serve as the basis for an alternative C3 convertase (C3(H_2O)Bb), which is able to cleave C3.

Several mAbs to neoepitopes in C3a and C3a-desArg (inactivated C3a where the terminal arginine residue has been cleaved off by carboxypeptidase N) were described by Burger *et al.* (28,29) and one of these (H466) has been used in a quantitative EIA specific for this anaphylatoxin (30). A similar antibody and EIA was described by Nilsson *et al.* (31). Hartmann *et al.* described several anti-C3a neoepitope antibodies and the mAb 2900 was used to design a quantitative C3a assay based on a combination of chromatographic and immunoassay procedures (32).

Some mAbs described by Hack *et al.* (33) identified neoepitopes expressed after hydrolysis of the internal thioester. These neoepitopes were detected both in the C3a (anti-C3–5), C3c (anti-C3–9), and C3d portion (anti-C3–11) of the intact C3(H_2O) molecule. The fact that they were also expressed in the activation fragments C3b, iC3b, and their further degradation products is consistent with the structural similarity between C3(H_2O) and C3b. The anti-C3–5 mAb was further used to detect iC3 in normal human plasma (42). A series of other mAbs to neoepitopes of the C3b fragment and its degradation products have been described (26,34–39,43) of which several are expressed in more than one fragment. Some of these antibodies have been used to design EIAs for quantitation of C3 activation products as described in detail in the original papers (44,45).

A recommended terminology for the activation products detected by antibodies reacting with more than one fragment is proposed: the terms C3bc and C3bd should be used when the antibody identifies the C3c and C3d fragments, respectively, and still reacts with the precursors iC3b, C3b, and/or iC3. The same terminology should be used for the C4 activation products (C4bc and C4bd) (21).

4.2.2 Factor B

After binding to C3b or C3(H_2O) factor B is cleaved to Ba and Bb by factor D. Neoepitopes are exposed both in the Ba (40,41) and Bb fragments (41) and the respective antibodies have been used in studies to quantify these fragments. Factor D is secreted and circulates in activated form *in vivo* and is thus probably not a candidate for neoepitope expression.

An assay to detect alternative pathway activation based on complex formation between C3b, Bb, and properdin (C3b(Bb)P) has been described using antibodies to C3 and properdin not specific for neoepitopes (24). Factor B and its activation fragments have also been specifically detected without mAbs to activation-dependent epitopes though still avoiding non-specific fractionation of the samples prior to testing (26). This was accomplished by specific depletion of factor B from the sample by immunomagnetic separation using beads which had been conjugated with mAbs to Bb or Ba prior to detection of Ba and Bb, respectively. Reviews on mAbs to activation-dependent epitopes in components of C3 and the alternative pathway are recommended for further reading (41,46).

Protocol 3 summarizes the specific equipment and essential details for the quantitation of C3 activation products. A detailed list of the equipment and methodology is given in *Protocol 2*.

Protocol 3. Sandwich EIA for the quantitation of complement C3 activation fragments C3b, iC3b, and C3c (C3bc)

Equipment and reagents

- See *Protocol 2*
- PBS as coating buffer
- Washing and incubation buffer: PBS containing 0.1% Tween 20
- Standard: pool of normal human serum activated with zymosan (Sigma) (10 mg/ml serum, incubate for 1 h at 37 °C, centrifuge for 45 min at 10 000 *g*)
- EDTA
- mAb bH6 (34) (similar mAbs (listed in *Table 3*) can be obtained from Quidel or other sources)
- Rabbit anti-human C3c (Behringwerke)
- Peroxidase-conjugated anti-rabbit Ig (Amersham)

Method

1. Coat ascitic fluid of mAb bH6, 1/10 000 diluted in PBS (or other mAb in appropriate dilution), overnight at 4 °C.
2. Wash.
3. Apply samples diluted in incubation buffer supplemented with 10 mM EDTA for 1 h at 4 °C; test and reference samples 1/150 diluted, standard serum 1/800 to 1/51 200 diluted.
4. Wash.
5. Apply detection antibody anti-C3c, 1/10 000 diluted in incubation buffer for 45 min at 37 °C.
6. Wash.
7. Apply conjugate anti-rabbit Ig, 1/1000 diluted in incubation buffer for 45 min at 37 °C.
8. Wash.
9. Apply substrate and read the plate.

4.3 The terminal pathway (*Table 4*)

Assembly of the terminal complement complex (TCC) during complement activation is different from activation of alternative and classical pathways as it is associated with considerable antigenic changes in the individual components C5, C6, C7, C8, and C9, but involves no enzymatic splitting of the components apart from the initiating cleavage of C5. These changes transform the hydrophilic properties of the native proteins into partly hydrophobic structures which permit the insertion of the nascent C5b–9 into lipid membranes. Consequently a number of native-specific epitopes become concealed whereas neoepitopes appear.

Native-specific mAbs have been characterized for most terminal complement proteins. In addition to their use for reliable quantitation of the unactivated

Table 4. Monoclonal antibodies to activation-dependent epitopes in the components of the terminal pathway

Antibody	Specificity	Reference
238.3	C5a-desArg; NE[a]	47
4A2E10E2, 3G3C4, 2H6A2,..	C5a-desArg; NE	48
269–10F7, ...	C5a/C5a-desArg; NE	49
2A5E3, ...	C5a/C5a-desArg; NE	50
C17/5	C5a, C5a-desArg; NE	51
Clone 568	C5; NRE[b]	52
N19–8, N20–9	C5; NRE	53
WU 6–4	C6; NRE	53
M1	C9; NRE	54
P40	C9; NRE	55
Poly C9-MA	C9 in C5b–9(m), SC5b–9, poly C9; NE	56
aE11/M0777	C9 in C5b–9(m), SC5b–9, poly C9; NE	57, DAKO
bC5	C9 in C5b–9(m), SC5b–9, poly C9; NE	57
3B1, 3D8, 2F3, 1A12	C9 in C5b–9(m), SC5b–9, poly C9; NE	58
056B-75/A209	C9 in C5b–9(m), SC5b–9, poly C9; NE	59, Quidel
1B4	C9 in C5b–9(m), SC5b–9, poly C9; NE	60
WU 7–2, WU 13–15	C9 in C5b–9(m), SC5b–9, poly C9; NE	53
X-11	C9 in C5b–9(m), SC5b–9, ?poly C9; NE	61, Biomedicals
B7	C9 in C5b–9(m), SC5b–9, poly C9; NE	62

[a] NE, neoepitope.
[b] NRE, native-restricted epitope.

molecule, they have been used to inhibit TCC formation *in vitro* since the structures represented by the epitopes might be essential for TCC formation in the fluid phase and also for its generation on membranes. Thus, these mAbs may provide possible therapeutic targets for *in vivo* interventions (63).

4.3.1 C5

C5 is unique among the terminal complement components as complement activation generates a biologically important chemotactically active split product, C5a. As for C3a, this anaphylatoxin is also under strict control of the ubiquitous carboxypeptidase N which converts C5a to the less potent but still biologically active C5a-desArg. Several mAbs specific for C5a/C5a-desArg have been described, some of which were obtained using rabbit C5a for immunization, but all cross-react with human C5a (50). Most of the mAbs also block the binding of C5a/C5a-desArg to its cellular receptor and can therefore be used for receptor studies. Two of the neutralizing anti-C5a mAbs were obtained by repeated competitive biopanning of a phage monovalent Fab display library (64). Two EIA appear to be superior to others for the quantitation of human C5a (48,51).

Despite the fact that C5a is cleaved from the α-chain, a mAb against the C5 β-chain was shown to be a powerful inhibitor of C5a liberation when added to the serum prior to complement activation (53) but it was not established whether this also reacted with C5 incorporated into human TCC. This was demonstrated for clone 568 which reacts with native C5 but not with C5 in the TCC (52).

4.3.2 C6

An EIA based on the native-restricted mAb anti-C6 WU 6–4 has been used to identify C6 deficient individuals whose sera were not completely devoid of C6 but contained low concentrations of this protein. In addition, the decrease of native C6 after *in vitro* complement activation indicated the presence of functionally active molecules which was confirmed by a simultaneous increase in TCC formation (65). When the mAb was added to serum before complement activation it inhibited TCC formation in the fluid phase and, to a lesser extent, on the membrane (53). Recent studies have revealed that WU 6–4 does not even react with the intermediate complex C5b6 (66).

4.3.3 C7 and C8

To date no mAb has been described which distinguishes between native C7 or C8 and their TCC-integrated form. For C8, however, a C8α-specific mAb has been reported which recognizes an epitope expressed only on free C8α–γ (67). This mAb inhibits the haemolytic activity of C8α–γ but has no effect on native or membrane-bound C8 (67).

4.3.4 C9

Two EIAs designed for the quantitation of non-activated C9 have been established using different native C9-specific mAbs (54,55). Of these two mAbs, one does not react with C9 adsorbed to plastic or blotted to nitrocellulose membranes (54) whereas the other does also bind under these conditions (55). Neither binds to poly C9 nor to C9 incorporated into the TCC. In addition, EIAs using both mAbs revealed complete C9 deficiencies within the detection limits of the EIA (55,68). Another three anti-C9 mAbs have been mentioned which strongly bound to native C9 in a sandwich EIA but failed to recognize C9 in the MAC on complement lysed ghosts (69). In studies for the detection of C9 in diseased tissues two of five anti-C9 mAbs failed to bind to C9 after its insertion into membranes (70).

The binding regions of all neoepitope-specific anti-TCC mAbs described so far are located on the C9 moiety of the TCC, with the exception of one mAb (aE11) which also cross-reacts with C8α within the nascent complex (71), which is likely to be a reflection of the fact that C8α is structurally and functionally related to C9. The predominant presence of the neoepitopes on C9 mirrors the marked conformational changes which C9 undergoes during TCC assembly but may also be due to the fact that it is the most abundant molecule in the TCC.

Despite the fact that the membrane-integrated form (C5b–9(m)) is structurally different from the fluid phase form (SC5b–9), especially with respect to the number of C9 molecules per complex, no mAb has been described so far which is able to distinguish between the two forms. Since vitronectin (S-protein) is also able to integrate into the membrane attack complex after generation of C5b–9(m), this cannot be used for discrimination.

For poly C9 the number of C9 molecules present may also play a role in the appearance and disappearance of activation-specific epitopes. Poly C9 can be made using zinc, generating much bigger complexes (with more C9 molecules) than by the method using magnesium. One mAb (X-11) failed to react to poly C9 generated by the latter method whereas the former was not used in these experiments (61). It is possible that mAbs will become available which can discriminate between C5b–9(m), SC5b–9, poly $C9_{(\text{too-few C9 molecules})}$, and poly $C9_{(\text{many C9 molecules})}$.

In any case, most of the other anti-TCC mAbs show differences, for example some precipitate C5b–9 complexes whereas others do not (58). In addition, some cross-react with animal sera (58), which is useful for animal studies, whereas others do not even cross-react with primate sera (61).

Sensitive EIAs, based on these neoepitope-specific mAbs which are able to detect TCC in EDTA–plasma have been described (15,53,59,60,72). TCC EIAs are superior in many circumstances, as a means of assaying complement activation, to assays quantifying the anaphylatoxin C5a:

(a) TCC has a much longer half-life *in vivo* than C5a due to immediate binding of the latter to its cell membrane receptor.

(b) Data from *in vitro* experiments suggest that terminal complement activation may also occur in the absence of C3 activation or C5a generation, by cleavage of C5 caused by enzymes released from injured tissues or by oxygen radicals.

(c) The stability of TCC *in vitro* is much higher than that of the early components.

Therefore, a TCC EIA is recommended for the assessment of terminal complement activation. Furthermore, an increase of TCC concentrations after *in vivo* or *in vitro* activation demonstrates that all terminal complement components are present in a functionally active form. This unique feature turns the immunochemical assay into a functional test.

Protocol 4 summarizes the specific equipment and essential details for the quantitation of the fluid phase terminal complement complex (TCC). A detailed list of the equipment and methodology is given in *Protocol 2*.

Protocol 4. Sandwich EIA for the quantitation of fluid phase terminal complement complex (TCC)

Equipment and reagents

- See *Protocol 2*
- Coating buffer consisting of 0.2 M sodium carbonate pH 10.6
- Blocking buffer: coating buffer containing 0.5% gelatin
- Washing and incubation buffer: PBS containing 0.05% Tween 20
- Standard: pool of normal human serum activated with baker's yeast (30 mg/ml plasma, incubate for 2 h at 37°C, centrifuge for 10 min at 10000 *g*, contains about 300–600 μg TCC/ml)
- EDTA (recommended)
- mAb WU 7–2 or WU 13–15 (53) (coating and detection antibodies and a reference sample are available from the authors upon request (R. W.); similar mAbs (listed in *Table 4*) can be obtained from other sources)
- Goat anti-C6, biotinylated
- Streptavidin–horse-radish peroxidase (Boehringer Mannheim, 1089152)

Method

1. Coat WU 7–2 or WU 13–15, 15 μg/ml in coating buffer, overnight at 4°C.
2. Block with blocking buffer for 30 min at room temperature.
3. Wash.
4. Apply samples diluted in incubation buffer preferably supplemented with 10 mM EDTA for 2 h at 4°C; human serum 1/20 diluted, human plasma 1/2 diluted, activated serum 1/400 diluted, standard activated serum 1/100 to 1/32000 diluted.
5. Wash.
6. Apply detection antibody goat anti-C6, biotinylated, 20 μg/ml in incubation buffer for 1 h at room temperature.
7. Wash.
8. Apply conjugate streptavidin–horse-radish peroxidase, diluted according to the manufacturer (usually 1/1000) in incubation buffer for 1 h at room temperature.
9. Wash.
10. Apply substrate and read the plate.

5. mAbs directed against complement control proteins (*Table 5*)

Complement is tightly controlled *in vivo* by a battery of fluid phase and membrane regulatory proteins (1). These proteins restrict complement activation at multiple stages in the pathway. In the fluid phase, C1 inhibitor (C1 INH)

Table 5. Monoclonal antibodies to complement regulatory proteins[a]

Antibody	**Specificity**	**Reference/comments**
KOK-12	C1 INH, complexed with target; NE[b]	73
KII	C1 INH, cleaved inactivated form; NE	74
4C3	C1 INH, complexed and inactivated; NE	75
nn[c]	C1 INH	CLB, p IgGx[d,e]
nn/A229	FH	Quidel, p IgGx
10–10	FH	Biogenesis, p IgGx
OX-23, OX-24	FH	Serotec, IgG1, T[f]
nn/A247	FI	Quidel, p IgGx, blocks
nn/A231	FI	Quidel, p IgGx, does not block
3R2–2/3R8	FI	Biogenesis, p IgGx
HYB61–1	FI	Statens Seruminstitut, IgG1, T
OX-21	FI	Serotec, IgG1, T
nn/A215	C4bp	Quidel, p IgGx
10–07	C4bp	Biogenesis, p IgGx
nn/A233	Properdin	Quidel, p IgGx, blocks
nn/A235	Properdin	Quidel, p IgGx, does not block
10–18, 10–24	Properdin	Biogenesis, p IgGx
HYB39–4/6	Properdin	Statens Seruminstitut, IgG1, T
nn/A237	Vitronectin (S-protein)	Quidel, p IgGx
1.110	Vitronectin (S-protein)	Biogenesis, IgG1, A[g]
nn/A241	Clusterin	Quidel, p IgGx
BRIC 216, BRIC 110	DAF	IBGRL, IgG1, T, blocks in combin.
BRIC 128	DAF	IBGRL, IgM, T
J4–48	MCP	Biogenesis/Serotec, p IgG1
E4.3	MCP	Serotec, IgG2a, A
E11	CR1	Seralab/Serotec, p IgG1
Mab 543	CR1	ATCC, hybridoma, IgG1
To5	CR1	DAKO, IgG1, T
BRIC 229	CD59	IBGRL, IgG2b, T, blocks
MEM 43	CD59	Biogen./Serotec, p IgG2a, blocks
YTH53.1	CD59	Serotec, rat IgG2b, blocks

[a]The list is not comprehensive and is restricted to those antibodies which are available commercially and of which the authors have personal experience.
[b]NE, neoepitope.
[c]nn, no name given for clone—catalogue number substituted when available.
[d]p, purified.
[e]x, subclass not stated.
[f]T, tissue culture supernatant.
[g]A, ascites.

dissociates activated C1, factor H (FH) acts as a cofactor for factor I (FI) cleavage of C3 in the convertases of the classical and alternative activation pathways, C4b binding protein acts as a cofactor for FI cleavage of C4 in the classical pathway convertase, and vitronectin (S-protein) and clusterin inhibit the assembly of the membrane attack complex. Properdin is unique in that it is a positive regulator, stabilizing the alternative pathway convertases and thus enhancing activation. On the membrane, decay accelerating factor (DAF), membrane cofactor protein (MCP), and complement receptor 1

(CR1) restrict the convertases of the activation pathways whereas CD59 inhibits membrane attack complex assembly. Each of the membrane inhibitors can additionally be found at low concentrations in biological fluids, although in some cases the significance of this finding remains uncertain. With the exception of vitronectin and clusterin, deficiencies of each of the fluid phase and membrane regulator proteins have been described and are associated with distinct clinical features.

Monoclonal antibodies have been produced against each of the fluid phase and membrane regulatory proteins and used to establish EIA protocols, to detect the regulators in tissues, and to quantify by flow cytometry their expression on cell membranes. With the exception of antibodies against C1 INH (see below), all the antibodies produced against regulatory proteins bind to the native molecule. Some of these antibodies bind near the active site of the regulator and block the inhibitory functions of the molecule. Most of the EIA protocols described have used monoclonal capture antibodies and polyclonal detection antibodies.

C1 INH dissociates activated C1 and forms complexes with C1r and C1s. Within these complexes neoepitopes appear, either in the complex (detected by mAb KOK-12) (73) or in the inactivated non-complexed form of C1 INH (mAb KII) (74). mAb KOK-12 has been used as a capture antibody to develop a non-separation assay for classical pathway activation complexes (C1 INH/C1r/C1s) and for activation complexes in the coagulation cascade in which C1 INH also plays a role (76). Another antibody, mAb 4C3, has been reported to recognize neoepitopes in both complexed and uncomplexed inactive C1 INH (75,77).

CD59 is present in urine, seminal plasma, amniotic fluid, breast milk, cerebrospinal fluid, tears, and (at very low levels) plasma. An example of an ELISA protocol for CD59 capable of measuring CD59 in these various fluids is given in *Protocol 5*.

Protocol 5. Sandwich EIA for the quantitation of CD59

Equipment and reagents

- See *Protocol 2*
- Coating buffer consisting of 0.2 M sodium carbonate pH 10.6
- Blocking buffer: PBS, containing 1% bovine serum albumin and 0.1% Tween 20
- Washing and incubation buffer: PBS containing 0.1% Tween 20
- Standards: purified CD59 isolated from urine or erythrocytes
- mAb YTH53.1 rat anti-CD59 (78) (coating and detection antibodies and a reference sample are available from the authors upon request (B. P. M.); similar mAbs (listed in *Table 5*) can be obtained from other sources)
- Rabbit anti-CD59
- Donkey anti-rabbit Ig–horse-radish peroxidase (Jackson Labs, code 711–035–152)

Method

1. Coat YTH53.1, 1 μg/ml in coating buffer, overnight at 4 °C.
2. Block with blocking buffer for 1 h at 37 °C.

Protocol 5. *Continued*

3. Wash.
4. Apply samples diluted in incubation buffer for 2 h at 37 °C: plasma, serum, cerebrospinal fluid 1/2 diluted; urine and other biological fluids 1/10 diluted; standards in range 1–1000 ng/ml.
5. Wash.
6. Apply detection antibody rabbit anti-CD59, 0.5 μg/ml in incubation buffer for 2 h at 37 °C.
7. Wash.
8. Apply conjugate donkey anti-rabbit Ig–horse-radish peroxidase, diluted according to the manufacturer (usually 1/1000) in incubation buffer for 2 h at 37 °C.
9. Wash.
10. Apply substrate and read the plate.

6. Allospecific mAbs (*Table 6*)

Allospecific mAbs are classified by their ability to exclusively react with one or more defined allotypes of that particular component. The application of these mAbs include the detection of homo- or heterozygous deficient subjects in family studies, the detection of gene duplications, and the assessment of the contribution of different sources of body fluids to a combined pool as in transplantation and transfusion studies. Allospecific mAbs have been characterized for C4, C3, and C7.

For C3 and C7 the allotype associated with a proline residue is not detected by the mAb whereas the leucine- (C3) or threonine- (C7) associated allotype is detected (81,83). The allospecific anti-C3 antibody (HAV 4–1) was discovered via its reaction pattern on immunoblots (80), whereas the allospecific anti-C7 antibody (WU 4–15) was found by comparing its reaction pattern with that of polyclonal anti-C7 IgG, in an EIA set-up where both were used as coating antibody (82,84).

Protocol 6 details the determination of the C7 M/N allotype.

Table 6. Allotype-specific monoclonal antibodies

Antibody	**Specificity**	**Reference**
AII 1	C4A	79
BII 1	C4B	79
HAV 4–1	C3 HAV 4–1 +	80,81
WU 4–15	C7 M	82,83

Protocol 6. Sandwich EIAs for the determination of the C7 M/N allotype

Equipment and reagents

- See *Protocol 2*
- Coating buffer consisting of 0.2 M sodium carbonate pH 10.6
- Blocking buffer: coating buffer containing 0.5% gelatin
- Washing and incubation buffer: PBS containing 0.05% Tween 20
- Standard serum of allotype C7 M, control sera with known C7 M/N phenotypes
- mAb WU 4–15 (for EIA M) (84) and goat anti-C7 (for EIA P) (coating and detection antibodies and reference samples are available from the authors upon request (R. W.); almost any good anti-C7 IgG may be used but no similar mAb exists)
- Goat anti-C7, biotinylated
- Streptavidin–horse-radish peroxidase (Boehringer Mannheim, 1089152)

Method

1. Coat half of the wells with WU 4–15, 5 μg/ml in coating buffer and the other half with goat anti-C7, 20 μg/ml in coating buffer, overnight at 4°C.
2. Block with blocking buffer for 30 min at room temperature.
3. Wash.
4. Apply sera or plasma 1/2500 diluted in incubation buffer for 1 h at room temperature.
5. Wash.
6. Apply detection antibody goat anti-C7, biotinylated, 20 μg/ml in incubation buffer for 1 h at room temperature.
7. Wash.
8. Apply conjugate streptavidin–horse-radish peroxidase, diluted according to the manufacturer (usually 1/1000) in incubation buffer for 1 h at room temperature.
9. Wash.
10. Apply substrate and read the plate. Calculate ratios for each sample by dividing the C7 concentration obtained with EIA M by the one obtained with EIA P. Samples with a ratio between 0.75 and 1.25 define C7 M subjects, whereas ratios between 0.35 and 0.65, or less than 0.02 identify C7 MN or C7 N subjects, respectively.

The Rodgers 1,2-specific mAbs 99H7 and VlaD2 recognize most C4A allotypes but also some C4B allotypes, whereas the Chido 1-specific mAbs 2B12, 1217, and 1228 are reactive with most C4B allotypes, but also some C4A allotypes—thus, both groups of mAbs are allotype-specific for a panel of allotypes (85–87).

More recently, anti-peptide mAbs have been obtained from mice immunized with C4A or C4B-specific peptides containing the specific amino acid residues 1101–1106. These mAbs AII 1 and BII 1 react with C4A or C4B allotypes, respectively (79).

References

1. Morgan, B. P. (1994). In *Immunochemistry* (ed. C. J. van Oss and M. H. V. van Regenmortel), p. 903. Marcel Decker, New York.
2. Mollnes, T. E. and Harboe, M. (1993). *Immunologist*, **1**, 43.
3. Morgan, B. P. and Walport, M. J. (1990). *Immunol. Today*, **12**, 301.
4. Densen, P. (1993). In *Complement in health and disease* (ed. K. Whaley, M. Loos, and J. Weiler), p. 173. Kluwer, Lancaster.
5. Colten, H. R. and Rosen, F. S. (1992). *Adv. Immunol.*, **10**, 785.
6. Figueroa, J. E. and Densen, P. (1991). *Clin. Microbiol. Rev.*, **4**, 359.
7. Würzner, R., Orren, A., and Lachmann, P. J. (1992). *Immunodef. Rev.*, **3**, 123.
8. Morgan, B. P. (1994). *Eur. J. Clin. Invest.*, **24**, 219.
9. Morgan, B. P. (1995). *Crit. Rev. Clin. Lab. Sci.*, **32**, 265.
10. Whaley, K. (1985). *Methods in complement for clinical immunologists*. Churchill-Livingstone, Edinburgh, UK.
11. Harrison, R. A. and Lachmann, P. J. (1986). In *Handbook of experimental immunology*, Vol. 1, *Immunochemistry* (ed. D. M. Weir), p. 39.1. Blackwell, Oxford.
12. Oppermann, M., Höpken, U., and Götze, O. (1992). *Immunopharmacology*, **24**, 119.
13. Mollnes, T. E., Garred, P., and Bergseth, G. (1988). *Clin. Exp. Immunol.*, **73**, 484.
14. Mollnes, T. E. (1989). *Complement Inflamm.*, **6**, 134.
15. Mollnes, T. E., Lea, T., Froland, S., and Harboe, M. (1985). *Scand. J. Immunol.*, **22**, 197.
16. Würzner, R., Oppermann, M., Zierz, R., Baumgarten, H., and Götze, O. (1990). *J. Immunol. Methods*, **126**, 231.
17. Golan, M. D., Burger, R., and Loos, M. (1982). *J. Immunol.*, **129**, 445.
18. Matsumoto, M. and Nagaki, K. (1986). *J. Immunol.*, **137**, 2907.
19. Ichihara, C., Nakamura, T., Nagasawa, S., and Koyama, J. (1986). *Mol. Immunol.*, **23**, 151.
20. Kolb, W. P., Latham, A. L., Morrow, P. R., and Tamerius, J. D. (1988). *Complement Inflamm.*, **5**, 214.
21. Wolbink, G. J., Bollen, J., Baars, J. W., Tenberge, R. J. M., Swaak, A. J. G., Paardekooper, J., *et al.* (1993). *J. Immunol. Methods*, **163**, 67.
22. Maeda, S., Takamaru, Y., Fukatsu, J., and Nagasawa, S. (1993). *Biochem. J.*, **289**, 503.
23. Stenbaek, E. I., Koch, C., Barkholt, V., and Welinder, K. G. (1986). *Mol. Immunol.*, **23**, 879.
24. Zilow, G., Sturm, J. A., Rother, U., and Kirschfink, M. (1990). *Clin. Exp. Immunol.*, **79**, 151.
25. Zwirner, J., Dobos, G., and Götze, O. (1995). *J. Immunol. Methods*, **186**, 55.
26. Oppermann, M., Baumgarten, H., Brandt, E., Gottsleben, W., Kurts, C., and Götze, O. (1990). *J. Immunol. Methods*, **133**, 181.

27. Heinz, H. P. and Loos, M. (1989). *Complement Inflamm.*, **6**, 166.
28. Burger, R., Bader, A., Kirschfink, M., Rother, U., Schrod, L., Worner, I., *et al.* (1987). *Clin. Exp. Immunol.*, **68**, 703.
29. Burger, R., Zilow, G., Bader, A., Friedlein, A., and Naser, W. (1988). *J. Immunol.*, **141**, 553.
30. Zilow, G., Naser, W., Rutz, R., and Burger, R. (1989). *J. Immunol. Methods*, **121**, 261.
31. Nilsson, B., Svensson, K. E., Inganas, M., and Nilsson, U. R. (1988). *J. Immunol. Methods*, **107**, 281.
32. Hartmann, H., Lubbers, B., Casaretto, M., Bautsch, W., Klos, A., and Kohl, J. (1993). *J. Immunol. Methods*, **166**, 35.
33. Hack, C. E., Paardekooper, J., Smeenk, R. J., Abbink, J., Eerenberg, A. J., and Nuijens, J. H. (1988). *J. Immunol.*, **141**, 1602.
34. Garred, P., Mollnes, T. E., Lea, T., and Fischer, E. (1988). *Scand. J. Immunol.*, **7**, 319.
35. Nilsson, B., Nilsson Ekdahl, K., Avila, D., Nilsson, U. R., and Lambris, J. D. (1990). *Biochem. J.*, **268**, 55.
36. Tamerius, J. D., Pangburn, M. K., and Müller-Eberhard, H. J. (1982). *J. Immunol.*, **128**, 512.
37. Burger, R., Deubel, U., Hadding, U., and Bitter Suermann, D. (1982). *J. Immunol.*, **129**, 2042.
38. Iida, K., Mitomo, K., Fujita, T., and Tamura, N. (1987). *Immunology*, **62**, 413.
39. Lachmann, P. J., Pangburn, M. K., and Oldroyd, R. G. (1982). *J. Exp. Med.*, **156**, 205.
40. Oppermann, M. and Götze, O. (1994). *Mol. Immunol.*, **31**, 307.
41. Kolb, W. P., Morrow, P. R., and Tamerius, J. D. (1989). *Complement Inflamm.*, **6**, 175.
42. Hack, C. E., Paardekooper, J., and Van Milligen, F. (1990). *J. Immunol.*, **144**, 4249.
43. Nilsson, B., Svensson, K. E., Borwell, P., and Nilsson, U. R. (1987). *Mol. Immunol.*, **24**, 487.
44. Aguado, M. T., Lambris, J. D., Tsokos, G. C., Burger, R., Bitter Suermann, D., Tamerius, J. D., *et al.* (1985). *J. Clin. Invest.*, **76**, 1418.
45. Garred, P., Mollnes, T. E., and Lea, T. (1988). *Scand. J. Immunol.*, **27**, 329.
46. Garred, P., Mollnes, T. E., and Kazatchkine, M. D. (1989). *Complement Inflamm.*, **6**, 205.
47. Takeda, J., Kinoshita, T., Takata, Y., Kozono, H., Tanaka, E., Hong, K., *et al.* (1987). *J. Immunol. Methods*, **101**, 265.
48. Bergh, K. and Iversen, O. J. (1992). *J. Immunol. Methods*, **152**, 79.
49. Larrick, J. W., Wang, J., Fendly, B. M., Chenoweth, D. E., Kunkel, S. L., and Deinhart, T. (1987). *Infect. Immunol.*, **55**, 1867.
50. Bergh, K. and Iversen, O. J. (1989). *Scand. J. Immunol.*, **29**, 333.
51. Oppermann, M., Schulze, M., and Götze, O. (1991). *Complement Inflamm.*, **8**, 13.
52. Mollnes, T. E., Klos, A., Tschopp, J. (1988). *Scand. J. Immunol.*, **28**, 307.
53. Würzner, R., Schulze, M., Happe, L., Franzke, A., Bieber, F. A., Oppermann, M., *et al.* (1991). *Complement Inflamm.*, **8**, 328.
54. Mollnes, T. E. and Tschopp, J. (1987). *J. Immunol. Methods*, **100**, 215.
55. Takata, Y., Moriyama, T., Fukumori, Y., Yoden, A., Shima, M., and Inai, S. (1989). *J. Immunol. Methods*, **117**, 107.

56. Falk, R. J., Dalmasso, A. P., Kim, Y., Tsai, C. H., Scheinman, J. I., Gewurz, H., *et al.* (1983). *J. Clin. Invest.*, **72**, 560.
57. Mollnes, T. E., Lea, T., Harboe, M., and Tschopp, J. (1985). *Scand. J. Immunol.*, **22**, 183.
58. Hugo, F., Jenne, D., and Bhakdi, S. (1985). *Biosci. Rep.*, **5**, 649.
59. Kolb, W. P., Morrow, P. R., Jensen, F. C., and Tamerius, J. D. (1988). *Complement*, **5**, 213.
60. Kusunoki, Y., Takekoshi, Y., and Nagasawa, S. (1990). *J. Pharmacobiodyn.*, **13**, 454.
61. Würzner, R., Xu, H., Franzke, A., Schulze, M., Peters, J. H., and Götze, O. (1991). *Immunology*, **74**, 132.
62. Kemp, P. A., Spragg, J. H., Brown, J. C., Morgan, B. P., Gunn, C. A., and Taylor, P. W. (1992). *J. Clin. Lab. Immunol.*, **37**, 147.
63. Würzner, R. (1993). In *Activators and inhibitors of complement* (ed. R. B. Sim), p. 167. Kluwer Academic Publishers, Doordrecht, The Netherlands.
64. Ames, R. S., Tornetta, M. A., Jones, C. S., and Tsui, P. (1994). *J. Immunol.*, **152**, 4572.
65. Würzner, R., Orren, A., Potter, P., Morgan, B. P., Ponard, D., Späth, P., *et al.* (1990). *Clin. Exp. Immunol.*, **83**, 430.
66. Würzner, R., Mewar, D., Fernie, B. A., Hobart, M. J., and Lachmann, P. J. (1995). *Immunology*, **85**, 214.
67. Doglio, L. T., Gawryl, M. S., and Lint, T. F. (1988). *J. Immunol.*, **141**, 2079.
68. Zoppi, M., Weiss, M., Nydegger, U. E., Hess, T., and Späth, P. J. (1990). *Arch. Intern. Med.*, **150**, 2395.
69. Laine, R. O., Tamerius, J. D., Kolb, W. P., and Esser, A. F. (1989). *Complement Inflamm.*, **6**, 358.
70. Morgan, B. P., Sewry, C. A., Siddle, K., Luzio, J. P., and Campbell, A. K. (1984). *Immunology*, **52**, 181.
71. Tschopp, J. and Mollnes, T. E. (1986). *Proc. Natl. Acad. Sci. USA*, **83**, 4223.
72. Hugo, F., Krämer, S., and Bhakdi, S. (1987). *J. Immunol. Methods*, **99**, 243.
73. Nuijens, J. H., Huijbregts, C. C., Eerenberg Belmer, A. J., Abbink, J. J., Strack van Schijndel, R. J., *et al.* (1988). *Blood*, **72**, 1841.
74. Nuijens, J. H., Huijbregts, C. C., van Mierlo, G. M., and Hack, C. E. (1987). *Immunology*, **61**, 387.
75. de Agostini, A., Schapira, M., Wachtfogel, Y. T., Colman, R. W., and Carrel, S. (1985). *Proc. Natl. Acad. Sci. USA*, **82**, 5190.
76. Cugno, M., Nuijens, J., Hack, E., Eerenberg, A., Frangi, D., Agostoni, A., *et al.* (1990). *J. Clin. Invest.*, **85**, 1215.
77. de Agostini, A., Patston, P. A., Marottoli, V., Carrel, S., Harpel, P. C., and Schapira, M. (1988). *J. Clin. Invest.*, **82**, 700.
78. Davies, A., Simmons, D. L., Hale, G., Harrison, R. A., Tighe, H., Lachmann, P. J., *et al.* (1989). *J. Exp. Med.*, **170**, 637.
79. Reilly, B. D., Levine, P., Rothbard, J., and Skanes, V. M. (1991). *Complement Inflamm.*, **8**, 33.
80. Koch, C. and Behrendt, N. (1986). *Immunogenetics*, **23**, 322.
81. Botto, M., Fong, K. Y., So, A. K., Koch, C., and Walport, M. J. (1990). *J. Exp. Med.*, **172**, 1011.
82. Würzner, R., Hobart, M. J., Orren, A., Tokunaga, K., Nitze, R., Götze, O., *et al.* (1992). *Immunogenetics*, **35**, 398.

83. Würzner, R., Fernie, B. A., Jones, A. M., Lachmann, P. J., and Hobart, M. J. (1995). *J. Immunol.*, **154**, 4813.
84. Würzner, R., Nitze, R., and Götze, O. (1990). *Complement Inflamm.*, **7**, 290.
85. O'Neill, G. J. (1984). *Vox Sang.*, **47**, 362.
86. Chrispeels, J., Bank, S., Rittner, C., and Bitter-Suermann, D. (1989). *J. Immunol. Methods*, **125**, 5.
87. Doxiadis, G. and Grosse-Wilde, H. (1990). *Complement Inflamm.*, **7**, 269.

9

Assays for complement receptors

ISTVÁN BARTÓK and MARK J. WALPORT

1. Introduction

The complement system is a group of about a dozen cell surface molecules and 20 glycoproteins present in the plasma of vertebrates. The first complement-mediated activity to be described was destruction of bacteria by fresh serum. This lytic activity of serum was composed of a heat stable component, antibody, and heat labile 'complementary' proteins. Complement has a complex series of effector activities which fall into three broad categories. The first category of effector activities follow the binding of the major complement opsonins, C3b and C4b and their catabolic products, to three types of complement receptor, complement receptors types 1, 2, and 3 (CR1, CR2, and CR3) located on a wide variety of cell types. The consequences of ligation of these receptors include phagocytosis of opsonized particles, activation of leucocytes and the transport of immune complexes. The interactions of complement with these three receptors forms the major focus of this chapter. The second category of effector activities of complement is the activation of inflammatory mechanisms by the interaction of the anaphylatoxins, C5a and C3a, with specific receptors present on leucocytes. The third category of effector activities results from the insertion of the membrane attack complex of complement into cell membranes. The consequences of this are lysis, particularly of bacteria and non-nucleated cells, and cellular activation by sublytic doses of membrane attack complex.

The major complement receptors fall into three protein superfamilies and are summarized in *Tables 1* and *2*. CR1 and CR2 are members of a large family of proteins containing a short consensus repeat sequence. This family of proteins contains several other complement control proteins, including Factor H and C4-binding protein. CR3 (CD11b/CD18) and CR4 (CD11c/CD18) are members of the β2-integrin family, of which the third member is LFA-1 (CD11a, CD18). The C5a receptor is a member of a large family of cell surface receptors containing seven transmembrane spanning domains, which includes other receptors for chemotactic molecules such as the f-met-leu-phe receptor.

The interaction of these receptors with their ligands is extremely complex.

Table 1. Characteristics of human complement receptors for large fragments of C3[a]

Receptor	Other names	Ligand specificity	Cellular expression
CR1	CD35; C3b/C4b receptor	C3b > C4b ≫ iC3b (soluble and surface bound)	High expression: B cells, neutrophils, eosinophils, monocytes, kidney podocytes, and follicular dendritic cells. Low expression: tissue macrophages. Very low expression: erythrocytes and some T cell clones.
CR2	CD21; EBV receptor	C3d region of iC3b, C3dg, and C3d (soluble and surface bound) Non-complement: gp350 of EBV and CD23	High expression: B cells and follicular dendritic cells. Low expression: pharyngeal epithelial cells. Very low expression: thymocytes and some T cell clones.
CR3	CD11b/CD18; Mac-1	iC3b (surface bound only) Non complement: ICAM-1, LPS, fibrinogen, and β-glucan (cell activation temporarily increases affinity)	Neutrophils, monocytes, macrophages, eosinophils. High expression: $CD8^+$ T cells, $CD5^+$ B cells, monocytes, neutrophils, eosinophils, and NK cells. Low expression: macrophages.
CR4	CD11c/CD18; p150/95	iC3b and fibrinogen	Tissue macrophages, monocytes, neutrophils, eosinophils, $CD8^+$ T cells, NK cells, and activated B cells.
CR5	This receptor has not been characterized extensively.	C3d region of fluid phase iC3b, C3dg, and C3d	Low expression: neutrophils and platelets.

[a]For more information consult recent review articles (1–5).

Specific factors affecting the receptors that need to be considered are the numerical expression, surface organization, and activation state of the receptor molecule. In the case of CR1, the surface organization of the receptor differs according to the cell type, for example CR1 is expressed in clusters on erythrocytes and singly on other cell types. Receptor numbers are also subject to complex regulation. There is an inherited polymorphism of numerical expression of CR1 on erythrocytes. On other cell types surface expression is regulated according to the state of activation of the cell. In neutrophils, for example, there are intracellular granule stores of CR1, allowing rapid upregulation of surface CR1 numbers following cellular activation. In the case

Table 2. Characteristics of other complement receptors

Receptor	Ligand	Cellular expression
C1qR	C1q collagen region	High expression: B cells, fibroblasts, neutrophils, and monocytes. Low expression: platelets.
C3a/C4aR	C3a, C4a	High expression: mast cells and eosinophils. Low expression: monocytes and neutrophils.
C5aR	C5a	High expression: neutrophils, monocytes, and mast cells.

of the β2-integrins, the affinity of the receptor for ligand increases as well as the number of cell surface receptors following cellular activation. The majority of complement receptors also bind a number of different complement and non-complement ligands (*Table 1*) and this provides additional complexity in the analysis of receptor function both *in vitro* and *in vivo*.

In this chapter, the methods of assay of human CR1, CR2, and CR3 are summarized.

2. Identification of complement receptors using fluorescence-labelled antibodies

There is a large range of monoclonal antibodies specific for each of the complement receptors CR1 to CR4 (a selection is summarized in *Table 3*). These are useful for the antigenic identification of the receptors and can be used to enumerate receptors approximately by immunofluorescence and more precisely by radioligand binding assay.

CR1 and CR3 show inherited structural polymorphisms and in the case of CR3 one allotype is defined by the monoclonal antibody, 2.184 (14). In the following three sections of this chapter protocols are given for the analysis by

Table 3. Blockade of complement ligands by mAbs[a]

Receptor	Available mAbs	Ligand	Reference
CR1	Efficient antibody blockade best achieved with rabbit polyclonal antibodies; monoclonal antibodies 3D9 and 1B4 also block CR1	C3b/C4b	6 7 8
CR2	OKB7	C3d	9
	OKB7, B2, and 21A/5	EC3bi	10
CR3	MN41, 2LPM19c, 5A4.c5, TMG 65, CBRM1/29	EC3bi	11
CR4	3.9, HC1/1, and BL-444	EC3bi	12

[a] Blockade of non-complement ligands on CR2 and CR3/CR4: refer to ref. 13 and *Leukocyte typing V*.

immunofluorescence of CR3 on neutrophils and the quantitation by radioligand binding assay of CR1 numbers on erythrocytes.

2.1 Isolation of human neutrophils

Human neutrophils should be isolated from fresh blood anticoagulated by chelation of calcium using sodium citrate. During the isolation procedure the presence of autologous plasma helps to keep the cells in good condition and therefore Ca^{2+}-containing buffers should be avoided.

Protocol 1. Isolation of human neutrophils

Equipment and reagents

- 3.8% sodium citrate
- Human blood
- 50 ml plastic tube
- Dextran (M_r 515 000) (Sigma)
- HBSS: Hanks' balanced salts without Ca/Mg (Gibco)
- Percoll (Pharmacia)
- Pasteur pipette

Method

1. Take 35 ml of human blood and transfer into a 50 ml tube containing 4 ml of 3.8% sodium citrate.
2. Spin at 400 *g* for 20 min at 20 °C.
3. Aspirate supernatant plasma but leave 5 ml on the top of the cells. Spin aspirated plasma at 1500 *g* for 10 min at 20 °C to produce platelet-poor plasma, and store until use (steps 7, 8, and 12).
4. Take cells and make up to 45 ml with Hanks' without Ca/Mg. Add 5 ml of 6% dextran (M_r 515 000) in saline and mix gently.
5. Store for sedimentation of red blood cells for 20 min at 37 °C.
6. After sedimentation of red blood cells take supernatant containing leucocytes and spin at 450 *g* for 6 min at 20 °C.
7. Take cell pellet, mix with 2 ml of autologous platelet-poor plasma (refer to step 3), and transfer into a 15 ml tube.
8. Make 2 ml of 42% (v/v) and 2 ml of 51% (v/v) Percoll gradient using 90% stock in saline as follows. Mix 840 μl of 90% Percoll with 1160 μl of platelet-poor plasma (from step 3) for 42% Percoll, and 1020 μl of 90% Percoll with 980 μl of platelet-poor plasma for 51% Percoll in a separate tube.
9. Take the 15 ml tube containing the cell suspension. Put an empty Pasteur pipette into the tube, through which the Percoll will be layered underneath the cell suspension. Using a syringe or a 1 ml pipette, load the 42% Percoll through the Pasteur pipette without disturbing the position of the pipette and follow with 51% Percoll. It is essential to avoid air bubble formation at the neck of the Pasteur

pipette to enable the Percoll to pass smoothly through the Pasteur pipette.

10. Close the top of the Pasteur pipette using your index finger and remove it gently so that it does not leak and disturb the gradient.
11. Spin the cells at 200 *g* for 11 min at 20°C in a well balanced centrifuge. Make sure the brake is turned off as rapid slowing of the centrifuge will disturb the interface between the Percoll layers.
12. Aspirate the neutrophil cell fraction from the interface between the 51% and 42% Percoll with a Pasteur pipette, mix with the remaining platelet-poor plasma, and make up to 15 ml with Hanks' without Ca/Mg. Spin at 450 *g* for 6 min at 20 °C.
13. Wash cell pellet once with 15 ml of Hanks' without Ca/Mg to remove plasma, and once with or without Ca/Mg depending on the further work.

2.2 Assay of cell surface receptors

A sample protocol is given for fluorescent labelling of neutrophil CR3 suitable for visualization using fluorescence microscopy or flow cytometry.

Protocol 2. Fluorescence assay of cell surface receptors

Equipment and reagents

- 2LPM19c anti-CR3 monoclonal antibody (or alternative anti-CR3 antibody) (MoAb) (Dako)
- Non-specific mouse antibody as negative control
- FITC-labelled anti-mouse IgG (Dako)
- Neutrophil cell suspension: 10^6 cell/ml (see *Protocol 1*)
- 1% FCS in PBS
- 1% paraformaldehyde in water
- 1.5 ml plastic tubes
- Fluorescence microscope

Method

1. Transfer 50 μl of cell suspension into a 1.5 ml tube, add 10 μl of 2LPM19c (500 μg/ml) MoAb, and the same volume of the non-specific antibody into a second tube as a negative control. Mix the cells by gentle pipetting, and incubate for 40 min at 4°C.
2. Add 1 ml of ice-cold PBS containing 1% FCS and mix by pipetting. Centrifuge cells for 2 min at 200 *g*. Discard supernatant by pipetting, and repeat washing two more times.
3. Add 100 μl of 1/50 diluted FITC-labelled secondary antibody to the cell pellet, and mix gently by pipetting. Cover tubes with silver foil to protect from light, and incubate cells for another 40 min at 4°C.
4. Add 1 ml of ice-cold PBS containing 1% of FCS. Wash cells three

Protocol 2. *Continued*

times as in step 2, then pellet cells, and discard the last washing buffer.

5. Resuspend cells in 200 μl of 1% paraformaldehyde. Cover tubes with silver foil and store at 4 °C (less than three to five days).
6. The sample can then be analysed using a fluorescent microscope or flow cytometer.

Notes:

(a) If several samples are tested, an ELISA plate is preferable instead of plastic tubes. During centrifugation use a plate holder and pellet cells by a 2 min centrifugation at 200 *g*.

(b) Because of the fast quenching of fluorescence under the light, once the labelled antibody is added to the cells protect samples from the light. For the same reason, do not leave labelled cells under the microscope for longer than necessary without moving to the next field.

(c) Whenever possible, use incident light and objective lenses with high (× 40 or more) magnification, because in contrast to ordinary light it gives a much brighter picture.

(d) If cheaper FITC-labelled antibody is used, the cell pellet may be contaminated with fluorescent crystals resulting in a poor quality picture under the fluorescence microscope. In this case prior to use, centrifugation of the antibody for 10 min at 10 000 *g* in a microcentrifuge may eliminate the problem.

3. Radioligand binding assay using C3b dimers to enumerate CR1

A method is given for studying the quantitative binding of C3b to CR1. In these binding studies serial dilutions of [^{125}I]ligand with known specific activity are incubated with the receptor-bearing cells. In order to determine non-specific binding in a set of parallel samples, binding of radiolabelled ligand is inhibited by the presence of unlabelled ligand in 100-fold excess, or alternatively by receptor blockade using a neutralizing antibody. After allowing the reaction to equilibrate, cells are separated from unbound radioactivity by centrifugation through an oil phase, followed by measuring the cell-bound and free radioactivity in a γ-counter. From these data the concentration of the free ligand, and the number of the bound molecules may be calculated and further analysed according to Scatchard. This analysis is a simple graphical method of modelling ligand–receptor interactions, and of calculating the binding constants, and the number of cell surface receptor molecules.

3.1 Binding of radiolabelled ligand to CR1

CR1 binds monomeric ligand with extremly low affinity in comparison with dimeric or multimeric C3b (15–17). However the preparation of C3b dimers is relatively straightforward (18) and a protocol is given here for measurement of the binding of C3b dimers to erythrocyte CR1. The normal range of CR1 on human erythrocytes is as low as 350–1000 molecules per cell, therefore the binding assay requires much higher cell concentrations than in the case of other cell types with a higher density of receptors (for example neutrophils which express 10- to 50-fold higher levels of CR1 than erythrocytes).

CR1 has previously been shown to exhibit non-cooperative binding of dimeric ligand with a single binding constant (K_d = 9.5–30 nM depending on the conditions) (15,16,19–23). However, we recently found that human erythrocytes incubated with highly purified dimerized C3b showed two binding constants with $K_{d1} = 7 \pm 3$ nM and $K_{d2} = 21 \pm 4$ nM (24). Although it is straightforward in principle to quantitate the binding of C3b dimers to CR1, a number of factors must be considered. While in practice complete saturation is difficult to achieve due to the limited concentration of highly purified and labelled ligand, it is necessary to offer concentrations of C3b dimers sufficiently high to reach the level at which specific binding begins to plateau (*Figure 1b*). Although CR1 numbers are much lower on erythrocytes than on other cell types, erythrocytes do offer certain advantages for studying receptor–ligand interactions. The absence of receptor internalization and the stable number of cell surface receptors means that binding studies can be performed at 37°C. At this temperature the rate of ligand association with, and dissociation from the receptor is four to six times higher than at 4°C, and equilibrium binding can nearly be achieved in 30 min. On neutrophils binding studies must be undertaken at 4°C because first, receptor numbers are unstable due to the presence of an intracellular pool, and secondly, internalization of surface receptors follows ligation.

Protocol 3. Isolation of human erythrocytes

Equipment and reagents

- Human blood containing 0.38% sodium citrate (stored at 4°C for less than one week)
- 50 ml conical tube (Falcon)
- PBS (Oxoid)
- Centrifuge

Method

1. Take 30 ml of blood, transfer into a 50 ml conical tube, and add 500 U sodium heparin or sodium citrate to 0.38% final concentration.
2. Centrifuge cells at 550 *g* for 20 min. Discard supernatant and the white cell layer (buffy coat) from the top of the erythrocytes.

Protocol 3. *Continued*

3. Add PBS up to 50 ml and resuspend cells again. Spin the cells down at 800 *g* for 8 min. Discard supernatant, and repeat washing until supernatant becomes clear, but at least three times, in order to eliminate lysed erythrocytes.
4. After the last wash resuspend pellet in 20–30 ml buffer chosen according to the planned experiment.

Protocol 4. Binding assay

Equipment and reagents

- Human erythrocytes from 2–5 ml of whole blood
- 1.5 ml plastic tubes
- 0.4 ml plastic Eppendorf tube
- Oil mixture of 40% dinonyl phthalate (Di-'isononyl' phthalate) (Fluka Chemie AG) in dibutyl phthalate (Di-*n*-butyl phthalate) (BDH)
- ^{125}I-labelled dimerized C3b (specific activity from 0.2–0.9 mCi/mg)
- Complement fixation test diluent (CFT) (Oxoid) containing 1% BSA and 3 mM NaN_3 pH 7.2
- 20% rabbit immune serum containing anti-CR1 neutralizing antibodies in CFT/BSA/NaN_3
- Slow overhead tube rotator
- Coulter counter
- γ-counter

Method

1. Transfer 2 ml of erythrocytes (refer to *Protocol 3*) into 10 ml plastic tube. Pellet cells in a centrifuge at 550 *g* for 5 min. Discard supernatant and resuspend cells in 10 ml PBS. Repeat wash until supernatant becomes clear to eliminate lysed cells.
2. Resuspend cells in 5 ml of CFT containing 1% of BSA and 3 mM NaN_3, and check cell concentration in a Coulter counter. Dilute cells in the same buffer to 2×10^9/ml.
3. Transfer 100 μl of cells into a 1.5 ml plastic tube. Make ten tubes for samples and ten tubes for control. Add 50 μl buffer into the samples or 50 μl of polyclonal anti-CR1 into the control tubes respectively. Rotate cells in a slow rotator for 30 min at 37 °C.
4. Add a further 100 μl of serial dilutions of ^{125}I-labelled C3b dimer ranging from 90 nM to 0.2 nM and rotate for 30 min at 37 °C on a slow overhead rotator.
5. Make one set of triplicates of 200 μl of oil in 0.4 ml plastic tubes for the samples and one set for the control tubes. After 30 min incubation transfer three 50 μl aliquots of suspension on to the oil phase of the triplicate tubes.
6. Separate cells from the buffer by spinning down in a microcentrifuge at 10000 *g* for 2 min. After centrifugation cells are pelleted in the

bottom of the oil phase while the aqueous phase, containing the free ligand, is on the top of the oil phase.

7. Freeze the tubes at -70°C and then separate the cells from the buffer by cutting the tube with wire clippers and transfer both parts separately into 2 ml plastic tubes.
8. Measure the radioactivity of the samples in a γ-counter.

3.2 Calculation of data

From these data it is possible to calculate the number of bound molecules per cell, and the concentration of free ligand, and these data can be plotted according to the method of Scatchard to determine the dissociation constant.

Data of a typical binding assay are summarized in *Table 4*.

From these data the specific binding, and the corresponding concentration are calculated as shown in *Table 5*.

The specific activity of $C3b_2$ is 714636 c.p.m./μg, therefore each c.p.m. reading represents 2.408×10^6 C3b dimers (calculated on the basis of a M_r of a C3b dimer of 350 kDa). The sum of *Table 4*, columns 1 and 2 represents the total amount of radiolabelled $C3b_2$ molecules in the 50 μl reaction. *Table 5*, column 1 shows the concentration of $C3b_2$ molecules in the reaction volume during the incubation calculated from the sums of *Table 4*, columns 1 and 2.

It is essential to calculate the specifically-bound counts by subtracting non-specific binding in the presence of blocked receptors (*Table 4*, column 3) from the total bound counts (*Table 4*, column 1). To do this accurately we plot the cell-bound radioactivity in the presence of receptor blockade (*Table 4*, column 3) against the sum of bound and unbound radioactivity (*Table 4*,

Table 4. Measured data of binding assay

1 Bound c.p.m.	2 Free c.p.m.	3 In the presence of receptor blockade bound c.p.m.	4 In the presence of receptor blockade free c.p.m.
25 199	1 102 025	11 193	1 047 638
20 739	772 258	7057	735 848
13 532	365 741	3665	362 387
9194	183 672	1896	183 371
6598	99 733	1069	104 342
4182	45 048	604	53 953
2745	24 729	284	28 684
1889	14 342	146	14 135
938	7027	66	7453
593	4151	38	4473
336	2281	10	2513

Table 5. Calculated data of binding assay

1 Input nM	2 Specific bound c.p.m.	3 Free nM	4 Bound molecules per cell	5 Bound/ free ratio
90.1	14119	88.1	479	5.43×10^9
63.4	12944	61.8	439	7.11×10^9
30.3	9804	29.2	333	1.14×10^{10}
15.4	7298	14.7	248	1.69×10^{10}
8.5	5553	8.0	188	2.36×10^{10}
3.9	3698	3.6	125	3.48×10^{10}
2.2	2475	2.0	84	4.25×10^{10}
1.3	1730	1.2	59	5.12×10^{10}
0.6	860	0.6	29	5.19×10^{10}
0.4	547	0.3	19	5.59×10^{10}
0.2	310	0.2	11	5.76×10^{10}

columns 3 and 4) (*Figure 1a*). By linear regression the slope of the non-specific binding = 0.00983. This slope is then used to calculate non-specific binding for each sample as follows. Non-specific binding is the total amount of $C3b_2$ offered (*Table 4*, columns 1 and 2) multiplied by 0.00983, and this value is subtracted from the total bound (*Table 4*, column 1). *Table 5*, column 2 presents the results.

The next step is to calculate the number of specifically-bound molecules of $C3b_2$ per cell. Since each c.p.m. represents 2.408×10^6 molecules (see above), and in the 50 μl (0.2 vol. of total) reaction volume there were 7.1×10^7 cells, the number of specific-bound molecules per single cell (*Table 5*, column 4) is determined by multiplying the data in column 2 by 2.408×10^6 and dividing by 7.1×10^7. The bound/free ratio is calculated in column 5 by dividing the number of bound $C3b_2$ molecules per single cell (column 4) by the concentration of free C3b2 (column 3).

3.3 Scatchard plot analysis

In order to determine the binding constant and the number of binding sites on the cells, a Scatchard plot is perfomed of the number of bound molecules per cell on the abscissa against the ratio of bound/free (*Table 5*, columns 4 and 5) on the ordinate. If the fitted curve is linear it represents single binding affinity.

As shown in *Figure 2*, the data displayed results in a curvilinear plot, best modelled by a two binding site model of $C3b_2$ binding. Using non-linear curve fitting computer programs (such as Statgraph) from the data of *Table 5* it is possible to determine the binding parameters. It is also possible by manual analysis to divide the data of *Figure 2a* into two different affinity components, and to plot separately the high (last seven rows of data of *Table 5*, columns 4 and 5) and low affinity data (first four rows in columns 4 and 5) (*Figure 2b* and *c*). In this way, the fitting of the data can be performed by simple

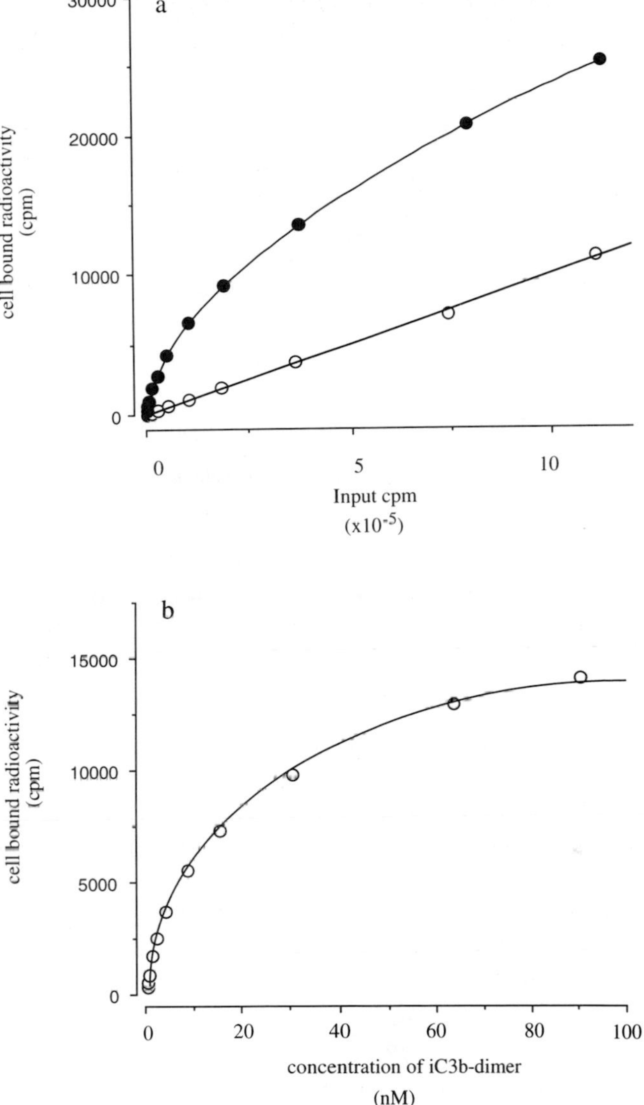

Figure 1. Binding of dimerized [^{125}I]C3b to human erythrocytes. (a) Total (●) and non-specific (○) binding. (b) Transformation of data shown in part (a) to illustrate specific binding of C3b dimers to erythrocytes, which shows saturation at high input concentrations.

linear regression analysis. The number of bound molecules per cell can be extrapolated by the fitted linear curve; the intersection with the × axis equals the number of binding sites per cell. The *y* axis intersection equals the bound/free ratio. The binding constant is determined by the ratio of the intersections:

$$K_d = \frac{x \text{ axis intersection}}{y \text{ axis intersection}}$$

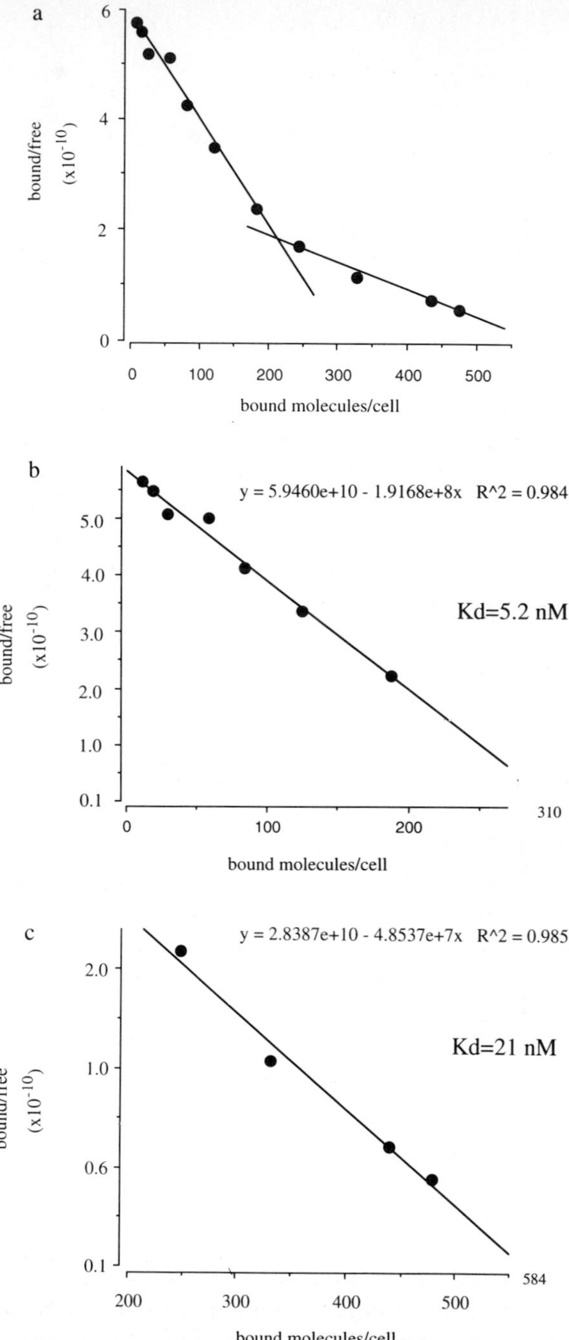

Figure 2. Scatchard plot analysis of binding data. (a) Scatchard analysis of data shown in *Figure 1*. (b) The high affinity component is plotted by linear regression. (c) The low affinity component is plotted by linear regression. X axis intersection equals the extrapolated number of bound molecules per cell.

In the case of the data shown in *Figure 2b*:

$$K_d = \frac{310}{5.946 \times 10^{10}} = 5.2 \text{ nM}$$

4. Complement receptor production and surface expression

Two general approaches may be applied to study the biosynthesis and structure of complement receptors by gel electrophoresis. The first is immunoblotting using solubilized cell membranes run on polyacrylamide gels, blotted, and probed using monoclonal or polyclonal antibodies. This approach is relatively insensitive for receptors expressed at low concentrations in cell membranes. The second approach, which is more sensitive and will be described in more detail, is to surface label cell membrane proteins, immunoaffinity purify the protein of interest, and then run the protein on polyacrylamide gel and visualize the product using autoradiography. Two approaches to surface labelling are iodination and biosynthetic labelling using [^{35}P]methionine and/or cysteine. Protocols are given here for surface labelling and biosynthetic labelling of CR1.

4.1 Immunoprecipitation of surface CR1

In this protocol human erythrocytes are used as a source of CR1. Because CR1 numbers on erythrocytes are low, high cell numbers are needed in the protocol. CR1 is also very sensitive to proteolytic cleavage and great care is needed to keep reagents cold and to use protease inhibitors as described. An indirect immunoprecipitation is used in order to optimize the recovery of the tiny concentrations of surface-labelled CR1. CR1 is first bound using a mouse monoclonal anti-CR1, followed by polyclonal rabbit anti-mouse IgG, and finally immobilized on beads coated with Staphylococcal protein A.

Protocol 5. Immunoprecipitation of surface CR1

Equipment and reagents

- $Na^{125}I$
- Lactoperoxidase (Sigma)
- Glucose oxidase (Sigma)
- α-D-glucose (BDH)
- Nonidet P-40 (BDH)
- Pepstatin (Sigma)
- Iodoacetamide (Sigma)
- PMSF (Sigma)
- E11 mAb (Sera-Lab)
- Rabbit anti-mouse IgG (Dako)
- SpA–Sepharose (Sigma)
- 10% Staphylococcus cell suspension (formalin treated) (Sigma)
- 6% SDS–PAGE
- X-ray film and cassette (Kodak)
- Coulter counter
- 1 ml containing 5×10^9 human RBC
- Electrophoretic apparatus for SDS–PAGE

Protocol 5. *Continued*

Method

1. Transfer the human red blood cells (5×10^9) into a 10 ml conical tube.
2. Spin down at 550 *g* for 5 min at 4°C. Resuspend cells in 10 ml of cold PBS and wash them two more times.
3. After the last wash resuspend pellet in 2 ml of 5 mM α-D-glucose in PBS made just prior to use. Add 1 mCi of ^{125}I, mix with 50 μl of 1 mg/ml lactoperoxidase and 150 μl of glucose oxidase, then incubate on ice for 40 min.
4. Quench the reaction by adding 100 μl of 50 mM KI and 10 mM tyrosine in PBS. (Alternatively you can block the enzyme by adding 38 μl of 1% NaN_3 for 5 min.)
5. Wash the cells three times in cold PBS containing 5 mM KI and 2% BSA.
6. After radiolabelling of the surface proteins, lyse the pellet of the cells in 5 ml of H_2O containing 2 mM PMSF, 3 mM EDTA, 1 μM pepstatin, and 20 mM iodoacetamide for 5 min on ice.
7. Add another 5 ml of 2 × saline containing the same enzyme inhibitors as above. Transfer samples into an ultracentrifuge tube and spin down at 33 000 *g* for 20 min at 4°C.
8. Take pellet of stroma and incubate with 2 ml of PBS containing 1% Nonidet P-40, 2 mM PMSF, 3 mM EDTA, 1 μM pepstatin, and 20 mM iodoacetamide (pH 7.2), and rotate for 5 min at 4°C.
9. Transfer samples into two 1.5 ml Eppendorf tubes and spin down the insoluble fraction in a microcentrifuge at 10 000 *g* for 2 min.
10. Take supernatant and in order to eliminate non-specific binding mix with 40 μl of SpA–Sepharose (1:1 vol. in PBS containing protease inhibitors), and 40 μl of formalin-treated Staphylococcus cell suspension, then incubate for 1 h or overnight in a cold room on a slow rotator.
11. Pellet resin and cell suspension by 1 min centrifugation at 10 000 *g* at 4°C.
12. Mix supernatant with 60 μl of of E11 mAb (50 μg/ml) and incubate on ice for 1 h or overnight.
13. Add 20 μl of rabbit anti-mouse IgG (150 μg/ml) and incubate on ice for 1 h.
14. Add 50 μl of SpA–Sepharose beads (1:1 vol. in PBS containing enzyme inhibitors as above), and incubate in a cold room on a slow rotator for 1 h. Pellet resin in a cold room by 1 min centrifugation at 10 000 *g* and resuspend in 1.5 ml of cold PBS. Transfer into an

Eppendorf tube and wash three times in cold PBS at 10 000 *g* for 1 min.

15. Take pellet of beads and mix in 25 μl of PBS and 25 μl of 2 × loading buffer for SDS–PAGE.
16. To elute immunoprecipitated CR1, boil the samples for 2 min in a water-bath, and spin in a microcentrifuge for 1 min at room temperature.
17. Take supernatant and load on to a 6% polyacrylamide gel.
18. Run the gel until the dye front has reached the bottom of the gel and dry in a gel dryer.
19. In a dark-room transfer gel into an X-ray film cassette containing an intensifying screen and cover with film.
20. Store the casette at −70°C for a week, then leave at room temperature for approx. 1 h to equilibrate the temperature of the film.
21. Develop film. If necessary incubate gel with a new film for shorter or longer times as required. (Incubation time should be ideally less than two weeks.)

Notes:

(a) After dissolving D-glucose there is a spontaneous isomerization of the hydrolysed molecules to L-glucose and therefore the efficiency of the radioiodination is better if α-D-glucose is dissolved immediately prior to use, in order to minimize isomerization.

(b) Depending on the antibodies used in steps 11–12, further calibration of the antibodies may be necessary to identify the optimal ratios of antigen: first antibody : second antibody.

4.2 Biosynthetic labelling of CR1

In this sample protocol cultured human monocyte cells are used as a source of CR1 receptors. If non-adherent cells are used, the cell suspension should contain ~ 5 × 10^5 cell/ml. The incubation time during protein synthesis, or pulse chase for shed receptors will vary depending on the state of activation and the type of the cells.

An important aspect of metabolic labelling is to optimize the incorporation of radiolabelled amino acids into the proteins of interest. During the incorporation of radiolabelled amino acids, instead of methionine- and cysteine-free medium, it is possible to use ordinary medium containing fetal calf serum. However, to increase sensitivity, it is best to use methionine- and cysteine-free medium. In some protocols, dialysed serum is also used in order to further restrict exposure of the cells to unlabelled methionine and cysteine. However if the cells are incubated for a relatively long period and starved of methionine and cysteine, the rate of protein synthesis may be reduced.

Therefore it is our practice to use methionine- and cysteine-free medium with unmodified fetal calf serum.

TRAN^{35}S-Label contains both methionine and cysteine. One disadvantage of using cysteine is that it can bind to proteins via free SH groups or by disulfide interchange. Proteins which are chemically rather than biosynthetically labelled may create artefactual bands in non-reduced PAGE gels; it is therefore necessary to run reduced gels in order to eliminate this artefact.

There may be problems during the immunoprecipitation steps caused by non-specific protein binding to the resin beads. This may be a particular problem if, at the end of the coupling of antibody to the resin to be used for immunoprecipitation, the remaining active groups were blocked by ethanolamine or glycine, causing the introduction of charged groups. Non-specific binding can be minimized by increasing the NaCl concentration to 0.5 M, which overcomes charge effects.

The signal from the specific immunoprecipitated radiolabelled protein bands may be very weak. There are several ways to try to overcome this problem. Usually the problem originates because of the very low energy of the β-emitting ^{35}S isotope. 'Pre-flashing' of the X-ray film can be used to increase the sensitivity of the film. A second approach is to treat the gel with Amplify (Amersham), which causes secondary fluorescent light to be emitted at the radioactive site. In contrast to the β-rays from the ^{35}S isotope, this can pass through the film support, and a cassette with an intensifying screen should be used. The sensitivity of detection can be significantly improved by using a combination of these measures.

Protocol 6. Biosynthetic labelling of CR1

Equipment and reagents

- Monocyte culture approaching confluence on a 25 cm^2 flask
- TRAN^{35}S-Label (ICN Biomedicals Inc.)
- DMEM: Dulbecco's medium with glucose, without glutamine, cystine, methionine, and cysteine (ICN Biomedicals Inc.) supplemented with 10% FCS
- DMEM supplemented with 10% FCS and 2 mM glutamine
- HBSS: Hanks' balanced salts (Gibco)
- Iodoacetamide (Sigma): 200 mM in water
- Phenylmethylsulfonyl fluoride (PMSF) (Sigma): 100 mM in ethanol or isopropanol
- PBS containing 0.5 mM EDTA pH 7.2
- PBS containing 0.5 M NaCl pH 7.2
- Minicon B15 concentrator (Amicon)
- PD-10 column (Pharmacia) equilibrated with PBS/EDTA
- Anti-CR1–Sepharose 4B resin in PBS/EDTA (50%, v/v)
- IgG–Sepharose 4B resin in PBS/EDTA (50%, v/v)
- Lysis buffer (sterile): 10 mM Tris containing 2% Triton X-100, 150 mM NaCl, 20 μg/ml SBTI, 40 mM benzamidine–HCl, 5 μg/ml pepstatin A, 5 μg/ml leupeptin, and prior to use 2 mM iodoacetamide and 0.5 mM PMSF
- Liquid Scintillator NE 260 for aqueous phase (NE Technology Ltd.)
- Biomax film and cassette (Kodak)
- Electrophoretic apparatus for SDS–PAGE

Method

1. Discard medium and wash cells in 10 ml sterile Hanks'. Remove Hanks' and add 5 ml of DMEM without methionine and cysteine. Add 0.5–1.0 mCi TRANS^{35}S-Label and culture cells under normal conditions for 2 h.

2. Separate medium from the cells; it may be relevant to analyse this in the case of secreted proteins. Supplement with iodoacetamide to 2 mM final concentration and incubate at 37 °C for 15 min to inhibit the formation of [^{35}S]cysteine adducts with protein disulfide bridges. Store at 4 °C.
3. Wash the cells rapidly in Hanks' medium previously equilibrated at 37 °C in an incubator. Add 5 ml of lysis buffer to the cells and incubate them for 30 min at 37 °C.
4. Vortex cell lysate vigorously in the flask and transfer into a Minicon concentrator to reduce the volume for application to a PD-10 column. Leave at 4 °C to concentrate to 2.5 ml (usually less than 1 h). Transfer concentrated lysate to the top of a PD-10 column equilibrated with PBS/EDTA in order to separate cell lysate from free label.
5. Collect the first 2.5 ml eluate which may contain some radioactive contamination, and discard it. Add 3.5 ml PBS/EDTA to the column in order to elute protein fraction of the cell lysate and collect the 3.5 ml elution volume. This fraction contains ~ 95% protein content of the cell lysate in PBS/EDTA. Discard the column which will have retained > 95% of free TRAN^{35}S-Label. Free label also has to be removed from culture medium if this is to be analysed (step 2) by desalting on the PD-10 column.
6. Transfer 1 ml of protein fraction into a 1.5 ml plastic tube and add 200 μl of IgG–Sepharose. Fix on a slow overhead rotator and rotate at 4°C for 2 h to adsorb non-specific binding.
7. Pellet resin in microcentrifuge at 10 000 *g* for 20 sec. Transfer supernatant on to pellet of 50 μl of anti-CR1–Sepharose (50%, v/v) and increase salt concentration to approximately 0.5 M by adding ~ 1/10 vol. of 5 M NaCl, in order to further decrease non-specific binding. Gently resuspend resin and rotate at 4°C for a further 2 h.
8. Pellet resin as above and discard supernatant. Wash pellet in 1 ml of PBS containing 0.5 M NaCl four times, followed by washing once in 1 ml of water, and once in PBS.
9. Discard supernatant after the last washing and add 30 μl of loading buffer containing β-mercaptoethanol. After a 1.5 min boiling in a water-bath, load samples on to a 7.5% SDS–PAGE.
10. After electrophoresis dry the gel and in a dark-room put into an X-ray cassette covered by a film. Make sure that the emulsified side of the film is facing the gel. Develop the film after a week. Using size markers in the same gel, CR1 should appear as a single band at 150 kDa apparent molecular weight. If necessary according to the amount of the radiolabelled proteins in the gel, change exposure time with a new film.

In order to analyse protein secreted into the medium the following modification may be applied: instead of lysing the cells at step 3, wash them in Hanks', then culture for a further 2–4 h in 5 ml of ordinary medium. Separate the cells and the medium, and follow *Protocol 6* from step 2. Desalt and immunoprecipitate supernatants in the same way as cell lysate. It is sensible to monitor each step by measuring radioactivity of 10 μl of each fraction by scintillation in a β-counter; this can be informative when troubleshooting.

5. Rosette formation assays

Rosette formation is a sensitive technique for modelling the adhesion of complement-coated particles to receptor-bearing cells. Due to the large number of bridges formed between the target and effector cells, the assay is very sensitive and is one of the most widely used assays in studies of complement receptors. Sheep erythrocytes bearing defined fragments of complement C3 are usually used as indicator cells for rosetting to cells expressing complement receptors. The usual methods of coupling C3 to sheep erythrocytes cause the C3 to be deposited in small clusters rather than in a random distribution, and this further enhances adhesion to the effector cells (17).

5.1 Generation of fixed fragments on sheep erythrocytes

C3 is covalently bound to sheep erythrocytes by two cycles of C3 addition. The first cycle attaches a small amount of randomly deposited C3b using trypsinized C3 or by classical pathway activation. The second cycle is an amplification step, using a nickel-stabilized C3 convertase formed by the addition of purified factor B, D, and further C3. In the second step small clusters of C3b molecules are formed at the sites of the C3b deposited during the first cycle; therefore the number of clusters can be controlled by adjusting the concentration of the C3 in the first step.

5.1.1 Binding of first cycle of C3b to sheep erythrocytes using trypsin

The trypsinization step to couple C3b to SRBC is very inefficient as only a small amount of cleaved C3 binds covalently to the cell surface. In order to optimize this step, it is important to use highly concentrated (10–15 mg/ml) haemolytically active C3. Due to multiple potential trypsin cleavage sites in C3, further digestion can occur after the first cleavage leading to the desired C3a and C3b fragments. Because of this it is essential to optimize the cleavage reaction of C3 by trypsin to achieve the most efficient binding of C3b to the cell membrane without over-digestion. The optimal trypsin concentration and time may differ between trypsin batches and it is usually necessary to recalibrate the first binding step reaction when a new batch of trypsin is opened.

Protocol 7. Generation of fixed C3 fragments on sheep erythrocytes using trypsin

Reagents

- Blood group II sheep erythrocytes (TCS Biologics Ltd.)
- C3, haemolytically active, 15 mg/ml in PBS
- Soybean trypsin inhibitor (Sigma)
- Trypsin (Sigma)
- GVB: 0.1% gelatin in veronal buffer, 14 mS, pH 7.4
- GVB–Ni: 0.15 mM nickelous chloride in GVB pH 7.4
- PBS pH 7.2

Method

1. Wash 1×10^{10} sheep E with PBS in a 10 ml tube. Resuspend the cells in 1 ml of PBS and transfer into a 1.5 ml plastic tube. After pelleting the cells at 3000 *g* for 1 min, mix with 140 μl of PBS containing C3 (15 mg/ml), and transfer to a 37 °C water-bath for 3 min to equilibrate the temperature. Then add 10 μl of pre-warmed trypsin (1 mg/ml in 1 mM HCl) for 45 sec.
2. Stop enzymatic cleavage by mixing 20 μl of soybean trypsin inhibitor (SBTI) (1 mg/ml) and transfer reaction into ice box.
3. Add 1 ml of ice-cold 0.1% gelatin-containing veronal buffer (GVB) and centrifuge at 3000 *g* for 1 min. Discard supernatant and resuspend cells in 1.5 ml ice-cold GVB and pellet. Repeat washing three more times with the same buffer, and once with ice-cold GVB containing 0.15 mM nickelous chloride.
4. In order to form Ni-stabilized convertase, to amplify C3b deposition, follow *Protocol 8,* steps 8–13.

5.1.2 Binding of first cycle of C3b to sheep erythrocytes using classical pathway activation

This is a very efficient and simple procedure to make EAC3b. Use frozen aliquots of C3-depleted or C3-deficient serum. To produce C3-depleted serum refer to (25) and (26).

Protocol 8. Generation of fixed C3 fragments on sheep erythrocytes using classical pathway activation

Reagents

- Rabbit haemolytic serum (TCS Biologics Ltd.)
- Complement fixation test diluent (CFT) (Oxoid) pH 7.2
- 10% of blood group 'ii' sheep erythrocytes (TCS Biologics Ltd.) in CFT
- C3 (haemolytically active), 2–4 mg/ml in CFT
- GVB: 0.1% gelatin in veronal buffer, 14 mS, pH 7.4
- GVB–Ni: 0.15 mM nickelous chloride in GVB pH 7.4
- Purified factor B, factor D, factor I, and factor H

Protocol 8. *Continued*

Method

1. Mix 450 μl of rabbit haemolytic serum with 10 ml CFT containing 10% SRBC in a scaled conical tube and incubate at 4°C for 30 min.
2. Chill in ice box, then centrifuge at 550 *g* for 8 min at 4°C. Resuspend cell pellet in 10 ml of ice-cold CFT and centrifuge again. Repeat washing in the same way at least three times or until supernatant becomes clear.
3. Discard last supernatant and check volume of cell pellet (EA). Make up 10% (v/v) cell suspension in CFT.
4. Centrifuge 500 μl of 10% EA (~ 10^9 cells) in an Eppendorf tube at 3000 *g* for 1 min, resuspend cells in 500 μl of 20% C3-deficient serum in CFT, and incubate at 37°C for 5 min. Chill in ice box.
5. Add 1 ml of ice-cold CFT. Centrifuge the cells at 3000 *g* for 1 min and wash the cells in CFT two more times. After the last wash resuspend cells in 150 μl of CFT.
6. Add 50 μl of isolated C3 (0.05–4 mg/ml in CFT depending on the required cluster number per cell), and incubate for 10 min at 37°C with frequent shaking. Chill in ice box.
7. Add 1 ml ice-cold GVB and centrifuge at 3000 *g* for 1 min. Remove supernatant, wash cells twice in the same buffer, and once in ice-cold GVB–Ni.
8. Pellet the cells and add 0.5 ml cold GVB–Ni containing 45 μg factor B and 116 ng factor D. In order to form Ni-stabilized convertase, incubate cells for 2 min at 37°C in a water-bath.
9. Add 1 ml ice-cold GVB–Ni and spin the cells at 3000 *g* for 1 min. Remove supernatant and wash the cells twice in the same way in cold GVB–Ni.
10. Pellet cells and add 300 μl of cold GVB–Ni containing 120 μg C3, and mix. Incubate cells in 37°C water-bath for 20 min to form clusters of C3b molecules at the site of previously introduced C3.
11. Chill cells in ice box and add 1 ml of cold GVB–Ni. Centrifuge cells and remove supernatant. Wash cells one more time in the same buffer and remove supernatant.
12. Resuspend cells in cold BDVEA (6 mS) (refer to *Protocol 13*) and inactivate Ni-stabilized convertases by 90 min 37°C incubation (or 10 min at 37°C and overnight at 4°C).
13. If further digestion of C3 is needed, pellet cells again and resuspend in 1 ml of Hanks' buffer. Add 10 μl of factor I (1.0 mg/ml) and 20 μl of factor H (2.5 mg/ml). Mix the cells and incubate for 1 h at 37°C. Wash cells as above in cold Hanks' or PBS according to the test for which you wish to use the cells.

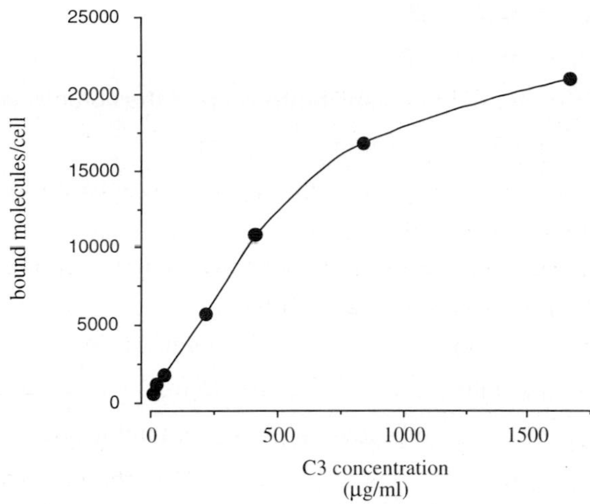

Figure 3. Bound C3b on sheep erythrocytes as a function of C3 concentration in the first binding step. Enumeration of surface-bound C3b was carried out according to *Protocol 10.*

5.2 Enumeration of complement fragments on sheep erythrocytes

5.2.1 Radio-iodination of antibodies

Rat monoclonal anti-C3d (Clone 3), anti-C3c (Clone 4), and anti-C3g neoantigen (Clone 9) can be used to identify specific fragments of C3 bound to cells and other particles (27,28). Iodobead labelling is used to radiolabel MoAbs reacting with different fragments of C3 for use in enumeration of fixed C3 fragments on sheep red blood cells (*Protocols 7* and *8*).

Protocol 9. Radiolabelling of antibodies

Equipment and reagents

- Iodobead (Pierce & Warriner)
- MoAbs to C3d (e.g. Clone 3), C3c (e.g. Clone 4), and C3g neoantigen (e.g. Clone 9)
- $Na^{125}I$, carrier-free (Amersham)
- 1% BSA in PBS
- PD-10 columns (Pharmacia)
- 19 G hypodermic and butterfly needles
- 50 ml syringe
- 1.5 ml plastic tubes
- Disposable spectrophotometer cuvettes for UV wavelengths

Method

1. Remove plunger from the 50 ml syringe and fix on a ring stand above a PD-10 column.
2. Punch a hole in the cap of the column with a 19 G hypodermic needle.
3. Place 19 G butterfly needle into the hole and connect to the syringe.

Protocol 9. *Continued*

4. Fill the syringe with PBS.
5. Cut off the end of the plastic bottom tip of the column with scissors.
6. Let 25 ml of PBS run through the column.
7. Put 50 μl of 2 mg/ml monoclonal antibody into an Eppendorf tube containing one Iodobead.
8. Mix with 50 μl of PBS to neutralize the alkaline sodium iodide.
9. Add 250 μCi of $Na^{125}I$ to each 100 μg of monoclonal antibody, and mix with pipetting up and down with a yellow tip.
10. Cap the tube tightly and incubate for 10 min at room temperature.
11. Place PD-10 column above a rack containing ten 1.5 ml plastic tubes.
12. In order to separate the majority of excess free iodine, place reaction onto the top sintered glass filter of a PD-10 column. To prevent sample dilution it is important to let the buffer run down to the surface of the filter before and after applying the sample.
13. Remove the bottom cap of the column to allow buffer to drip into an Eppendorf tube. Add 850 μl of PBS to the column and collect the first millilitre effluent in the first Eppendorf tube. Wait until the last drop leaves the column then move rack to position the next tube under the column. In this way collect ten 1 ml fractions by adding 1 ml aliquots of buffer to the column.
14. Monitor each tube directly or count a 5 μl sample from each tube in a γ-counter.
15. Pool contents of the tubes containing first radioactive peak. The peak of protein-bound activity is usually found between 2.5–6 ml, whereas, depending on the excess of sodium iodide, a second peak of protein-free radioactivity may be found at 7–9 ml.
16. Check the protein concentration using a spectrophotometer.
17. In order to determine the specific activity of the radiolabelled monoclonal antibodies, precipitate 5 μl of sample as follows. Transfer 5 μl of sample into a 1.5 ml tube containing 0.4 ml of PBS/BSA. Precipitate with 1 ml 10% TCA for 30 min at 4°C. Centrifuge at 10 000 *g* in a microcentrifuge for 20 min at 4°C.
18. Transfer 0.7 ml supernatant into another 1.5 ml tube and measure the radioactivity of both the aspirated supernatant and the remaining half of the supernatant which contains the protein pellet, in a γ-counter.
19. Subtract the activity of the aspirated 0.7 ml supernatant from the

activity of the tube containing both the pellet and the remaining 0.7 ml of supernatant to identify the protein-bound activity. The specific activity of the radiolabelled antibody can then be calculated using the protein concentration and the protein-bound activity.

20. Add 1/30 vol. of 30% (w/v) BSA in PBS to the sample, and 1/100 vol. of 300 mM sodium azide, and store at 4°C.

After gel filtration on the PD-10 column, the sample is usually diluted to 2–3 ml, and the protein concentration may be below an accurately measurable concentration using a spectrophotometer, especially if a small amount of protein (50–100 μl of 1 mg/ml or less) has been used for labelling. This causes difficulty in calculating an accurate specific activity. In this case 1 μl of the radiolabelled sample should be taken before gel filtration on the PD-10 column and stored in 0.4 ml of PBS/BSA, and precipitation of protein-bound counts should be performed as described in *Protocol 9*, step 17. The supernatant should be discarded and the pellet washed twice in 1 ml of 10% TCA. The protein-bound radioactivity of the 1 μl reaction can then be counted, and the specific activity calculated on the basis of the known protein concentration in the labelling mixture (see steps 7–9). Protein-bound radioactivity is separated from unbound on a PD-10 column as described in steps 11–15 and the protein concentration in the peak fraction can now be calculated using the measured specific activity. It is prudent to undertake a further TCA precipitation of the gel filtered protein to check whether separation of bound from free iodine was complete in the peak fraction (if separation is complete there should be no activity in the supernatant). If some free iodine remains the percentage of protein-bound activity should be calculated and the concentration of the protein corrected accordingly. For example, in the case of 90% protein-bound activity, the calculated concentration should be multiplied by 0.9.

5.2.2 Enumeration of surface-bound C3 fragments

The number of C3 fragments bound per cell can be determined by the binding of radiolabelled antibodies of known specific activity. Because the Ab to Ag ratio is 1:1 in the case of the three rat monoclonal antibodies used in this protocol, each bound antibody represents a single bound C3 fragment. If only C3b fragments are bound to the erythrocytes, the binding of Clone 3 and Clone 4 are equal whilst Clone 9 binding is negligible. If all of the C3b is digested to iC3b, the binding of the three monoclonal antibodies is equal, but when iC3b is further digested to C3d only Clone 3 reacts with the cells. Using these three monoclonal antibodies at saturating concentrations it is therefore possible to characterize the numbers and state of C3 fragments bound to cells or other particles.

Protocol 10. Enumeration of surface-bound C3 fragments

Equipment and reagents

- Radiolabelled Clone 3, Clone 4, and Clone 9 (specific activity: 1–3 mCi/mg)
- Sheep red blood cells with fixed C3 fragments (5×10^7/ml)
- Sensitized sheep red blood cells (5×10^7/ml)
- PBS
- 0.4 ml plastic tube
- Oil mixture (40% of dinonyl phthalate in dibutyl phthalate)
- Slow overhead rotator
- γ-counter

Method

1. Transfer 400 μl of cell suspension into a 1.5 ml plastic tube. Add 10 μl of radiolabelled antibody at 200 μg/ml, and fix tube onto the rotator. As a control use sheep red blood cells without C3 fragments. Incubate cells for 20 min at 20 °C.
2. Separate unbound radioactivity by layering two 200 μl aliquots of sample over duplicates of 200 μl of oil and spin down in a microcentrifuge at 10 000 *g* for 2 min.
3. Freeze tubes at −70 °C and cut tubes with a wire stripper between cell pellet and supernatant. Transfer cell pellet into a new tube and measure radioactivity in a γ-counter.
4. Subtract radioactivity of non-specific binding (sample cells without C3 fragments).
5. From the specific activity of the labelled antibodies, calculate how many molecules are represented by 1 c.p.m. based on Avogadro's number = 6×10^{23} molecules per mole, and a molecular weight of IgG of 1.6×10^5.
6. Because in 200 μl there are 1×10^7 cells, the radioactivity per cell can be determined by dividing the specific bound activity by 1×10^7.
7. The number of bound molecules is determined by multiplying radioactivity per cell by the number of molecules represented by 1 c.p.m.

5.3 Rosette formation

We give here examples of two protocols for receptor-dependent rosetting of C3-coated indicator cells. These assays may be adapted to study other receptor–ligand interactions. The principle is to incubate receptor-bearing cells with a 50–100 times excess of ligand-bearing indicator cells. Rosettes are defined as receptor-bearing cells with at least three attached indicator cells. Rosette formation depends on the density of ligand and receptor and on the affinity of the interaction between ligand and receptor.

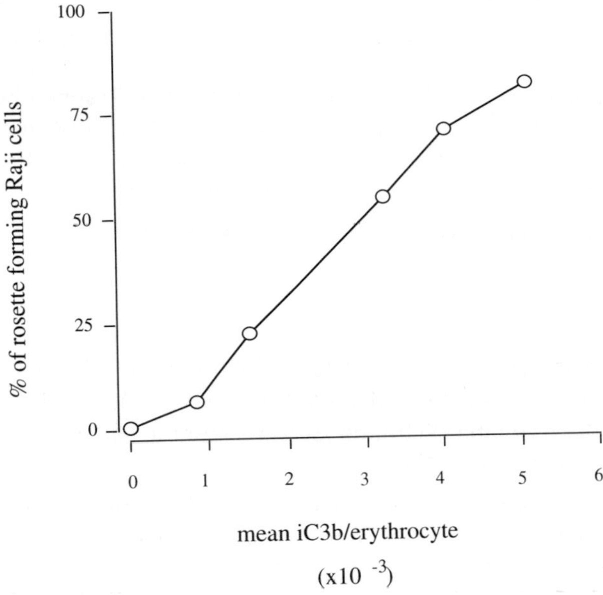

Figure 4. Density-dependent rosette formation of EiC3b with Raji cells. The per cent of rosette forming Raji cells increases in parallel with the number of iC3b molecules per erythrocyte.

5.3.1 Rosette formation by CR2-bearing cells

CR2 is able to react with iC3b, C3dg, and C3d, and also Epstein–Barr virus. We give a protocol for studying the binding of iC3b-coated indicator cells to CR2 on Raji cells. These transformed cells are CR2 positive and CR1 negative. If using other B cells which also carry CR1 it is then essential to block CR1-dependent rosetting using an inhibitory antibody.

The advantage of using iC3b as a ligand is that indicator cells bearing this molecule can be used to study binding to CR1, CR2, and CR3. The disadvantage is that many cells bear more than one type of iC3b receptor and therefore appropriate inhibitors and controls must be used to establish conditions for specific binding to each individual receptor type.

Protocol 11. Rosette formation of CR2-bearing cells

Equipment and reagents

- Raji cells
- U-bottom 2 ml plastic tube
- Hanks' (Flow Laboratories)
- Hepes (Flow Laboratories)
- Human serum albumin (HSA) (Sigma)
- EiC3b 2.5×10^8 cell/ml
- Hanks' containing 0.1 M Hepes and 0.2 % human serum albumin
- iC3b 100 μg/ml
- Haemocytometer

Protocol 11. *Continued*

Method

1. Harvest Raji cells from 25 cm^2 tissue culture flask. Transfer cells into a 10 ml scaled plastic tube and centrifuge at 450 *g* for 6 min. Discard supernatant and resuspend cells in 10 ml of Hanks' buffer. Repeat washing two more times and discard the last supernatant.
2. Resuspend cells in 2 ml of Hanks' containing 0.1 M Hepes, 0.2% human serum albumin, and count cell concentration using a haemocytometer. Dilute cells to 5×10^6 cells/ml in the same buffer.
3. Transfer 25 μl of Raji cells into a 2 ml U-bottom plastic tube and mix with 25 μl indicator cells (2.5×10^8 EiC3b/ml, refer to *Protocol 8*). Add 50 μl of buffer or as a negative control 50 μl of 100 μg/ml iC3b in the same buffer to inhibit CR2-dependent rosette formation, then incubate samples for 10 min at 37 °C.
4. Centrifuge cells in a slow centrifuge at 15 *g* for 5 min at room temperature to stabilize contacts between the cells. Turn the tube until the surface of the buffer reaches the cell pellet and mix cells by rotating the tube gently around the axis.
5. Cut off 1–2 mm from the top of a yellow tip to increase the diameter of the hole. Transfer 5–10 μl of cells into haemocytometer by gentle pipetting in order not to break cell contacts.
6. Put haemocytometer under × 40 magnification objective lens and count the free and rosette-forming Raji cells in a microscope. Move to the next field and continue until at least 200 Raji cells are counted.
7. Calculate the number of Raji cells in rosettes as a per cent of the total number of the counted cells.

5.3.2 Rosette formation of CR3-bearing cells

Both cell surface numbers and the binding affinity of CR3 on neutrophils temporarily increase after cell activation. As a consequence rosette formation rises to a maximum at 15 min after neutrophil activation, and then decreases (29). The presence of 0.5–5 mM Ca^{2+} and Mg^{2+} is essential during rosette formation because CR3 ligand binding is dependent on the presence of bivalent cations. Conversely, the use of 10 mM EDTA to chelate Ca^{2+} and Mg^{2+} completely abolishes CR3-dependent rosette formation.

Several precautions must be undertaken when performing rosetting assays with neutrophils. Because neutrophils bear both CR1 and CR3 as well as Fc receptors, appropriate controls must be performed to ensure the specificity of the rosetting reaction. Secondly neutrophils express cell surface protease activity and the buffer must be supplemented with protease inhibitors to avoid proteolytic digestion of iC3b to C3d.

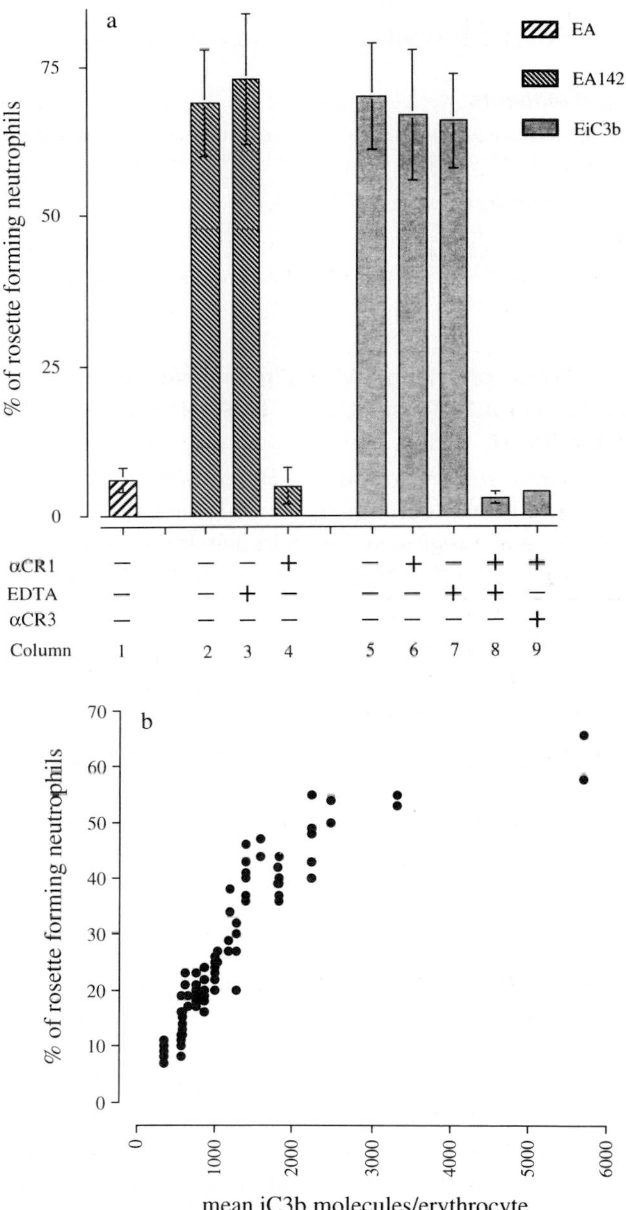

Figure 5. Rosette formation by neutrophils with erythrocyte preparations bearing different complement intermediates. (a) In columns 2 to 4 is shown CR1-dependent rosetting of neutrophils with EC4b; rosetting is inhibited by anti-CR1 (column 4) but not by EDTA (column 3). In columns 5 to 9 is shown CR1- (columns 7 and 9) and CR3-dependent (columns 6 and 8) rosetting of neutrophils with EiC3b. (b) The per cent of CR3-dependent rosette forming neutrophils increases in parallel with the number iC3b molecules per erythrocyte. Reproduced from ref. 24, with permission.

Protocol 12. Rosette formation of CR3-bearing cells

Equipment and reagents

- *N*-Formyl-L-methionyl-L-leucyl-L-phenylalanine (FMLP) (Sigma) 10^{-4} M in glacial acetic acid/NaOH at pH 5–7
- HBSS: Hanks' balanced salts (Flow Laboratories)
- HBSS without Ca/Mg (Flow Laboratories)
- Hepes (Flow Laboratories)
- 20% rabbit immune serum containing anti-CR1 neutralizing antibodies
- Human serum albumin (HSA) (Sigma)
- Soybean trypsin inhibitor (Sigma)
- Isolated neutrophils
- EiC3b
- 2 ml U-bottom plastic tubes

Method

1. Thaw one aliquot of frozen FMLP and transfer 10 μl into 1 ml of Hanks' containing 0.1 M Hepes, 0.2% HSA. Neutralize pH by adding ~ 3 μl of 4 M NaOH.
2. Make a neutrophil suspension at 5×10^6 cells/ml concentration (refer to *Protocol 1*) in Hanks' containing 0.1 M Hepes, 0.5% human serum albumin (HSA), and 1 mg/ml soybean trypsin inhibitor (SBTI). Transfer 25 μl of cells into a 2 ml U-bottom tube and activate cells at 37 °C for 3 min by adding 2.5 μl of 10^{-6} M FMLP.
3. Add 25 μl of 20% rabbit immune serum containing blocking anti-CR1 antibodies and 25 μl of 2.5×10^8 EC3bi (see *Protocol 8*) in the same buffer as above. Incubate mixture for 7 min in a 37 °C water-bath.
4. Centrifuge samples in a slow centrifuge at 15 *g* for 5 min at room temperature. Turn the tube until the surface of the buffer reaches the cell pellet and mix cells gently by rotating the tube around the axis.
5. Cut off 1–2 mm from the top of a yellow tip to increase the diameter of the hole. Transfer 5–10 μl of cells into a haemocytometer by gentle pipetting without breaking cell contacts.
6. Put haemocytometer onto a microscope under × 40 magnification objective lens and count the free and rosette-forming neutrophils. Move to the next field and continue until at least 200 neutrophils are counted.
7. Calculate the number of neutrophils in rosettes as a per cent of the total number of the counted cells:

   $$\%\text{ of rosette-forming neutrophils} = \frac{\text{number of rosettes}}{\text{number of rosettes} + \text{number of free neutrophils}}$$

When using adherent cells such as monocytes, macrophages, etc. it is possible to carry out rosette formation '*in situ*' on cells attached to a solid surface, e.g. tissue culture dish. In this case the excess of indicator cells is gently washed out, before enumerating rosettes under an inverted microscope (30).

6. Complement receptor-dependent phagocytosis

Complement receptors can mediate phagocytosis of opsonized particles. Neutrophils can phagocytose iC3b-coated latex particles by both CR1- and CR3-dependent mechanisms. Specific receptor-mediated phagocytosis by either of these receptors therefore requires the blockade of the other receptor using antibodies or cation chelation to block CR3-dependent uptake.

6.1 Preparing C3bi-coated particles

In this protocol a method for passive adsorption of iC3b to fluorescence-labelled latex beads is given. For further protocols for binding proteins to beads the reader is referred to the particle manufacturer and to refs 31–33.

Protocol 13. Preparing iC3b-coated latex particles

Equipment and reagents

- Fluorobrite plain YG 1 micron microspheres (Polysciences Inc.)
- 2% human serum albumin (HSA) (Sigma) in PBS
- iC3b 1.5 mg/ml in PBS
- BDVEA: 3.5 mM veronal buffer containing 1% BSA, 3.2% dextrose, 20 mM EDTA, 0.2% NaN_3, 6 mS, pH 7.4

Method

1. Transfer 16.3 μl of Fluorobrite microspheres into a 1.5 ml plastic tube.
2. Add 300 μl 1.5 mg/ml of iC3b in PBS and rotate on a slow overhead rotator at 37 °C for 20 min.
3. Block remaining binding sites by a further 20 min incubation at 37 °C after adding 300 μl of 2% HSA. Alternatively rotate overnight at 4 °C.
4. Transfer tube into a microcentrifuge and pellet microspheres at 10 000 *g* for 30 sec.
5. Remove supernatant and resuspend pellet in 1.5 ml BDVEA. Wash microspheres two more times in the same way.
6. After last washing, resuspend pellet in 300 μl of BDVEA, cover with aluminium foil to protect from light, and store at 4 °C. The concentration of microspheres should be 2.5×10^9/ml.

After adsorption of the iC3b, the density of the bound molecules can be tested using radiolabelled anti-C3 antibodies using a modification of *Protocol 10*. In our hands, incubation of 16.3 μl of Fluorobright in 300 μl of 1.5 mg/ml iC3bi resulted in $\sim 10^4$ molecules/microspheres.

6.2 Phagocytosis of C3bi-coated fluorescent microspheres

In this sample protocol, the phagocytic activity of f-met-leu-phe-activated neutrophils is assayed. In order to assay specifically phagocytosis by neutrophils mediated by CR3 it is necessary to block neutrophil CR1; this is best achieved using a polyclonal rabbit anti-CR1 antibody. The length of the activation time is based on the peak of rosette formation mediated by activated CR3 (17).

Protocol 14. CR3-dependent phagocytosis

Equipment and reagents

- Human neutrophil cell suspension at 5 × 10^6/ml concentration
- iC3b-coated microspheres prepared according to *Protocol 13*
- 10% rabbit immune serum containing anti-CR1 neutralizing antibodies in HBSS, 0.1 M Hepes, 0.2% HSA, and 1 mg/ml SBTI
- 2% human serum albumin (HSA) (Sigma) in PBS
- BDVA: 3.5 mM veronal buffer containing 1% BSA, 3.2% dextrose, 20 mM EDTA, 0.2% NaN_3, 6 mS, pH 7.4
- *N*-Formyl-L-methionyl-L-leucyl-L-phenylalanine (FMLP) (Sigma) 10^{-4} M in glacial acetic acid/NaOH at pH 5–7
- HBSS: Hanks' balanced salts (Gibco)
- HBSS containing 0.1 M Hepes, 0.2% HSA, and 1 mg/ml soybean trypsin inhibitor (SBTI)
- HBSS without Ca^{2+}/Mg^{2+} containing 20 mM EDTA, 0.1 M Hepes, 0.2% HSA, 1 mg/ml SBTI
- 40 μg/ml 2LPM19c anti-CR3 monoclonal antibody (MoAb) (Dako) in HBSS containing 0.1 M Hepes, 0.2% HSA, and 1 mg/ml SBTI
- 37.8% Percoll in HBSS without Ca^{2+}/Mg^{2+} containing 0.2 M Hepes, 0.2% HSA, and 1 mg/ml SBTI

Method

1. Dilute 10 μl of 10^{-4} M FMLP in 1 ml HBSS containing 0.1 M Hepes. Adjust pH to neutrality with ~ 3 μl of 4 M NaOH.
2. Activate 25 μl of neutrophil suspension in HBSS supplemented with Hepes, HSA, and SBTI by mixing with 2.5 μl of FMLP (10^{-6} M prepared in step 1), and incubate in a 37 °C water-bath for 3 min in a 1.5 ml plastic tube.
3. Add 25 μl of anti-CR1, 25 μl of microspheres (2.5 × 10^9/ml in HBSS containing Hepes, HSA, and SBTI), 25 μl of buffer or, as a negative control, 25 μl of anti-CR3, and leave in 37 °C water-bath for 15 min without mixing.
4. Layer cell suspension over 1 ml of 37.8% Percoll and separate unbound microspheres by a 10 min centrifugation at 200 *g*.
5. Discard fluorobead containing supernatant, and resuspend cell pellet in 100 μl of PBS.
6. Pipette 10–20 μl of cells onto a microscope slide or haemocytometer and cover.Under fluorescent microscope count microspheres phagocytosed by 200 neutrophils. (See remarks about fluorescent microscope in *Protocol 2*, step 6, and notes.)

While the concentration of the Percoll gradient in this protocol is the same as used for isolation of the neutrophils, instead of autologous serum Hepes is used to balance the pH. For simplicity to make up 37.8% Percoll gradient, one can dilute 420 μl of 90% Percoll to 1 ml in the buffer. The actual concentration of the microspheres can be tested throughout by a standard curve of fluorescence intensity, measured in a fluorimeter, e.g. Cytofluor 2300 (Millipore).

7. Conclusion

In this review we have concentrated on providing protocols suitable for the study of the interactions between the three major complement receptors, CR1, CR2, and CR3, and their ligands. Many of these methods can be adapted in a straightforward manner for the analysis of the interactions between other cell surface receptors and their ligands.

References

1. Sim, R. B., Malhotra, V., Day, A. J., and Erdei, A. (1987). *Immunol. Lett.*, **14**, 183.
2. Dierich, M. P., Schulz, T. F., Eigentler, A., Huemer, H., and Schwable, W. (1988). *Mol. Immunol.*, **25**, 1043.
3. Arnaout, M. A. (1990). *Blood*, **75**, 1037.
4. Fearon, D. T. and Ahearn, J. M. (1990). *Curr. Top. Microbiol. Immunol.*, **153**, 83.
5. Ross, G. D. (1993). In *Clinical aspects of immunology* (ed. P. J. Lachmann, Sir Keith Peters, F. S. Rosen, and M. J. Walport), Vol. 1, p. 241. Blackwell Scientific Publications, Boston.
6. Ross, G. D., *et al.* (1995). In *Leucocyte typing V. White cell differentiation antigens. Proceedings of the fifth international workshop and conference*, Boston, USA, 3–7 November 1993 (ed. S. F. Schlossman, *et al.*), Vol. 1, p. 871. Oxford University Press, Oxford.
7. Madi, N., Paccaud, J. P., Steiger, G., and Schifferli, J. A. (1991). *Clin. Exp. Immunol.*, **84**, 9.
8. Edberg, J. C., Kimberly, R. P., and Taylor, R. P. (1992). *Eur. J. Immunol.*, **22**, 1333.
9. Rao, P. E., Wright, S. D., Westberg, E. F., and Goldstein, G. (1985). *Cell. Immunol.*, **93**, 549.
10. Vetvicka, V. and Ross, G. D. (1995). In *Leucocyte typing V. White cell differentiation antigens. Proceedings of the fifth international workshop and conference*, Boston, USA, 3–7 November 1993 (ed. S. F. Schlossman, *et al.*), Vol. 1, p. 520. Oxford University Press, Oxford.
11. Diamond, M. S., Garcia, A. J., Bickford, J. K., Corbi, A. L., and Springer, T. A. (1993). *J. Cell. Biol.*, **120**, 1031.
12. Bilsland, C. A., Diamond, M. S., and Springer, T. A. (1994). *J. Immunol.*, **152**, 4582.

13. Aubry, J. P., Pochon, S., Graber, P., Jansen, K. U., and Bonnefoy, J. Y. (1992). *Nature*, **358**, 505.
14. Russ, G. R., Haddad, A. P., Tait, B. D., and d'Apice, A. J. (1985). *J. Clin. Invest.*, **76**, 1965.
15. Arnaout, M. A., Melamed, J., Tack, B. F., and Colten, H. R. (1981). *J. Immunol.*, **127**, 1348.
16. Arnaout, M. A., Dana, N., Melamed, J., Medicus, R., and Colten, H. R. (1983). *Immunology*, **48**, 229.
17. Hermanowski, V. A., Detmers, P. A., Gotze, O., Silverstein, S. C., and Wright, S. D. (1988). *J. Biol. Chem.*, **263**, 17822.
18. Kalli, K. R., Hsu, P. H., Bartow, T. J., Ahearn, J. M., Matsumoto, A. K., Klickstein, L. B., *et al.* (1991). *J. Exp. Med.*, **174**, 1451.
19. Wilson, J. G., Wong, W. W., Schur, P. H., and Fearon, D. T. (1982). *N. Engl. J. Med.*, **307**, 981.
20. Wong, W. W., Wilson, J. G., and Fearon, D. T. (1983). *J. Clin. Invest.*, **72**, 685.
21. Roberts, W. N., Wilson, J. G., Wong, W., Jenkins, D. J., Fearon, D. T., Austen, K. F., *et al.* (1985). *J. Immunol.*, **134**, 512.
22. Wilson, J. G., Jack, R. M., Wong, W. W., Schur, P. H., and Fearon, D. T. (1985). *J. Clin. Invest.*, **76**, 182.
23. Makrides, S. C., Scesney, S. M., Ford, P. J., Evans, K. S., Carson, G. R., and Marsh, H. J. (1992). *J. Biol. Chem.*, **267**, 24754.
24. Bartók, I and Walport, M. J. (1995). *J. Immunol.*, **154**, 5367.
25. Harrison, R. A. and Lachmann, P. J. (1986). In *Handbook of experimental immunology* (ed. D. M. Weir), Vol. 1, p. 39.20. Blackwell Scientific Publications, Oxford.
26. Stewart, J., Glass, E. J., Weir, D. M., and Daha, M. R. (1986). In *Handbook of experimental immunology* (ed. D. M. Weir), Vol. 2, p. 48.6. Blackwell Scientific Publications, Oxford.
27. Lachmann, P. J., Oldroyd, R. G., Milstein, C., and Wright, B. W. (1980). *Immunology*, **41**, 503.
28. Ross, G. D., Newman, S. L., Lambris, J. D., Devery, P. J., Cain, J. A., and Lachmann, P. J. (1983). *J. Exp. Med.*, **158**, 334.
29. Hermanowski, V. A., Van, S. J., Swiggard, W. J., and Wright, S. D. (1992). *Cell*, **68**, 341.
30. Wright, S. D. and Silverstein, S. C. (1982). *J. Exp. Med.*, **156**, 1149.
31. Lambris, J. D. and Ross, G. D. (1982). *J. Immunol.*, **128**, 186.
32. Ross, G. D. and Lambris, J. D. (1982). *J. Exp. Med.*, **155**, 96.
33. Ogle, J. D., Ogle, C. K., Noel, J. G., Hurtubise, P., and Alexander, J. W. (1985). *J. Immunol. Methods*, **76**, 47.

A1

List of suppliers

Agar Scientific Ltd., 66a Cambridge Road, Stansted, Essex CM24 8DA, UK.

Aldrich Chemical Co. Inc., 1001 W. St. Paul Avenue, Milwaukee, Wisconsin 53233, USA.

Aldrich Chemical Co., The Old Brickyard, Gillingham, Dorset SP8 4JL, UK.

America A/S, Winthersmollevej 1, DK 7700 Thisted, Denmark.

American National Can, Greenwich, CT 06836, USA.

American Type Culture Collection, 12301 Parklawn Drive, Rockville, Maryland 20852-1776, USA.

Amersham

Amersham International plc., Lincoln Place, Green End, Aylesbury, Buckinghamshire HP20 2TP, UK.

Amersham Corporation, 2636 South Clearbrook Drive, Arlington Heights, IL 60005, USA.

Amicon Inc., Cherry Hill Drive, Beverly, MA 01915, USA.

Amicon Ltd., Upper Mill, Stonehouse, Gloucestershire GL10 2BJ, UK.

Amplify, Amersham, Little Chalfont, Buckinghamshire, UK.

Anachem, Charles Street, Luton, Bedfordshire LU2 0EB, UK. (Also suppliers of Gilson pipettes)

Anderman

Anderman and Co. Ltd., 145 London Road, Kingston-Upon-Thames, Surrey KT17 7NH, UK.

Avanti Polar Lipids, 700 Industrial Park Drive, Alabaster, Alabama 35007, USA.

Bachem (Switzerland), Hauptstrasse 144, CH-4416 Bubendorf, Switzerland.

Baxter Diagnostics Inc., 1430 Waukegan Road, McGaw Park, IL 60085-6787, USA.

Baxter Diagnostics Inc., Wallingford Road, Compton, Newbury, Berkshire, UK.

Beckman Instruments

Beckman Instruments UK Ltd., Progress Road, Sands Industrial Estate, High Wycombe, Buckinghamshire HP12 4JL, UK.

Beckman Instruments Inc., PO Box 3100, 2500 Harbor Boulevard, Fullerton, CA 92634, USA.

Becton Dickinson, European HQ, Denderstraat 24, B-9320 Erenbodegem-Aalst, Belgium.

Becton Dickinson and Co., Between Towns Road, Cowley, Oxford OX4 3LY, UK.

Becton Dickinson and Co., 2 Bridgewater Lane, Lincoln Park, NJ 07035, USA.

Behringwerke, Marburg, Germany.

BIAcore Pty Ltd., Davy Avenue, Knowlhill, Milton Keynes MK5 8PH, UK.

Bio

Bio 101 Inc., c/o Statech Scientific Ltd., 6163 Dudley Street, Luton, Bedfordshire LU2 0HP, UK.

Bio 101 Inc., PO Box 2284, La Jolla, CA 92038/2284, USA.

Biogenesis, 7 New Fields, Stinsford Road, Poole, Dorset BH17 0NF, UK.

Biological Detection Systems, Pittsburgh, PA, USA.

Biomedicals, Rheinstrasse 28-32, CH-4302 Augst, Switzerland.

bio-Merieux, 69280 Marcy-l'Etoile, France.

Bio-Rad Laboratories

Bio-Rad Laboratories Ltd., Bio-Rad House, Maylands Avenue, Hemel Hempstead HP2 7TD, UK.

Bio-Rad Laboratories, Division Headquarters, 3300 Regatta Boulevard, Richmond, CA 94804, USA.

Biotecx Laboratories Inc., 6023, South Loop East, Houston, TX 77033-9980, USA.

Boehringer Mannheim

Boehringer Mannheim UK (Diagnostics and Biochemicals) Ltd., Bell Lane, Lewes, East Sussex BN17 1LG, UK.

Boehringer Mannheim Corporation, Biochemical Products, 9115 Hague Road, PO Box 504, Indianopolis, IN 46250-0414, USA.

Boehringer Mannheim Biochemica, GmbH, Sandhofer Str. 116, Postfach 310120 D-6800 Ma 31, Germany.

British Drug Houses (BDH) Ltd., Poole, Dorset, UK.

Calbiochem–Novabiochem (UK) Ltd., 3 Heathcoat Building, Highfields Science Park, University Boulevard, Nottingham NG7 2QJ, UK.

Calbiochem–Novabiochem Corporation, 10394 Pacific Court Centre, San Diego, CA 92121, USA.

Celltech Therapeutics Ltd., 216 Bath Road, Slough, Berkshire SL1 4EN, UK.

Central Labs Netherlands Red Cross (CNB), Plesmanlaan 125, 1066 CX Amsterdam, The Netherlands.

Chiron Technologies, 11055 Roselle St, San Diego, CA 92121, USA.

Chiron Technologies, PO Box 1415, Clayton South, Victoria 3169, Australia.

Chiron Technologies, 10 rue Chevreul, 92150 Suresnes, France.

Conair Churchill, Uxbridge, Middlesex, UK.

Coulter Electronics Ltd., Northwell Drive, Luton, Bedfordshire LU3 3RH, UK.

CP Pharmaceuticals Ltd., Ash Road North, Wrexham, Clwyd LL13 9UF, UK.

Dako A/S, Produktionsvej 42, DK-2000 Glostrup, Denmark.

DAKO Ltd., 16 Manor Courtyard, Hughenden Avenue, High Wycombe, Buckinghamshire HP13 5RE, UK.

DAKO Corporation, 6392 Via Real, Carpinteria, CA 93013, USA.

Dakopatts A/S, Produktionsvej 42, Postbox 1359, DK 2600 Glostrup, Denmark.

Difco Laboratories

Difco Laboratories Ltd., PO Box 14B, Central Avenue, West Molesey, Surrey KT8 2SE, UK.

Difco Laboratories, PO Box 331058, Detroit, MI 48232-7058, USA.

Du Pont

Dupont (UK) Ltd., Industrial Products Division, Wedgwood Way, Stevenage, Hertfordshire SG1 4QU, UK.

Du Pont Co. (Biotechnology Systems Division), PO Box 80024, Wilmington, DE 19880-002, USA.

Dynatech Laboratories Ltd., Daux Road, Billingshurst, West Sussex RH14 9SJ, UK.

European Collection of Animal Cell Culture, Division of Biologics, PHLS Centre for Applied Microbiology and Research, Porton Down, Salisbury, Wiltshire SP4 0JG, UK.

Falcon (Falcon is a registered trademark of Becton Dickinson and Co.)

Fisher Scientific Co., 711 Forbest Avenue, Pittsburgh, PA 15219-4785, USA.

Flow Cytometry Standards, PO Box 1336, 2302 Blt Leiden, The Netherlands.

Flow Laboratories, Woodcock Hill, Harefield Road, Rickmansworth, Hertfordshire WD3 1PQ, UK.

Fluka

Fluka–Chemie AG, CH-9470, Buchs, Switzerland.

Fluka Chemicals Ltd., The Old Brickyard, New Road, Gillingham, Dorset SP8 4JL, UK.

Gibco BRL

Gibco BRL (Life Technologies Ltd., Trident House, Renfrew Road, Paisley PA3 4EF, UK.

Gibco BRL (Life Technologies Inc.), 3175 Staler Road, Grand Island, NY 14072-0068, USA.

Halocarbon, PO Box 661, River Edge, NH 07661, USA.

C.A. Hendley (Essex) Ltd., Oakwood Hill Industrial Estate, Loughton, Essex, UK.

Arnold R. Horwell, 73 Maygrove Road, West Hampstead, London NW6 2BP, UK.

Hybaid

Hybaid Ltd., 111–113 Waldegrave Road, Teddington, Middlesex TW11 8LL, UK.

Hybaid, National Labnet Corporation, PO Box 841, Woodbridge, NJ 07095, USA.

HyClone Laboratories, 1725 South HyClone Road, Logan, UT 84321, USA.

ICN Biomedicals Inc., Costa Mesa, CA, USA.

ICN Pharmaceuticals Inc., 3300 Hyland Avenue, Costa Mesa, CA 92626, USA.

ICN Pharmaceuticals Ltd., Thame Park Business Centre, Wenman Road, Thame, Oxfordshire OX9 3XA, UK.

IGS, Nikon, Nippon Kogaku ICK, Tokyo, Japan.

International Biotechnologies Inc., 25 Science Park, New Haven, Connecticut 06535, USA.

International Blood Group Reference Laboratory (IBGRL), Dagger Lane, Elstree, Hertfordshire WD6 3BX, UK.

Invitrogen Corporation

Invitrogen Corporation, 3985 B Sorrenton Valley Building, San Diego, CA 92121, USA.

Invitrogen Corporation, c/o British Biotechnology Products Ltd., 410 The Quadrant, Barton Lane, Abingdon, Oxfordshire OX14 3YS, UK.

Jackson Immuno Research Laboratories Inc., 61–63 Dudley Street, Luton, Bedfordshire LU2 0NP, UK.

Jackson Immuno Research Laboratories, 827 W. Baltimore Pike, West Grove, PA 19390, USA.

Kabi Pharmacia Diagnostics, Gydevangen 21, 3450 Allerod, Denmark.

Kirkegaard and Perry Labs (KPL), 2 Cessna Court, Gaithersburg, MD 20879, USA.

Kodak: Eastman Fine Chemicals, 343 State Street, Rochester, NY, USA.

Labsystems Oy, PO Box 8, FIN-0-881 Helsinki, Finland.

Leo Pharmaceutical Products BV, Pampusalaan 186, 1382 JS Weesp, The Netherlands.

Life Sciences International (UK) Ltd., Unit 5, The Ringway Centre, Edison Road, Basingstoke, Hampshire RG21 6ZZ, UK. (Suppliers of Finnpipettes and Labsystems microtitre plates).

Life Technologies Inc., 8451 Helgerman Court, Gaithersburg, MN 20877, USA.

Litex A/S, Copenhagen, Denmark.

Merck Ltd. (BDH), Hunter Boulevard, Magna Park, Lutterworth, Leicestershire LE17 4XN, UK.

Merck Industries Inc., 5 Skyline Drive, Nawthorne, NY 10532, USA.

Merck, Frankfurter Strasse, 250, Postfach 4119, D-64293, Germany.

Millipore

Millipore (UK) Ltd., The Boulevard, Blackmoor Lane, Watford, Hertfordshire WD1 8YW, UK.

Millipore Corp./Biosearch, PO Box 255, 80 Ashby Road, Bedford, MA 01730, USA.

Molecular Bio-Products Inc., 9888 Waples Street, San Diego, CA 92121, USA.

Molecular Bio-Products Inc., distributor in the UK: Merck Ltd., BDH Laboratory Supplies, Poole BH15 1TDF, UK.

Molecular Devices Corporation, 3180 Porter Drive, Palo Alto, CA 94304, USA.

Molecular Probes, Eugene, OR, USA.

Molecular Probes Europe BV, Poort Bebrouw, Rijnsburgerweg 10, 2333 AA Leiden, The Netherlands.

NE Technology Ltd., Sighthill, Edinburgh, UK.

New England Biolabs (NBL)

New England Biolabs (NBL), 32 Tozer Road, Beverley, MA 01915-5510, USA.

New England Biolabs (NBL), c/o CP Labs Ltd., PO Box 22, Bishops Stortford, Hertfordshire CM23 3DH, UK.

Nikon Corporation, Fuji Building, 23 Marunouchi 3-chome, Chiyoda-ku, Tokyo, Japan.

Nordic Immunological Laboratories BV, Langestraat 55-61, PO Box 22, 5000 AA Tilburg, The Netherlands.

Novabiochem, Calbiochem-Novabiochem AG, Weidenmattweg 4, Postfach, CH-4448 Laufelfingen, Switzerland.

Nucleopore Inc., 7035 Commerce Circle, Pleasanton, California 94566, USA.

Nunc A/S, Postbox 280, Kamstrup, DK-4000 Roskilde, Denmark.

Nycomed UK Ltd., Nycomed House, 2111 Coventry Road, Sheldon, UK.

Omega Optical, Brattleboro, VT, USA.

Oxoid, Basingstoke, Hampshire, UK.

Perkin-Elmer

Perkin-Elmer Ltd., Maxwell Road, Beaconsfield, Buckinghamshire HP9 1QA, UK.

Perkin-Elmer Ltd., Post Office Lane, Beaconsfield, Buckinghamshire HP9 1QA, UK.

Perkin Elmer-Cetus (The Perkin-Elmer Corporation), 761 Main Avenue, Norwalk, CT 0689, USA.

Pharmacia Biotech Europe Procordia EuroCentre, Rue de la Fuse-e 62, B-1130 Brussels, Belgium.

Pharmacia LKB Biotechnology AB, S-75182 Uppsala, Sweden.

Pharmingen, 10975 Torreyana Road, San Diego, CA 92121, USA.]

Phase Sep, Deeside, Clwyd, UK.

Pierce, 3747 N Meridian Road, PO Box 117, Rockford, IL 61105, USA.

Pierce Europe BV, PO Box 1512, 3260 BA and Beijerland, Holland.

Polysciences Inc., Warrington, PA, USA.

Promega

Promega Ltd., Delta House, Enterprise Road, Chilworth Research Centre, Southampton, UK.

Promega Corporation, 2800 Woods Hollow Road, Madison, WI 53711-5399, USA.

Qiagen

Qiagen Inc., c/o Hybaid, 111–13 Waldegrave Road, Teddington, Middlesex TW11 8LL, UK.

Qiagen Inc., 9259 Eton Avenue, Chatsworth, CA 91311, USA.

Quidel, 10165 McKellar Court, San Diego, CA 92121, USA.

Rathburn Chemicals Ltd., Caberston Road, Walkerburn, Peebleshire, Scotland EH13 6AU, UK.

Rudolf Brand GmbH, PO Box 310, D-6980 Wertheim/Main, Germany.

Sarstedt Inc., PO Box 468, Newton, NC 28658, USA.

Sarstedt Inc., 68 Boston Road, Beaumont Leys, Leicester LE1 AQ, UK.

Schleicher and Schuell

Schleicher and Schuell Inc., Keene, NH 03431A, USA.

Schleicher and Schuell Inc., D-3354 Dassel, Germany. Schleicher and Schuell Inc., c/o Andermann and Company Ltd.

Scott Smith Electronics, Wimborne, Dorset, UK.

Semat Technical Ltd., St Albans, UK.

Seralab, Crawley Down, Sussex RH10 4FF, UK.

Serotec, 22 Bankside, Station Approach, Kidlington, Oxford OX5 1JE, UK.

Serotec distributed by Harlan Bioproducts for Science USA, PO Box 29171, Indianapolis, IN 46163, USA.

Shandon Scientific Ltd., Chadwick Road, Astmoor, Runcorn, Cheshire WA7 1PR, UK.

Sherwood Medical, Crawley, Sussex RH11 7YQ, UK.

Sherwood Medical, St Louis, MO 63103, USA.

Sigma Chemical Company

Sigma Chemical Company (UK), Fancy Road, Poole, Dorset BH17 7NH, UK.

Sigma Chemical Company, 3050 Spruce Street, PO Box 14508, St Louis, MO 63178-9916, USA.

SLT Labinstruments GmbH, Unterbergstrasse 1 A, 5082 Grodig, Austria.

Sorvall DuPont Company, Biotechnology Division, PO Box 80022, Wilmington, DE 19880-0022, USA.

Southern Biotechnology, Birmingham, AL, USA.

Statens Seruminstitut, Artillerivej 5, DK-2300 Copenhagen, Denmark.

Stratagene

Stratagene Ltd., Unit 140, Cambridge Innovation Centre, Cambridge Science Park, Milton Road, Cambridge, CB4 4GF, UK.

TCS Biologics Ltd., Botolph Claydon, Buckingham, MK18 2LR, UK.

Vector Laboratories, Burlingame, CA, USA.

Ventana Medical Systems, Tucson, AZ, USA.

Wallac Co. (UK), EG&G Instruments Ltd., 20 Vincent Avenue, Crownhill Business Centre, Crownhill, Milton Keyne MK8 0AB, UK.

Wallac Inc. (USA), 9238 Gaither Road, Baithesburg, Maryland 20877, USA.

Wallac Oy, PO Box 10, FIN-20101 Turku, Finland.
Whatman International, Whatman House, St Leonard's Road, Maidstone, Kent ME16 0LS, UK.
Whatman LabSates, PO Box 1359, Hillsboro, OR 97123-9981, USA.

Index